Atlas of Cardiac Innervation

Vasken Dilsizian • Jagat Narula
Editors

Atlas of Cardiac Innervation

Springer

Editors
Vasken Dilsizian, MD
Division of Nuclear Medicine
Department of Diagnostic Radiology
University of Maryland School of Medicine
Baltimore, MD, USA

Jagat Narula, MD, PhD
Division of Cardiology
Mount Sinai Medical Center
New York, NY, USA

ISBN 978-3-319-45798-7 ISBN 978-3-319-45800-7 (eBook)
DOI 10.1007/978-3-319-45800-7

Library of Congress Control Number: 2016960298

Printed on acid-free paper

This Springer imprint is published by Springer Nature
The registered company is Springer International Publishing AG
The registered company address is: Gewerbestrasse 11, 6330 Cham, Switzerland

Preface

The synthesis of molecular radiotracers in parallel with recent advances in hybrid imaging has made it possible to study and characterize cardiac anatomy, function, perfusion, metabolism, and innervation in vivo, with exceptional accuracy. The ability to image the shift in the primary source of myocardial energy production from fatty acids toward glucose utilization in the setting of reduced blood flow has helped explain the pathophysiology of hibernation and myocardial viability, as well as management of patients with chronic ischemic left ventricular dysfunction and heart failure for the assessment of myocardial viability. The neuronal component of the myocardium, however, has been sparingly evaluated. This might be an inadvertent oversight, or an apt omission due to its interaction with the abnormalities produced by other myocardial compartments, that have been more easily measured.

The heart and the brain have complex interconnected communications with the heart supplying blood to the brain and the brain exerting neuronal control over cardiac function. Some central nervous system and myopathies are associated and often determine patient outcome, while other cardiac neurological conditions are concurrent but not causally related. Remodeling of the cardiac innervation, for example, may play a critical role in the development of heart failure rather than being a response to the disease process. Imaging cardiac innervation may provide insight into central versus regional intrathoracic autonomic nervous system disorders. Understanding the neurohumoral basis of the diseased heart (e.g., overactivation of cardiac sympathetic efferent neurons and the renin-angiotensin system) may have important implications for treatment options.

Molecular imaging allows direct visualization and characterization of the neuronal component and function of living cardiac cells. It provides an entirely new and unanticipated window of opportunity for simultaneous assessment of cardiac structure and function, noninvasively, as well as image-guided therapy. The aim of the *Atlas of Cardiac Innervation* is to elucidate the role of neuronal component in normal and disease states and discuss various imaging targets and probes that are currently available in clinical practice. All contributors have made sincere efforts to include the latest developments in their chapters. The chapters are intended to provide the reader a firm foundation in cardiac neuronal imaging and image processing to effectively utilize these techniques in the clinical setting and/or in the research setting to develop new ones. Schematic diagrams, tables, and diagnostic algorithms are interspersed with color illustrations to emphasize key concepts in cardiovascular physiology, pathology, and innervation.

In the first two chapters (Chaps. 1 and 2), the principles of autonomic control in the regulation of cardiac function, sympathetic and parasympathetic innervation, and circulating neurohormones are presented in health and disease. Chapter 3 details the chemistry and biology of radiotracers designed to target changes in the myocardial sympathetic and parasympathetic innervation as a function of disease or treatment. The next three chapters (Chaps. 4, 5 and 6) address neuronal imaging in heart failure and reverse remodeling, as well as the future role of PET imaging and quantification of cardiac innervation. Chapters 7 and 8 discuss cardiac sympathetic innervation in ventricular arrhythmias and device therapy, and its role for guiding ablation of ventricular tachycardia. Chapter 9 covers conditions which affect the autonomic nervous system, from brain disorders to neuropathies, including diabetes mellitus. Chapter 10 examines the role of myocardial blood flow and cardiac neuronal imaging in denervation and reinnervation in cardiac transplant recipients.

Extraordinary advances in basic sciences and molecular imaging techniques in recent years have enabled scientists to address classic questions of cardiovascular discipline. Targeted imaging of cardiac innervation and the use of image-guided therapy will further improve the management of heart failure by identifying patients for whom the response to medical, device, or ablation therapy would be optimal or perhaps not beneficial at all, as we move closer to personalized medicine. It would not be an overstatement to say that molecular imaging, particularly the neuronal component of the myocardium, will revolutionize research in many areas of cardiovascular diseases. In the next century, innovative neuronal imaging strategies will propel the field from diagnostic to image-guided therapeutic procedures. It is our hope that the *Atlas of Cardiac Innervation* will serve as a foundation for clinicians and electrophysiologists and foster cross-fertilization among investigators from various disciplines.

Baltimore, MD, USA Vasken Dilsizian, MD
New York, NY, USA Jagat Narula, MD, PhD

Contents

Contributors

Olujimi A. Ajijola, MD Ronald Reagan UCLA Medical Center, Los Angeles, CA, USA

Jeffrey L. Ardell Ronald Reagan UCLA Medical Center, Los Angeles, CA, USA

J. Andrew Armour Ronald Reagan UCLA Medical Center, Los Angeles, CA, USA

John M. Canty Jr., MD University at Buffalo/Jacobs School of Medicine and Biomedical Sciences, Department of Medicine/Cardiovascular Medicine, Buffalo, NY, USA

Ignasi Carrió, MD Hospital de la Santa Creu i Sant Pau, Barcelona, Spain

Wengen Chen, MD Department of Diagnostic Radiology and Nuclear Medicine, University of Maryland School of Medicine, Baltimore, MD, USA

Ray W. Chui, MS Ronald Reagan UCLA Medical Center, Los Angeles, CA, USA

Timm Dickfeld, MD Division of Cardiology, Department of Medicine, University of Maryland School of Medicine, Baltimore, MD, USA

Vasken Dilsizian, MD Department of Diagnostic Radiology and Nuclear Medicine, University of Maryland School of Medicine, Baltimore, MD, USA

John T. Duell, MD Division of Cardiology, Department of Medicine, University of Maryland School of Medicine, Baltimore, MD, USA

William C. Eckelman Molecular Tracer, Bethesda, MD, USA

James A. Fallavollita, MD University at Buffalo/Jacobs School of Medicine and Biomedical Sciences, Department of Medicine/Cardiovascular Medicine, Buffalo, NY, USA

Stanley F. Fernandez, MD University at Buffalo/Jacobs School of Medicine and Biomedical Sciences, Department of Medicine/Cardiovascular Medicine, Buffalo, NY, USA

Albert Flotats, MD Hospital de la Santa Creu i Sant Pau, Department of Nuclear Medicine, Barcelona, Spain

Wataru Fujita, MD Kanazawa Medical University, Department of Cardiology, Uchinada, Japan

Myron C. Gerson, MD University of Cincinnati Medical Center, Division of Cardiovascular Health and Disease, Department of Internal Medicine, Cincinnati, OH, USA

Henry Gewirtz, MD Division of Cardiology, Department of Medicine, Harvard Medical School, Massachusetts General Hospital, Boston, MA, USA

Avishay Grupper, MD Mayo Clinic, Division of Cardiovascular Diseases, Rochester, MN, USA

David M. Harris, MD University of Cincinnati College of Medicine, Division of Cardiovascular Health and Disease, Cincinnati, OH, USA

Arnold F. Jacobson, MD Icahn School of Medicine at Mount Sinai, Department of Medicine, New York, NY, USA

Kouji Kajinami, MD Kanazawa Medical University, Department of Cardiology, Uchinada, Japan

Thomas Klein, MD Providence Sacred Heart Medical Center, Department of Medicine, Spokane, WA, USA

Sudhir S. Kushwaha, MD Mayo Medical Center, Cardiovascular Division, Rochester, MN, USA

Ichiro Matsunari, MD Saitama Medical University Hospital, Division of Nuclear Medicine, Department of Radiology, Iruma-gun, Japan

Jagat Narula, MD Division of Cardiology, Icahn School of Medicine at Mount Sinai, New York, NY, USA

Pradeep S. Rajendran, BS Ronald Reagan UCLA Medical Center, Los Angeles, CA, USA

Kalyanam Shivkumar, MD Ronald Reagan UCLA Medical Center, Los Angeles, CA, USA

Mark F. Smith University of Maryland School of Medicine, Department of Diagnostic Radiology and Nuclear Medicine, Baltimore, MD, USA

Marmar Vaseghi, MD, MS Ronald Reagan UCLA Medical Center, Los Angeles, CA, USA

1

Anatomy and Molecular Basis of Autonomic Innervation of the Heart

Wengen Chen and Vasken Dilsizian

Introduction

The heart is innervated extensively by sympathetic and parasympathetic nerves of the peripheral autonomic nervous system, as well as by sensory nerves. Most sympathetic neurons use norepinephrine as a primary neurotransmitter. Acetylcholine is the main neurotransmitter released by preganglionic and postganglionic vagal nerve terminals, which wrap around the heart and activate the parasympathetic nervous system. Sympathetic and parasympathetic systems exert opposite effects on the heart to regulate the contractile rate and force. Sympathetic nerves increase both heart rate (positive chronotropy) and contractile function (positive inotropy), whereas parasympathetic nerves diminish heart rate (bradycardia) and attenuate sympathetic effects on contractile function. Under normal conditions, the two systems are well balanced to maintain a normal response to external stimulation.

Sympathetic nerves are not distributed homogeneously in the ventricle. The basal inferior region has less innervation compared with the other regions of the left ventricular myocardium [1]. The sympathetic nerve fibers display an epicardial-to-endocardial gradient in the heart [2]. Maintenance of this physiologic innervation gradient is required to sustain a physiologic repolarization gradient across the ventricular walls. Collapse of the innervation gradient may have an adverse effect on the electrical phenotype of the ventricular wall and cause ventricular arrhythmia.

Several radiotracers have been developed for functional imaging of cardiac sympathetic tone. For example, to target the neurotransmitter norepinephrine, ^{123}I *meta*-iodobenzylguanidine (^{123}I-*m*IBG) and ^{11}C-hydroxyephedrine (^{11}C-HED) were developed. Both radiotracers mimic the neuronal transport and storage process of norepinephrine and represent cardiac sympathetic activity. ^{123}I-*m*IBG is a single-photon emitter and is imaged by using planar or single photon emission computed tomography (SPECT). ^{11}C-HED is a positron emitter and is imaged by using positron emission tomography (PET) or PET/CT hybrid imaging.

Many neuronal factors are involved in sympathetic nerve growth, development, and regeneration after injury, although detailed molecular signaling and regulation mechanisms are not fully understood. Understanding changes and regeneration in sympathetic innervation is more important clinically in the diseased heart than in the normal heart. For example, one of the characteristic neurohormonal changes during heart failure is activation of the sympathetic nervous system. In acute-phase or early heart failure, this activation may preserve cardiovascular homeostasis promptly and even restore cardiac function. However, persistent activation of the sympathetic nervous system in a decompensated heart would be extremely toxic and ultimately would lead to progressively worsening heart function [3]. It is well known that in chronic heart failure, cardiac adrenoceptor signaling and function are significantly deranged and the adrenergic reserve of the heart is diminished [4–6]. Imaging with ^{123}I-*m*IBG or ^{11}C-HED has repeatedly shown the utility of ^{123}I-*m*IBG cardiac scanning in identifying heart failure patients with an increased risk of adverse cardiac events [7–9]. It has been shown that ^{123}I-*m*IBG imaging can predict sudden cardiac death and total cardiac mortality [10]. Similarly, myocardial

V. Dilsizian, J. Narula (eds.), *Atlas of Cardiac Innervation*, DOI 10.1007/978-3-319-45800-7_1

sympathetic denervation quantified by using ^{11}C-HED PET imaging identifies patients with ischemic cardiomyopathy who are at high risk for sudden cardiac death [11].

Distribution of Autonomous Nervous System in the Heart

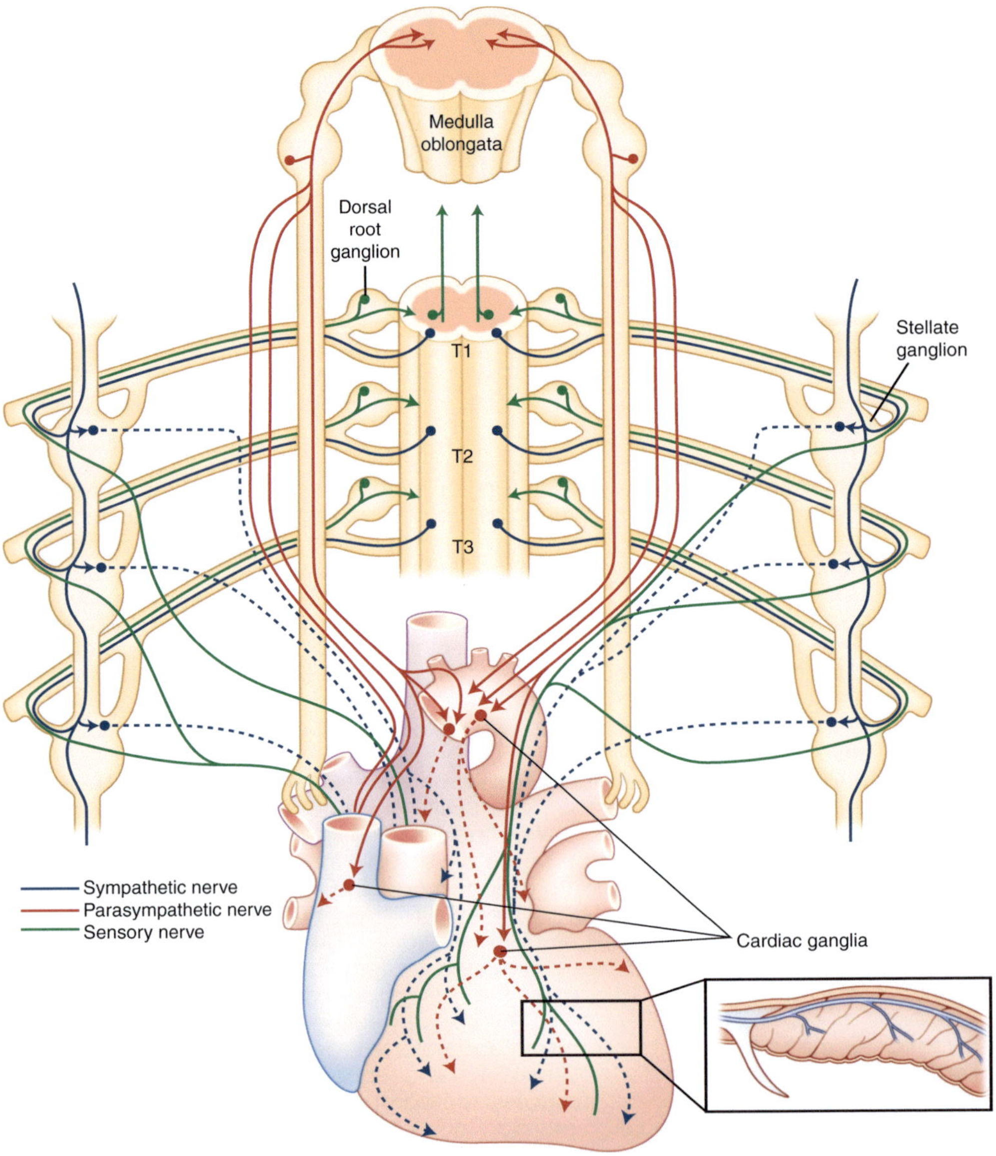

Figure 1-1. Anatomy and distribution of the cardiac nervous systems. The cardiac sympathetic nerve ends (*blue*) are projected from sympathetic neurons in the stellate ganglia, which are bilateral to the thoracic vertebra. The stellate ganglia originate from the spinal cord (dorsal root ganglia or preganglia). The cardiac parasympathetic nerves (*red*) extend from parasympathetic neurons in the cardiac ganglia, which are located at the base of both atria, and are direct branches of the vagus nerve in the human from the brainstem (10th cranial verve). The sensory nerves (*green*) project to the upper thoracic dorsal horn via dorsal root ganglia, which are responsible for pain perception and initiation of a protective response during cardiac injury. The inset indicates the transverse section of the heart and demonstrates the distribution of sympathetic nerve fibers within the left ventricle. The sympathetic nerve fibers run in the epicardial area and then individually dive into the myocardial wall, and display an epicardial-to-endocardial gradient in the heart [2]. Maintenance of this physiologic innervation gradient is required for sustaining a physiologic repolarization gradient across the ventricular walls. Collapse of the innervation gradient may have an adverse effect on the electrical phenotype of the ventricular wall, resulting in arrhythmia (Data from Kimura et al. [12]).

Sympathetic Neuronal Synapse in the Heart

Figure 1-2. Sympathetic neuronal synapse in the heart. The sympathetic neuronal transmitter norepinephrine (*NE*) is synthesized from tyrosine. First, it is converted to dopamine by cytoplasmic enzymes. Dopamine then is transported to intraneuronal vesicles, where NE is synthesized and stored. Upon neuronal stimulation, the vesicles fuse with the presynaptic membrane and release the NE into the cleft. The released NE then binds to the postsynaptic α- and β-adrenergic receptors, which are G-protein–coupled receptors, to transduce signals to improve excitation–contraction coupling of the myocardium and to increase heart rate and force. Cleft NE also activates the presynaptic α_2-adrenergic receptors to inhibit further NE release. The effect of the NE is terminated by two mechanisms: approximately 80% of the NE is taken up to the presynaptic area by an ATP-dependent active process via a transporter called human norepinephrine transporter 1 (hNET1; uptake-1 system), whereas the reminder spills over into the nonneuronal tissue and bloodstream (uptake-2 system). Thus, several molecules in this pathway may serve as targets for the functional imaging of sympathetic tone in the heart. For example, to target the neurotransmitter NE, ^{123}I-*m*IBG and ^{11}C-HED were developed. Both radiotracers mimic the neuronal transport and storage process of NE and represent cardiac sympathetic activity. hNET1 also may be an ideal target to represent the uptake-1 system activity in the heart. *AC* adenyl cyclase, *AMP* adenosine monophosphate, *cAMP* cyclic adenosine monophosphate, *COMT* catechol-*O*-methyltransferase, *DA* dopamine, *DHPG* dihydroxyphenylglycol, *DOPA* dihydroxyphenylalanine, *MAO* monoamine oxidase, *NMN* normetanephrine (Data from Haider et al. [13]).

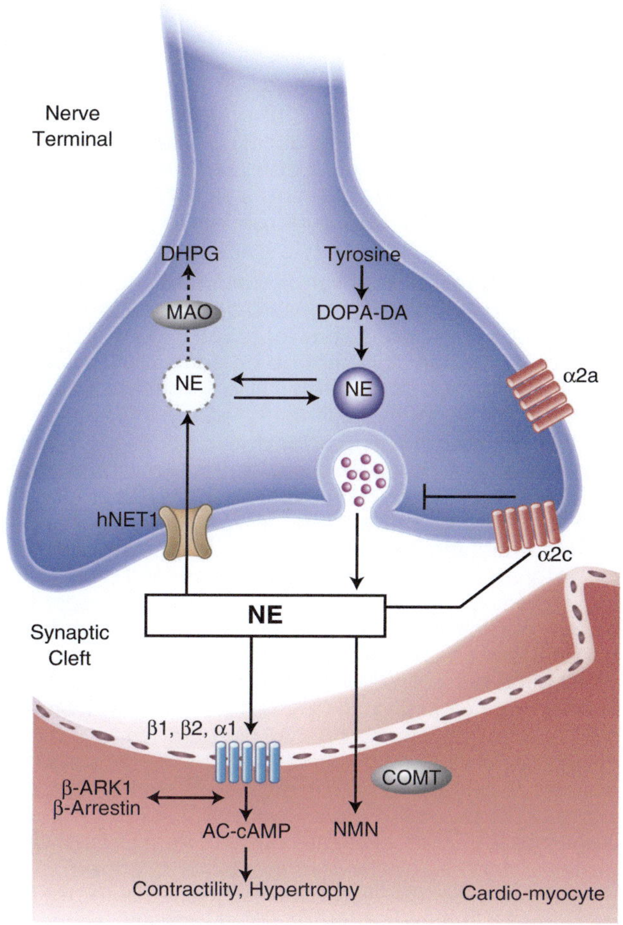

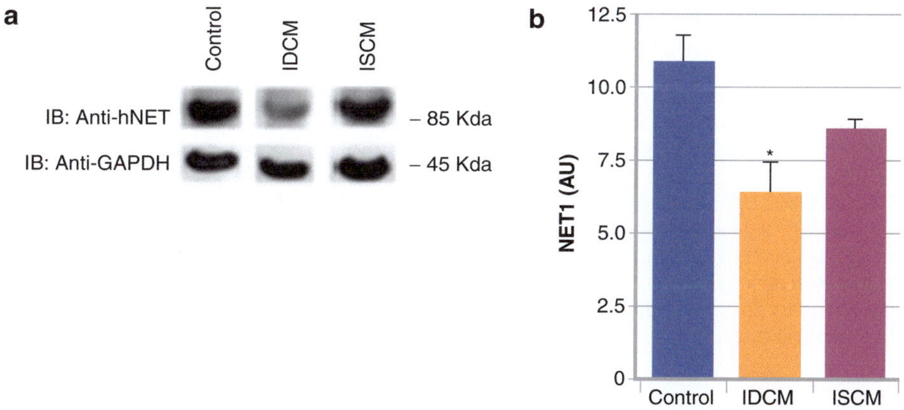

Figure 1-3. Down-regulation of the presynaptic hNET1 in heart failure. In patients with heart failure (ischemic or nonischemic), initially there is increased sympathetic activity with increased release of NE from the presynaptic vesicles as a compensatory reaction to contribute to increased cardiac contractility. (**a**, **b**) There is corresponding down-regulation of the hNET1 transporter (decreased uptake-1 system) in idiopathic dilated cardiomyopathy (IDCM) and ischemic cardiomyopathy (ISCM) [13], with a subsequent increase in quantities of NE in the synaptic cleft. Gradually, the compensatory mechanism is overwhelmed, and a persistent NE excess in the cleft eventually results in desensitization of the postsynaptic adrenergic receptors [5], myocyte apoptosis/myocellular loss [14], worsening heart failure, increased susceptibility to arrhythmia, and sudden cardiac death [15]. A small proportion of this NE spills into the bloodstream (increased uptake-2 system, with increasing plasma NE levels). These compensatory changes can be imaged with the NE analogue ^{123}I-*m*IBG as decreased retention of the radiotracer in the presynaptic area and increased washout. *GAPDH* glyceraldehyde-3-phosphate dehydrogenase, *IB* immunoblot. *$P<0.05$: intensity of the hNET1 bands mean SEM of four IDCM, four ISCM, and eight control hearts. Values were corrected by the respective values of GAPDH for each sample (Data from Haider et al. [13]).

Signal Transduction of the Postsynaptic Cardiac Adrenergic Receptors

The human genome encodes nine different adrenoceptor genes. They are grouped into three G-protein–coupled receptor (GPCR) families with three members each, namely the α_1-adrenoceptors (α_{1A}, α_{1B}, and α_{1D}), α_2-adrenoceptors (α_{2A}, α_{2B}, and α_{2C}), and β-adrenoceptors (β_1, β_2, and β_3) [16]. In the human heart, the β_1-adrenoceptor subtype is predominant, representing 75–80% of total adrenoceptor density. The β_2 subtype also is present, representing 15–18%, whereas β_3-adrenoceptors comprise the remaining 2–3% [17, 18]. The β_1 subtype mediates an increase in cardiac contractility, whereas the β_2 subtype is responsible for vasodilatation. These receptors are not just signal transducers but also components of a complex and highly regulated signaling machinery. Adrenoceptors consist of seven transmembrane (TM)-spanning α-helical domains, an extracellular region (N terminus, three extracellular loops), and an intracellular region (three intracellular loops, C terminus).

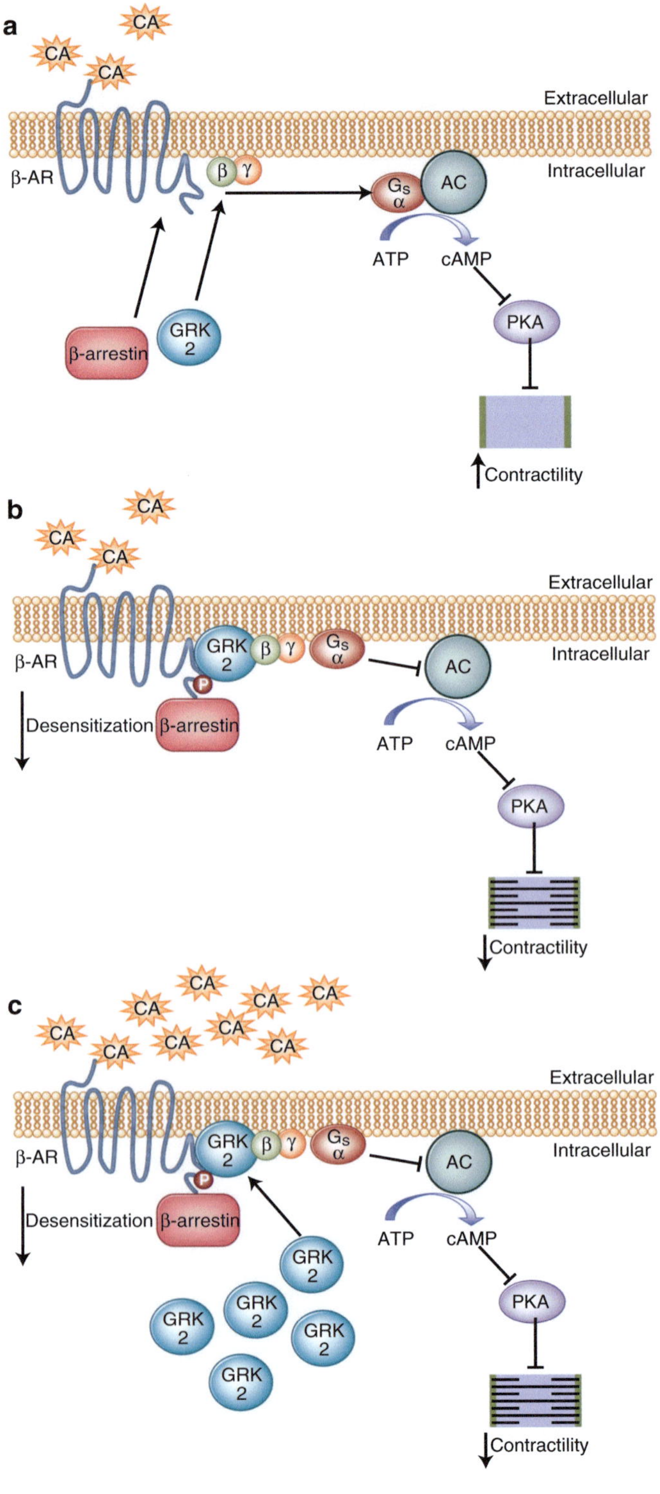

Figure 1-4. Signal transduction of cardiac myocyte contraction and its regulation by cardiac adrenergic receptors. Under normal conditions (**a**), upon catecholamine binding, adrenoceptors change conformation, couple to and activate Gαs, and thereby initiate various intracellular signaling cascades that ultimately lead to increased contractility by activating adenylate cyclase (AC) and protein kinase A (PKA). β-adrenoceptor signaling is subject to agonist-promoted desensitization (**b**), a loss of function as a result of uncoupling from the signal transducing G protein, which occurs within a few seconds and diminishes receptor response to continuous or repeated agonist stimulation. At the molecular level, this rapid process can be induced by receptor phosphorylation by a family of kinases, termed G-protein-coupled receptor kinases (GRKs). The cytosolic GRK translocates and anchors to the membrane by binding to Gβγ via its C terminus where it is able to interact with the agonist-occupied receptor and phosphorylate it, which begins the G protein uncoupling process. G protein activation is blocked by recruitment of β-arrestin molecules to the phosphorylated receptor. The β-arrestins then uncouple the receptor from its cognate G proteins, sterically hinder its further binding to them (functional desensitization), and subsequently target the receptor for internalization [19, 20]. In addition, receptors can be downregulated, a mechanism requiring several hours, by decreasing receptor synthesis or increasing receptor degradation or sequestration. In addition, β-adrenoceptors mRNA destabilization in response to agonist exposure may also occur [21]. After cardiac injury (**c**), GRKs levels are increased because of enhanced β adrenoceptor activation after stress-induced increases in catecholamines. The increase in GRKs help to prevent overstimulation of the β adrenoceptors initially, but over time a vicious cycle of chronically increased β adrenoceptor desensitization occurs and β1 downregulation [22], which lead to progressive worsening of the cardiac adrenergic and inotropic reserves, the hallmark of heart failure [23] (Data from Woodall et al. [24]).

Heterogeneity of Innervation in the Normal Heart

Clinical studies using ^{123}I-*m*IBG scintigraphy have demonstrated heterogeneous sympathetic distribution in normal hearts, particularly in the inferior region. Such decreased inferior *m*IBG activity was found to be more prevalent in older subjects and more evident in men than women [1]. The findings were confirmed by others who showed that in men, *m*IBG uptake in the inferior wall was inversely correlated with age. There was a 16% reduction in *m*IBG uptake in the 80-year-old age group compared with the 40-year-old age group [24]. Although the mechanism for this age-related decrease of *m*IBG in the inferior region of the left ventricular myocardium is not clear, it might be related to high parasympathetic activity in that area. In a study of *m*IBG uptake in high-level male athletes, the subset of athletes with sinus bradycardia (heart rate <50 bpm; mean age, 27 years) had significantly less inferior *m*IBG uptake (44±13%) than those with higher heart rates (heart rate >60 bpm; mean age, 34 years), who exhibited relatively preserved inferior *m*IBG uptake (72±11%, $P<0.01$) [25]. These findings support the notion that high parasympathetic activity, as characterized by sinus bradycardia, may contribute to the inferior *m*IBG abnormalities, as do diaphragmatic attenuation artifacts.

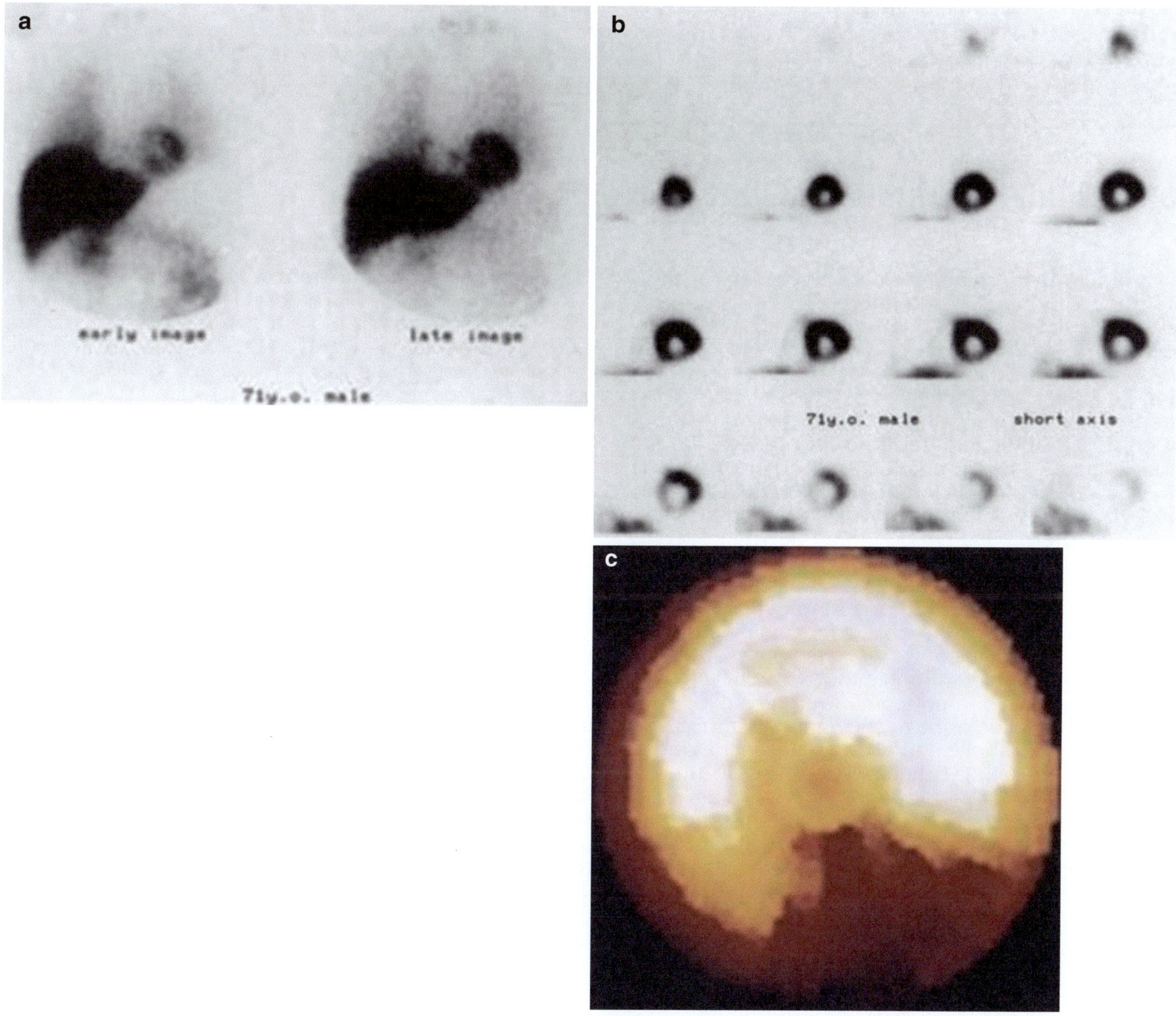

Figure 1-5. Heterogeneity of Innervation in the Normal Heart. The images show a 71-yr-old man with malignant lymphoma before adriamycin administration. High accumulation of tracer in the myocardium is shown on the early and the late planar images (**a**). On the short-axis SPECT images (**b**) and bull's-eye polar map (**c**), however, decreased *m*IBG uptake in the inferior region is noted (This research was originally published in JNM. Tsuchimochi et al. [1]. Figure 1.2. © by the Society of Nuclear Medicine and Molecular Imaging, Inc.).

Reinnervation in the Transplanted Heart

The transplanted heart lacks both sympathetic and parasympathetic innervation because the nerves are dissected during surgery. The absence of direct nerve stimulation leads to an inadequate balance between the sympathetic and parasympathetic systems. In the absence of parasympathetic stimulation, heart rate and myocardial contractility are both increased in the transplanted heart [26, 27]. On the other hand, the lack of sympathetic denervation and norepinephrine release prevents the heart rate from increasing enough to meet stress or exercise demands (chronotropic incompetency). The denervated heart becomes dependent on circulating norepinephrine for increasing the heart rate, contractility, and conduction via β_1-receptor stimulation [28], which is minimal and delayed. Both parasympathetic [29] and sympathetic [30] reinnervation has been observed in transplanted hearts. Although the time course of reinnervation and the extent of reinnervation in the transplanted heart may vary, clinical studies have reported partial cardiac reinnervation between 1 and 15 years after cardiac transplantation [31–33]. Reinnervation may occur earlier in younger donor hearts and with a shorter surgical transplantation (ischemic) time. Reinnervation of the transplanted heart results in subsequent improvement in both left ventricular function and exercise tolerance in recipients [30].

Through the use of ^{123}I-*m*IBG or ^{11}C-HED PET imaging, studies have demonstrated partial reinnervation after transplantation [34–36]. Reinnervation has been found primarily in the basal anteroseptal region and, to a lesser degree, in the inferobasal and apical regions [34, 37]. The midventricular region of the myocardium typically demonstrates less reinnervation than the basal region. The findings of heterogeneous reinnervation may be explained partly by the fact that sympathetic neurons travel along arterial structures; thus, the basal regions are reached first by the newly grown fibers.

Molecular Regulation of Cardiac Nerve Development

Molecular signaling and regulation of cardiac autonomic development and innervation are not well elucidated yet. Understanding the mechanisms involved in neuronal development and reinnervation after injury is important in managing the diseased heart, especially with regard to conditions such as life-threatening ventricular arrhythmias after infarction, which may be related to sympathetic nerve sprouting. Studies have shown that cardiac autonomic neurogenesis and function are regulated tightly by a plethora of neurotrophic factors, which are divided into two classifications: the neurotrophin and glial cell line–derived neurotrophic factor (GDNF) families. The neurotrophin family is composed of several factors, including nerve growth factor (NGF), brain-derived neurotrophic factor (BDNF), and neurotrophins 3 and 4/5 (NT3 and NT4/5), acting through the high-affinity tyrosine kinase receptors, tropomyosin receptor kinase (Trk), and lower-affinity neurotrophin receptor p75 (p75NTR). The GDNF family includes GDNF, neurturin, and artemin, which bind to GDNF family receptor-α (GFRα) and RET [38–40].

NGF, the prototypic member of the neurotrophin family, acts primarily through TrkA, which promotes growth, survival, and maintenance of sympathetic nerves [41, 42]. The level of NGF expression in the heart correlates approximately to the sympathetic innervation density. Overexpression of NGF in the mouse heart results in hyperinnervation and hyperplasia in stellate ganglia neurons [43]. On the other hand, sympathetic ganglion volume is reduced by 80% at postnatal day 3 in mice with a disruption of the NGF gene [41]. In mice lacking the NGF receptor TrkA, no neurons remain at postnatal day 9 [39, 44]. NGF mediates axonal growth and synapse formation during development [45]. It is required for complete peripheral innervation of sympathetic ganglia targets [46] and is necessary and sufficient for synapse formation within sympathetic ganglia [47].

Different from neurotrophic factors such as NGF, as mentioned above, which act as chemoattractants in cardiac nerve development, some factors work as chemorepellents that inhibit nerve growth and distribution during development. Studies have shown that Sema3a, a member of the semaphorin family, is such a chemorepellent, affecting sympathetic neural patterning in the developing heart [47]. *Sema3a* is expressed in the subendocardium but not in the subepicardium, in contrast to the epicardial-to-endocardial gradient of sympathetic innervation (Fig. 1.6). Cardiac-specific *Sema3a*-overexpression mice had reduced sympathetic innervation and attenuation of the epicardial-to-endocardial innervation gradient. These results indicate that cardiomyocyte-derived Sema3a plays a critical role in cardiac sympathetic innervation patterning by inhibiting neural growth.

The GDNF family also is involved in sympathetic nerve regeneration in addition to its effect on parasympathetic nerve development [48]. Artemin, a neurotrophic factor of the GDNF family, was shown to promote the development of sympathetic innervation along blood vessels by enhancing sympathetic axon growth [49, 50]. Cocultures of sympathetic ganglionic neurons and cardiomyocytes demonstrated that GDNF promotes sympathetic axon growth toward cardiomyocytes more potently than NGF, with morphologic and functional synapse formation with the concomitant increase of β_1-adrenergic receptors in cardiomyocytes [51, 52]. Under pathophysiologic conditions, the effect of GDNF was more potent than that of neurotrophic factors such as NGF, BDNF, or ciliary neurotrophic factor [53].

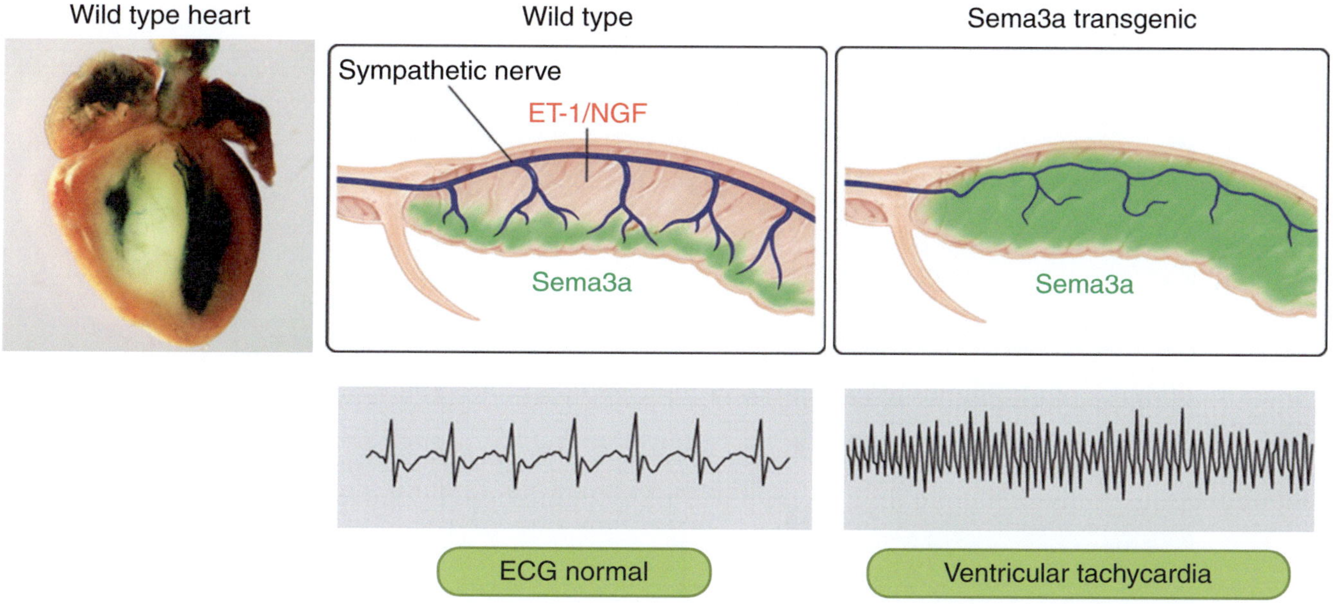

Figure 1-6. Regulation of cardiac innervation patterning and maintenance of an arrhythmia free heart. *Left*, X-gal staining (*green*) of *Sema3alacZ* hearts at E15 demonstrates strong *Sema3a* expression in the subendocardium. *Middle*, Cardiac sympathetic innervation shows an epicardial-to-endocardial transmural gradient. This patterning is established by the balance between ET-1/NGF and Sema3a expression in the heart. Note that NGF is expressed abundantly in the working myocardium, whereas Sema3a is expressed specifically in the subendocardium. *Right*, Appropriate Sema3a mediated sympathetic innervation patterning is critical for the maintenance of an arrhythmia-free heart. *Sema3a* Transgenic mice display disruption of innervation patterning and are highly susceptible to ventricular tachyarrhythmias (From Kimura et al. [**12**]; with permission).

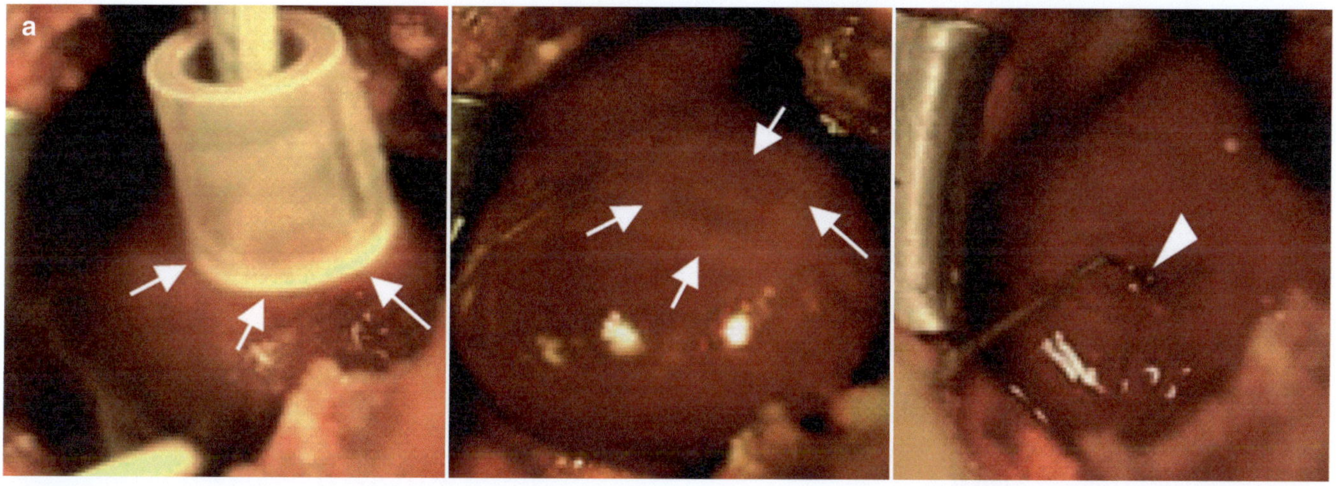

Figure 1-7. Re-innervation in a rat model of denervation by cryoinjury. (**a**) Induction of denervation in rat hearts in vivo. A ring-shaped denervation was induced by cryoinjury on the epicardial surface of the left ventricular free wall (*arrows in left and middle panels*). Ad-GDNF was injected into the inner area of the injured ring (*arrowhead in right*). Ad-GFP was injected in controls. (**b**) Representative pictures of axon growth in the ring-shaped denervated area 5 days after the creation of cryoinjury. The hearts were isolated and whole-mount labeled for neurofilament-M (NFM, DAB stain). In the control heart (*top*), axons were detected only sparsely in the denervated area (*arrows*). In the Ad-GDNF-injected heart (*bottom*), in contrast, axons grew abundantly across the denervated area (*arrows*). Arrowheads indicate the uninjured central area (*inner ring*). *Right* panels show magnified images of the rectangular zones (injured areas). Bars indicate 1 mm. (**c**) The percentage of the denervated area covered by axons (NFMpositive). Values are means±SD. *$p<0.05$ vs control ($n=5$). (**d**) Representative immunolabeling images of NFM (*green*), α-actinine (AA, *red*) and GDNF (*blue*) in the sections across the long axis of the rat hearts (denervated area). Note that GDNF was abundantly expressed in the myocardium, and the NFM-positive axons grew from the epicardial surface (*arrows*) into the mid myocardium in the AdGDNF heart (*bottom*). In the control heart (*top*), in contrast, GDNF was undetectable in the myocardium and the axons were recognized only scarcely on the epicardial surface. Bars indicate 50 mm (From Miwa et al. [51]).

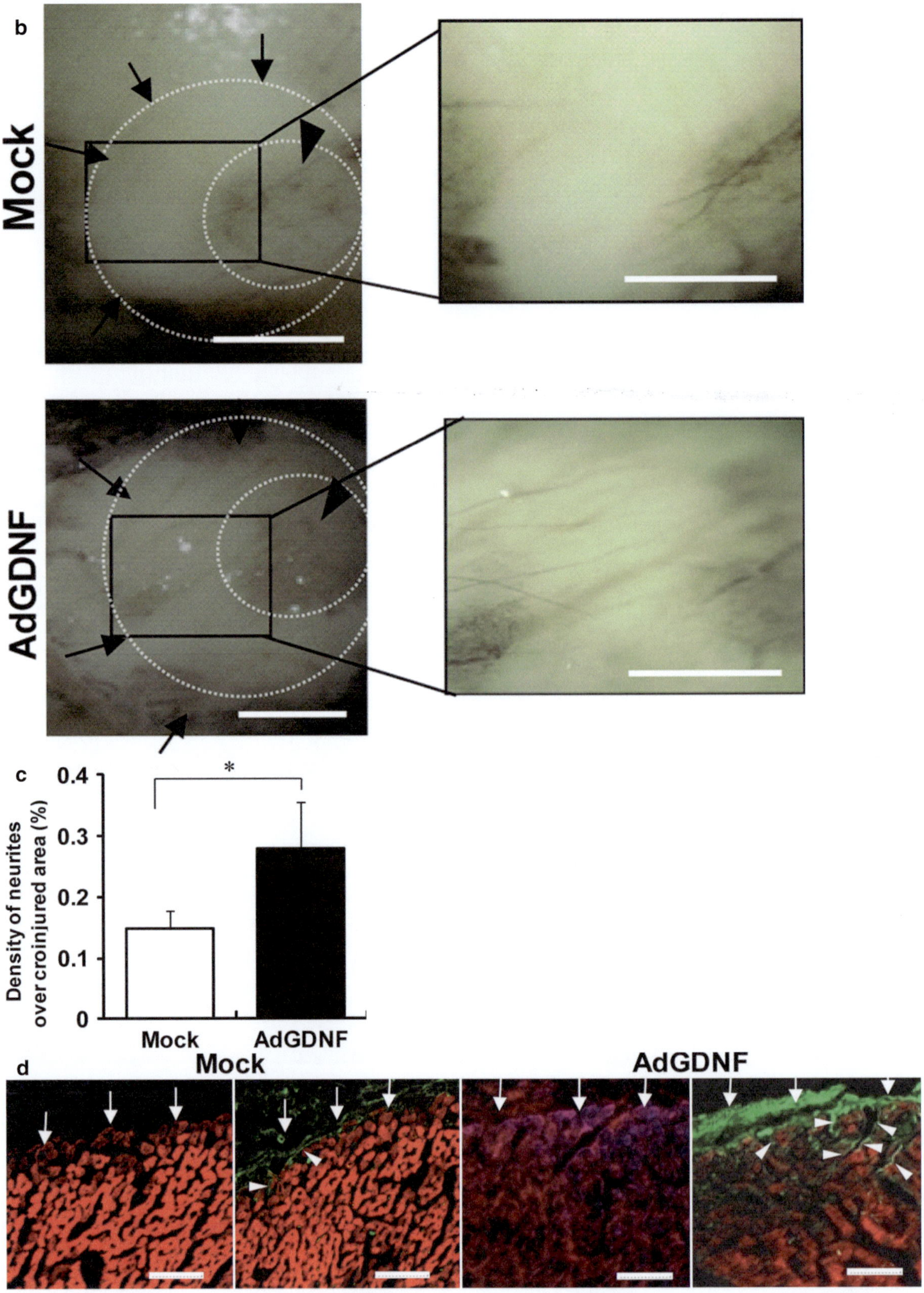

Figure 1-7. (continued)

Sympathetic Dysfunction in Cardiac Diseases

Compared with the normal heart, heterogeneity of sympathetic innervation in the diseased heart is more important clinically because it may cause ventricular arrhythmias and even sudden cardiac death. Imaging with ^{123}I-*m*IBG scintigraphy or ^{11}C-HED PET repeatedly has shown heterogeneous sympathetic innervation in diseased hearts. For example, after myocardial infarction, cardiac nerves undergo degenerative changes that result in heterogeneous innervations. The unbalanced sympathetic nerve innervation density may cause lethal arrhythmia [54].

Heart Failure

In the failing heart, cardiac sympathetic activity is increased, leading to pathophysiologic cardiac damage, depressed cardiac performance, and fatal arrhythmia. Although the underlying mechanisms are not fully understood, the phenomenon of increased innervation in the failing heart is associated with observations of decreased reuptake of norepinephrine into the presynaptic area (uptake-1 system) [55] and increased norepinephrine turnover or spillover in the synaptic cleft (uptake-2 system) [56]. This usually is reflected as decreased cardiac ^{123}I-*m*IBG uptake on imaging. It should be mentioned that decreased cardiac activity on ^{123}I-*m*IBG or ^{11}C-HED PET often is described inappropriately as cardiac denervation in the literature. A true denervation usually is the result of nerve death in a totally infarcted area with complete absence of ^{123}I-*m*IBG or ^{11}C-HED PET activity.

Studies repeatedly have shown the utility of ^{123}I-*m*IBG cardiac scanning in identifying heart failure patients with an increased risk of adverse cardiac events. A meta-analysis of 1755 patients from 18 studies confirmed that patients with a reduced heart-to-mediastinal (H/M) ratio have a poorer prognosis than those with a normal H/M ratio [8]. The ADMIRE-HF (AdreView Myocardial Imaging for Risk Evaluation in Heart Failure) study validated the independent prognostic value of the H/M ratio in patients with class II and III heart failure with left ventricular dysfunction [9]. The results showed that for patients with an H/M ratio less than 1.6, 2-year cardiac death and all-cause mortality were 11.2% and 16.1%, respectively, versus 1.8% and 3.0% for those with an H/M ratio ≥1.6. There was a progressive decline in both cardiac and all-cause mortality from greater than 20% for H/M less than 1.10–0% for H/M ≥1.8.

Cardiomyopathy

Dilated cardiomyopathy frequently is associated with regional neuronal dysfunction rather than a perfusion abnormality [57]. In patients with dilated cardiomyopathy, the inferobasal region is affected more commonly by neuronal dysfunction [58]. Diabetic cardiomyopathy often is associated with autonomic neuropathy. Imaging studies demonstrated a reduction in tracer uptake in the inferior wall of the left ventricle gradually spreading to adjacent segments. The extent of the reduced uptake was related to the severity of autonomic dysfunction as measured by conventional markers [59, 60]. Figure 1.8 shows an ^{11}C-HED PET image from a patient with diabetes.

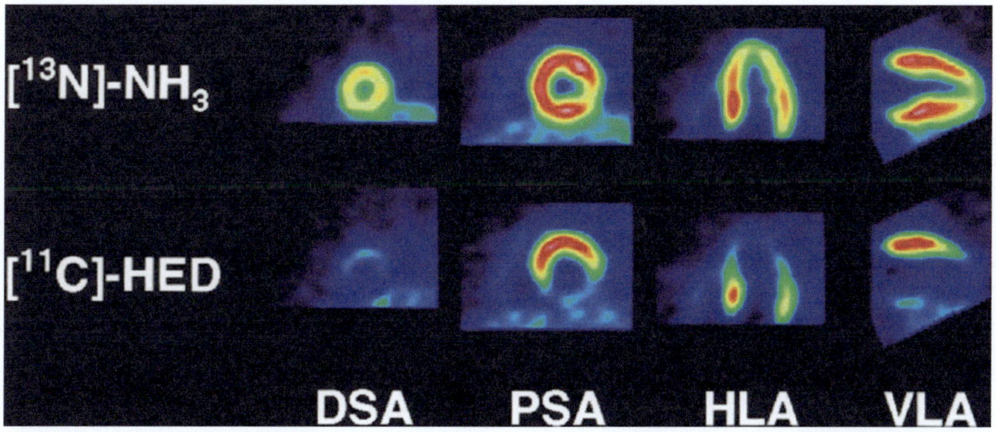

Figure 1-8. PET images of the left ventricle from a 21-year old woman who after 13 years of diabetes has symptoms from autonomic neuropathy (gastroparesis and postural hypotension) and abnormalities in all her autonomic function tests. Blood flow images appear normal (*top panels*), but abnormalities of ^{11}C-HED retention are extensive, with only the proximal cardiac segments being preserved (*bottom panels*). *DSA* distal short axis, *HLA* horizontal long axis, *PSA* proximal short axis, *VLA* vertical long axis (From Stevens et al. [61]; with permission).

Sudden Cardiac Death

Sudden cardiac death from ventricular arrhythmias remains the leading cause of death in developed countries [62, 63]. Alterations in cardiac autonomic regulation induced by cardiac diseases, such as myocardial ischemia and infarction, play an important role in the genesis of life-threatening arrhythmias. Changes in the balance of parasympathetic and sympathetic regulation of the heart during the disease process may contribute significantly to the induction of ventricular fibrillation [64, 65].

Increased cardiac sympathetic activity (decreased activity on ^{123}I-*m*IBG scintigraphy or ^{11}C-HED PET images) enhances the development of lethal cardiac arrhythmias. Sympathetic nerve sprouting and compensatory reinnervation following myocardial infarction alter regional electrical properties of the heart, thereby facilitating the formation of ventricular arrhythmias [64, 66, 67]. Interventions that reduce cardiac sympathetic activity have been shown to protect against arrhythmias. β-Adrenoceptor blockade has been shown to reduce cardiac mortality in patients recovering from myocardial infarction [68]. In these patients, β-adrenoceptor blockers reduced overall mortality by 20% and mortality due to sudden death by 30–50% [69]. β-Adrenoceptor blockers were most effective in reducing early (1 h to 7 days) cardiac mortality during myocardial infarction [70].

Reduction in parasympathetic control is associated with an increased risk for sudden death [65]. Electrical stimulation of the vagus nerves may reduce the ventricular fibrillation threshold and reduce the incidence of ventricular fibrillation [71]. Pretreatment with drugs that increase cholinergic receptor activation also has been shown to protect against ischemia-induced ventricular fibrillation in animal models [72].

Multiple large clinical trials have shown that LVEF is the only parameter used clinically to distinguish between high- and low-risk sudden cardiac death groups. Based on this, prophylactic placement of an implantable cardiac defibrillator (ICD) has a proven benefit in preventing sudden cardiac death and improving survival in patients with an LVEF lower than 35% [73, 74]. Nevertheless, most patients never require device therapy to prevent a lethal ventricular arrhythmia. The ability to identify the risk of arrhythmic death independent of LVEF might better target therapy among ICD candidates, as well as identify patients with LVEF greater than 35% who are at high risk of sudden cardiac death [75, 76]. Because sympathetic innervation inhomogeneity may create a myocardial substrate particularly vulnerable to the development of lethal ventricular arrhythmias and death [77], ^{123}I-*m*IBG imaging can predict sudden cardiac death and total cardiac mortality [10]. Recent studies consistently showed an association between *m*IBG defect and ventricular arrhythmias causing appropriate ICD therapy, as well as the composite of appropriate ICD therapy or cardiac death [78].

Other studies also demonstrated that myocardial sympathetic denervation quantified using ^{11}C-HED PET imaging could identify patients with ischemic cardiomyopathy at high risk for sudden cardiac death [11]. Thus, quantifying the extent of myocardial sympathetic defect may provide a novel approach to identifying a subgroup of patients with ischemic cardiomyopathy who would derive the most benefit from a primary prevention ICD.

References

1. Tsuchimochi S, Tamaki N, Tadamura E, et al. Age and gender differences in normal myocardial adrenergic neuronal function evaluated by iodine-123-MIBG imaging. J Nucl Med. 1995;36:969–74.
2. Ieda M, Fukuda K. Cardiac innervation and sudden cardiac death. Curr Cardiol Rev. 2009;5:289–95.
3. Rona G. Catecholamine cardiotoxicity. J Mol Cell Cardiol. 1985;17:291–306.
4. Bristow MR, Ginsburg R, Minobe W, et al. Decreased catecholamine sensitivity and beta-adrenergic-receptor density in failing human hearts. N Engl J Med. 1982;307:205–11.
5. Bristow MR, Ginsburg R, Umans V, et al. Beta 1- and beta 2-adrenergic-receptor subpopulations in nonfailing and failing human ventricular myocardium: coupling of both receptor subtypes to muscle contraction and selective beta 1-receptor down-regulation in heart failure. Circ Res. 1986;59:297–309.
6. Port JD, Bristow MR. Altered beta-adrenergic receptor gene regulation and signaling in chronic heart failure. J Mol Cell Cardiol. 2001;33:887–905.
7. Merlet P, Merlet P, Valette H, et al. Prognostic value of cardiac metaiodobenzylguanidine imaging in patients with heart failure. J Nucl Med. 1992;33:471–7.
8. Verberne HJ, Brewster LM, Somsen GA, et al. Prognostic value of myocardial 123I-metaiodobenzylguanidine (MIBG) parameters in patients with heart failure: a systematic review. Eur Heart J. 2008;29:1147–59.
9. Jacobson AF, Senior R, Cerqueira MD, et al. Myocardial iodine-123 meta-iodobenzylguanidine imaging and cardiac events in heart failure. Results of the prospective ADMIRE-HF (AdreView Myocardial Imaging for Risk Evaluation in Heart Failure) study. J Am Coll Cardiol. 2010;55:2212–21.
10. Tamaki S, Yamada T, Okuyama Y, et al. Cardiac iodine-123 metaiodobenzylguanidine imaging predicts sudden cardiac death independently of left ventricular ejection fraction in patients with chronic heart failure and left ventricular systolic dysfunction: results from a comparative study with signal-averaged electrocardiogram, heart rate variability, and QT dispersion. J Am Coll Cardiol. 2009;53:426–35.
11. Fallavollita JA, Heavey BM, Luisi Jr AJ, et al. Regional myocardial sympathetic denervation predicts the risk of sudden cardiac arrest in ischemic cardiomyopathy. J Am Coll Cardiol. 2014;63:141–9.
12. Kimura K, Ieda M, Fuluda K. Development, maturation, and transdifferentiation of cardiac sympathetic nerves. Circ Res. 2012;110:325–36.
13. Haider N, Baliga RR, Chandrashekhar Y, et al. Adrenergic excess, hNET1 down-regulation, and compromised mIBG uptake in heart failure poverty in the presence of plenty. JACC Cardiovasc Imaging. 2010;3:71–5.
14. Narula J, Haider N, Virmani R, et al. Apoptosis in myocytes in end-stage heart failure. N Engl J Med. 1996;335:1182–9.
15. Ellison KE, Stevenson WG, Sweeney MO, et al. Management of arrhythmias in heart failure. Congest Heart Fail. 2003;9:91–9.

16. Bylund DB, Eikenberg DC, Hieble JP, et al. International Union of Pharmacology nomenclature of adrenoceptors. Pharmacol Rev. 1994;46:121–36.
17. Brodde OE. Beta-adrenoceptors in cardiac disease. Pharmacol Ther. 1993;60:405–30.
18. Gauthier C, Tavernier G, Charpentier F, et al. Functional beta3-adrenoceptor in the human heart. J Clin Invest. 1996;98:556–62.
19. Reiter E, Lefkowitz RJ. GRKs and beta-arrestins: roles in receptor silencing, trafficking and signaling. Trends Endocrinol Metab. 2006;17:159–65.
20. Ferguson SS. Evolving concepts in G protein-coupled receptor endocytosis: the role in receptor desensitization and signaling. Pharmacol Rev. 2001;53:1–24.
21. Lohse MJ, Engelhardt S, Danner S, et al. Mechanisms of beta-adrenergic receptor desensitization: from molecular biology to heart failure. Basic Res Cardiol. 1996;91 Suppl 2:29–34.
22. Brodde OE. Beta-adrenergic receptors in failing human myocardium. Basic Res Cardiol. 1996;91 Suppl 2:35–40.
23. Eschenhagen T. Beta-adrenergic signaling in heart failure-adapt or die. Nat Med. 2008;14:485–7.
24. Woodall MC, Ciccarelli M, Woodall BP, et al. G protein–coupled receptor kinase 2, a link between myocardial contractile function and cardiac metabolism. Circ Res. 2014;114: 1661–70.
25. Estorch M, Estorch M, Serra-Grima R, et al. Myocardial sympathetic innervation in the athlete's sinus bradycardia: is there selective inferior myocardial wall denervation? J Nucl Cardiol. 2000;7:354–8.
26. Beckers F, Ramaekers D, Speijer G, et al. Different evolutions in heart rate variability after heart transplantation: 10-year follow-up. Transplantation. 2004;78:1523–31.
27. Gaer J. Physiological consequences of complete cardiac denervation. Br J Hosp Med. 1992;48:220–5.
28. Thompson CJ. Denervation of the transplanted heart: nursing implications for patient care. Crit Care Nurs Q. 1995;17:1–14.
29. Uberfuhr P, Frey AW, Fuchs A, et al. Signs of vagal reinnervation 4 years after heart transplantation in spectra of heart rate variability. Eur J Cardiothorac Surg. 1997;12:907–12.
30. Bengel FM, Bengel FM, Ueberfuhr P, et al. Clinical determinants of ventricular sympathetic reinnervation after orthotopic heart transplantation. Circulation. 2002;106:831–5.
31. Bengel FM, Ueberfuhr P, Schiepel N, et al. Effect of sympathetic reinnervation on cardiac performance after heart transplantation. N Engl J Med. 2001;345:731–8.
32. Uberfuhr P, Ziegler S, Schwaiblmair M, et al. Incomplete sympathic reinnervation of the orthotopically transplanted human heart: observation up to 13 years after heart transplantation. J Cardiothorac Surg. 2000;17:161–8.
33. Murphy DA, Thompson GW, Ardell JL, et al. The heart reinnervates after transplantation. Ann Thorac Surg. 2000;69:1769–81.
34. Bengel FM, Ueberfuhr P, Ziegler SI, et al. Serial assessment of sympathetic reinnervation after orthotopic heart transplantation. A longitudinal study using PET and C-11 hydroxyephedrine. Circulation. 1999;99:1866–71.
35. De Marco T, Dae M, Yuen-Green MS, et al. Iodine-123 metaiodobenzylguanidine scintigraphic assessment of the transplanted human heart: evidence for late reinnervation. J Am Coll Cardiol. 1995;25:927–31.
36. Estorch M, Campreciós M, Flotats A, et al. Sympathetic reinnervation of cardiac allografts evaluated by 123I-MIBG imaging. J Nucl Med. 1999;40:911–6.
37. Momose M, Momose M, Kobayashi H, et al. Regional cardiac sympathetic reinnervation in transplanted human hearts detected by 123I-MIBG SPECT imaging. Ann Nucl Med. 2000;14:333–7.
38. Suvanto P, Hiltunen JO, Arumäe U, et al. Localization of glial cell line-derived neurotrophic factor (GDNF) mRNA in embryonic rat by in situ hybridization. Eur J Neurosci. 1996;8:816–22.
39. Snider WD. Functions of the neurotrophins during nervous system development: what the knockouts are teaching us. Cell. 1994;77:627–38.
40. Baloh RH, Tansey MG, Lampe PA, et al. Artemin, a novel member of the GDNF ligand family, supports peripheral and central neurons and signals through the GFRalpha3-RET receptor complex. Neuron. 1998;21:1291–302.
41. Crowley C, Spencer SD, Nishimura MC, et al. Mice lacking nerve growth factor display perinatal loss of sensory and sympathetic neurons yet develop basal forebrain cholinergic neurons. Cell. 1994;76:1001–11.
42. Ieda M, Kanazawa H, Ieda Y, et al. Nerve growth factor is critical for cardiac sensory innervation and rescues neuropathy in diabetic hearts. Circulation. 2006;114:2351–63.
43. Hassankhani A, Steinhelper ME, Soonpaa MH, et al. Overexpression of NGF within the heart of transgenic mice causes hyperinnervation, cardiac enlargement, and hyperplasia of ectopic cells. Dev Biol. 1995;169:309–21.
44. Fagan AM, Fagan AM, Zhang H, et al. TrkA, but not TrkC, receptors are essential for survival of sympathetic neurons in vivo. J Neurosci. 1996;16:6208–18.
45. Glebova NO, Ginty DD. Heterogeneous requirement of NGF for sympathetic target innervation in vivo. J Neurosci. 2004;24:743–51.
46. Sharma N, Deppmann CD, Harrington AW, et al. Long-distance control of synapse assembly by target-derived NGF. Neuron. 2010;67:422–34.
47. Ieda M, Kanazawa H, Kimura K, et al. Sema3a maintains normal heart rhythm through sympathetic innervation patterning. Nat Med. 2007;13:604–12.
48. Hiltunen JO, Hiltunen JO, Laurikainen A, et al. GDNF family receptors in the embryonic and postnatal rat heart and reduced cholinergic innervation in mice hearts lacking ret or GFRalpha2. Dev Dyn. 2000;219:28–39.
49. Honma Y, Araki T, Gianino S, et al. Artemin is a vascular-derived neurotropic factor for developing sympathetic neurons. Neuron. 2002;35:267–82.
50. Damon DH, Teriele JA, Marko SB. Vascular-derived artemin: a determinant of vascular sympathetic innervation? Am J Physiol Heart Circ Physiol. 2007;293:H266–73.
51. Miwa K, Lee JK, Takagishi Y, et al. Axon guidance of sympathetic neurons to cardiomyocytes by glial cell line-derived neurotrophic factor (GDNF). PLoS One. 2013;8:e65202.
52. Shcherbakova OG, Hurt CM, Xiang Y, et al. Organization of beta-adrenoceptor signaling compartments by sympathetic innervation of cardiac myocytes. J Cell Biol. 2007;176:521–33.
53. Miwa K, Lee JK, Takagishi Y, et al. Glial cell line-derived neurotrophic factor (GDNF) enhances sympathetic neurite growth in rat hearts at early developmental stages. Biomed Res. 2010;31:353–61.
54. Chen LS, Zhou S, Fishbein MC, et al. New perspectives on the role of autonomic nervous system in the genesis of arrhythmias. J Cardiovasc Electrophysiol. 2007;18:123–7.
55. Backs J, Haunstetter A, Gerber SH, et al. The neuronal norepinephrine transporter in experimental heart failure: evidence for a posttranscriptional downregulation. J Mol Cell Cardiol. 2001;33:461–72.
56. Hasking GJ, Esler MD, Jennings GL, et al. Norepinephrine spillover to plasma in patients with congestive heart failure: evidence of increased overall and cardiorenal sympathetic nervous activity. Circulation. 1986;73:615–21.
57. Momose M, Kobayashi H, Iguchi N, et al. Comparison of parameters of 123I-MIBG scintigraphy for predicting prognosis

in patients with dilated cardiomyopathy. Nucl Med Commun. 1999;20:529–35.

58. Turpeinen AK, Vanninen E, Kuikka JT, et al. Demonstration of regional sympathetic denervation of the heart in diabetes. Comparison between patients with NIDDM and IDDM. Diabetes Care. 1996;19:1083–90.
59. Schnell O, Muhr D, Weiss M, et al. Reduced myocardial 123I-metaiodobenzylguanidine uptake in newly diagnosed IDDM patients. Diabetes. 1996;45:801–5.
60. Hattori N, Tamaki N, Hayashi T, et al. Regional abnormality of iodine-123-MIBG in diabetic hearts. J Nucl Med. 1996;37:1985–90.
61. Stevens MJ, Dayanikli F, Raffel DM, et al. Scintigraphic assessment of regionalized defects in myocardial sympathetic innervation and blood flow regulation in diabetic patients with autonomic neuropathy. J Am Coll Cardiol. 1998;31:1575–84.
62. Chugh SS, Reinier K, Teodorescu C, et al. Epidemiology of sudden cardiac death: clinical and research implications. Prog Cardiovasc Dis. 2008;51:213–28.
63. Zheng ZJ, Croft JB, Giles WH, et al. Sudden cardiac death in the United States, 1989 to 1998. Circulation. 2001;104:2158–63.
64. Cao JM, Fishbein MC, Han JB, et al. Relationship between regional cardiac hyperinnervation and ventricular arrhythmia. Circulation. 2000;101:1960–9.
65. Rubart M, Zipes DP. Mechanisms of sudden cardiac death. J Clin Invest. 2005;115:2305–15.
66. Cao JM, Chen LS, KenKnight BH, et al. Nerve sprouting and sudden cardiac death. Circ Res. 2000;86:816–21.
67. Fishbein MC, Chen PS, Chen LS, et al. Sympathetic nerve sprouting, electrical remodeling and the mechanisms of sudden cardiac death. Cardiovasc Res. 2001;50:409–16.
68. Held P, Yusuf S. Early intravenous beta-blockade in acute myocardial infarction. Cardiology. 1989;76:132–43.
69. Hjalmarson A, Elmfeldt D, Herlitz J, et al. Effect on mortality of metoprolol in acute myocardial infarction. A double-blind randomised trial. Lancet. 1981;2:823–7.
70. Norris RM, Barnaby PF, Brown MA, et al. Prevention of ventricular fibrillation during acute myocardial infarction by intravenous propranolol. Lancet. 1984;2:883–6.
71. Zuanetti G, De Ferrari GM, Priori SG, et al. Protective effect of vagal stimulation on reperfusion arrhythmias in cats. Circ Res. 1987;61:429–35.
72. De Ferrari GM, Mantica M, Vanoli E, et al. Scopolamine increases vagal tone and vagal reflexes in patients after myocardial infarction. J Am Coll Cardiol. 1993;22:1327–34.
73. Moss AJ, Zareba W, Hall WJ, et al. Prophylactic implantation of a defibrillator in patients with myocardial infarction and reduced ejection fraction. N Engl J Med. 2002;346:877–83.
74. Bardy GH, Lee KL, Mark DB, et al. Amiodarone or an implantable cardioverter-defibrillator for congestive heart failure. N Engl J Med. 2005;352:225–37.
75. Passman R, Goldberger JJ. Predicting the future: risk stratification for sudden cardiac death in patients with left ventricular dysfunction. Circulation. 2012;125:3031–7.
76. Lorvidhaya P, Lorvidhaya P, Addo K, et al. Sudden cardiac death risk stratification in patients with heart failure. Heart Fail Clin. 2011;7:157–74.
77. Tomaselli GF, Zipes DP. What causes sudden death in heart failure? Circ Res. 2004;95:754–63.
78. Boogers MJ, Borleffs CJ, Henneman MM, et al. Cardiac sympathetic denervation assessed with 123-iodine metaiodobenzylguanidine imaging predicts ventricular arrhythmias in implantable cardioverter-defibrillator patients. J Am Coll Cardiol. 2010;55:2769–77.

2 Neural Control of Cardiac Function in Health and Disease

Pradeep S. Rajendran, Ray W. Chui, Olujimi A. Ajijola, Marmar Vaseghi, J. Andrew Armour, Jeffrey L. Ardell, and Kalyanam Shivkumar

Introduction

The autonomic nervous system regulates all aspects of cardiac function [1]. Traditional dogma regarding autonomic control of cardiac function suggests that the heart is reciprocally regulated by the sympathetic and parasympathetic divisions of the autonomic nervous system, directly under the influence of the central nervous system. However, evidence gathered over the past several decades has shown that autonomic control of the heart is more complex [2]. The cardiac autonomic nervous system is composed of a series of interacting feedback loops consisting of intrinsic cardiac ganglia, extracardiac intrathoracic ganglia, the spinal cord, the brainstem, and higher centers [1]. Together, this neural network intricately regulates cardiac excitability and contractile function [1]. Thus, neurons involved in regulation of cardiac function are found from the level of the insular cortex [3, 4] to the heart [2]. At the organ level, regulation occurs via the intrinsic cardiac nervous system, a distributed network of ganglia and their interconnecting nerves [2].

Sudden cardiac death due to ventricular arrhythmias is one of the leading causes of mortality worldwide, resulting in an estimated four to five million deaths each year [5, 6]. Concepts regarding autonomic control of cardiac function have been revisited and advanced in recent years as it has become increasingly evident that autonomic dysregulation plays a major role not only in sudden cardiac death but also in the development and progression of most cardiovascular diseases [1–7]. Therefore, cardiac autonomic neuromodulation provides an important avenue of scientific inquiry and therapeutic intervention [8]. Therapies such as vagus nerve stimulation and bilateral cervicothoracic sympathetic decentralization, for example, have already shown promise in slowing the progression of heart failure [9] and reducing the incidence of ventricular arrhythmias [10, 11], respectively. The purpose of this chapter is to provide an overview of the cardiac autonomic nervous system in health and to outline the adverse remodeling that occurs in disease. Based on this foundation, emergent cardiac autonomic neuromodulation therapies are presented.

V. Dilsizian, J. Narula (eds.), *Atlas of Cardiac Innervation*, DOI 10.1007/978-3-319-45800-7_2

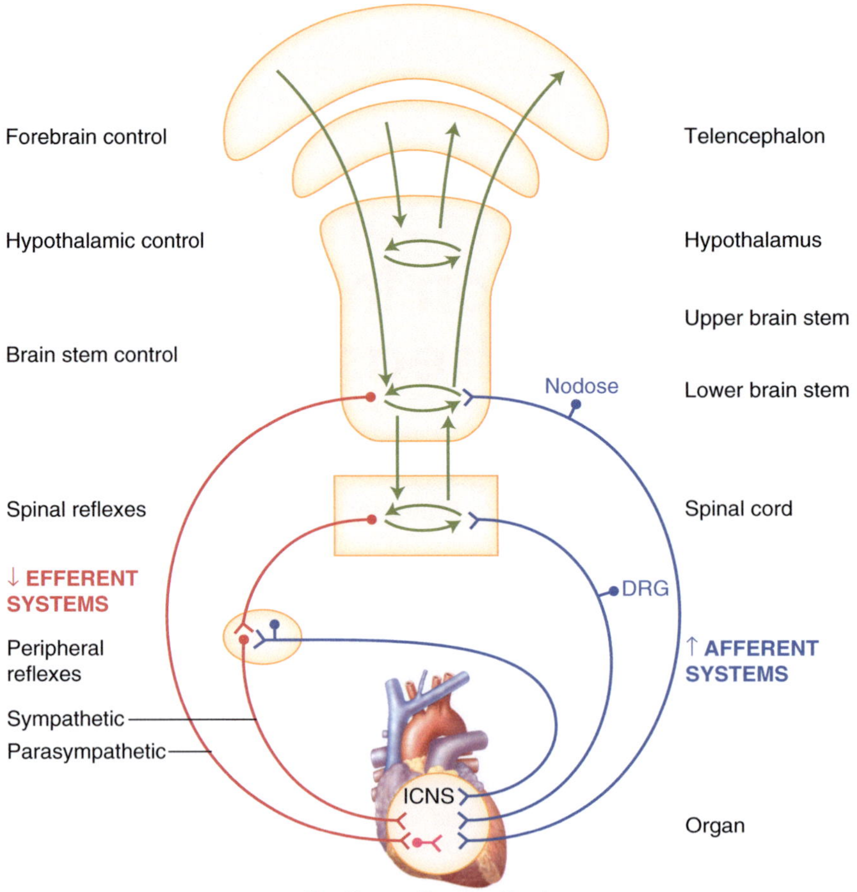

Figure 2-1. Hierarchy for cardiac autonomic control. Autonomic control of cardiac function is mediated by a series of interacting feedback loops from the level of the heart [2] to that of the insular cortex [3, 4]. Cardiac afferents provide beat-to-beat sensory information about cardiac muscle activity to the cardiac autonomic nervous system [1]. The processing of these afferent neural signals at multiple levels of the hierarchy provides a mechanism for fine-tuned regulation of efferent neural signals in normal and stressed states [1]. *DRG* dorsal root ganglia, *ICNS* intrinsic cardiac nervous system (Adapted from Jänig [12]).

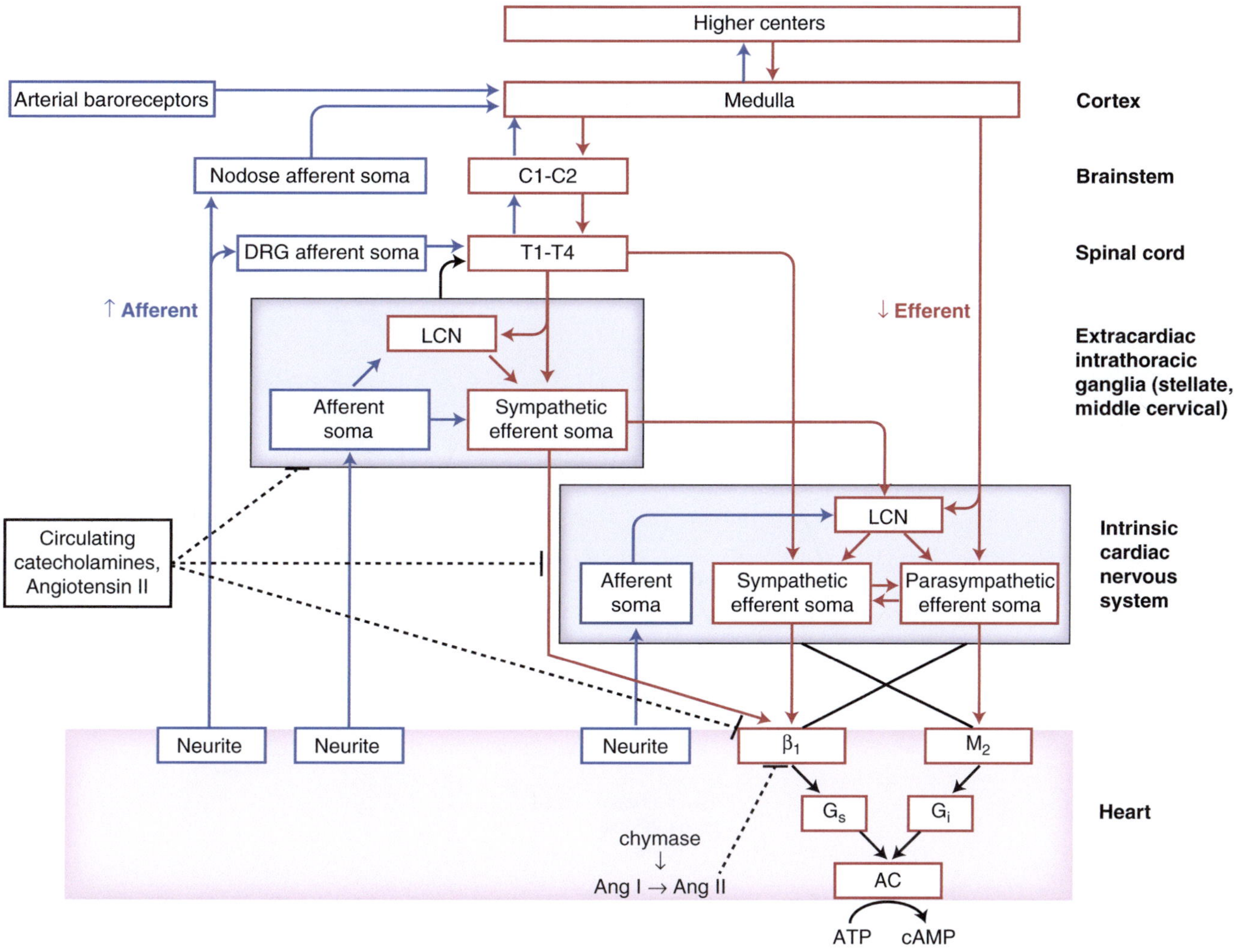

Figure 2-2. Functional organization of cardiac innervation. This schematic shows neural network interactions between central and peripheral aspects of the cardiac autonomic nervous system. *AC* adenylate cyclase, *Ang* angiotensin, *ATP* adenosine triphosphate, *C* cervical, *cAMP* cyclic adenosine monophosphate, *DRG* dorsal root ganglion, *LCN* local circuit neuron, *T* thoracic (Adapted from Fukuda et al. [1]).

Cardiac Motor Neurons: Efferent Control of Cardiac Function

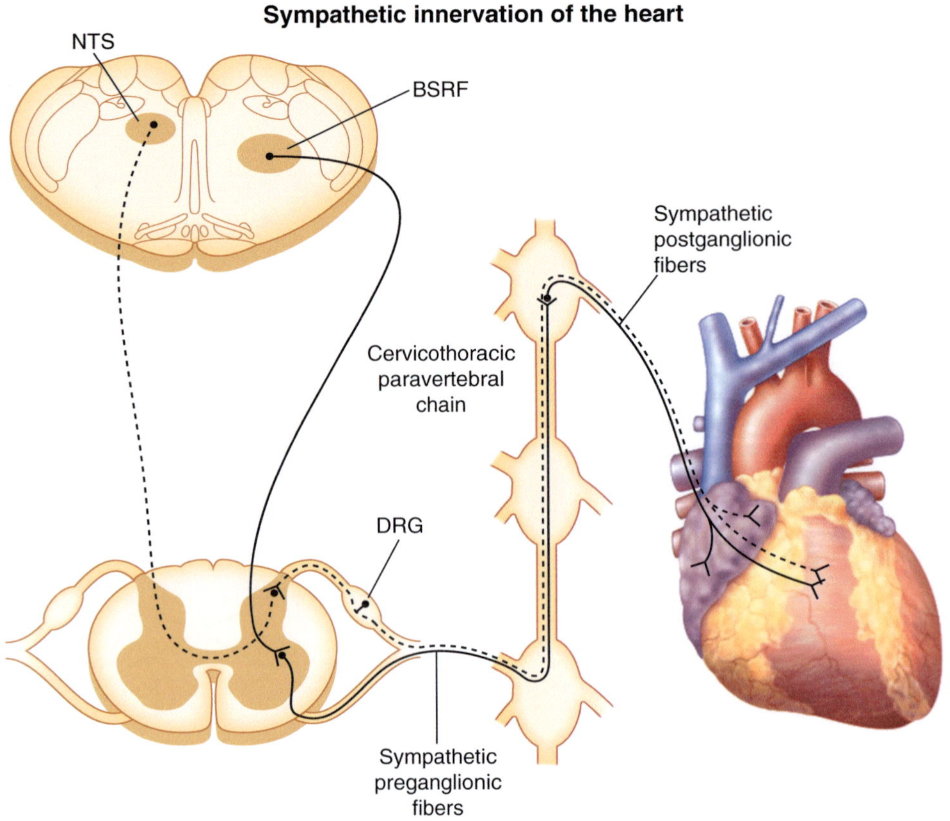

Figure 2-3. Cardiac sympathetic innervation. The sympathetic nervous system is one of the two divisions of the autonomic nervous system that regulates cardiac function, the other being the parasympathetic nervous system. This diagram illustrates the path of sympathetic nerve fibers to the heart (*solid line*). Sympathetic preganglionic neurons innervating the heart originate in the intermediolateral cell column between the first and fourth thoracic segments of the spinal cord [13]. These preganglionic neurons receive inputs from glutamatergic neurons of the brainstem reticular formation (*BSRF*), which includes the rostral ventrolateral medulla [14]. Preganglionic neurons course through the ventral rami and synapse on postganglionic neurons contained primarily within extracardiac intrathoracic ganglia. Traditionally, it was thought that cell bodies of cardiac sympathetic postganglionic neurons were restricted to the stellate ganglia [15]; however, more recent data demonstrate that they also are found in the superior, middle cervical [16], mediastinal [17], and even intrinsic cardiac ganglia [2]. Postganglionic neurons from these ganglia innervate the atrial and ventricular myocardium, as well as the coronary vasculature. Preganglionic neurons release acetylcholine, which binds to nicotinic acetylcholine receptors on postganglionic neurons. Postganglionic neurons in turn release norepinephrine, which binds to α- and β-adrenergic receptors on cardiac myocytes and the coronary vasculature. This initiates a signal transduction cascade that involves G proteins, cyclic adenosine monophosphate, and protein kinase A, resulting in changes in chronotropy, dromotropy, inotropy, and lusitropy [13]. Also depicted in this schematic is one of the paths through which cardiac afferent signals are transmitted to the central nervous system (*dashed line*). These bipolar neurons with cell bodies in the dorsal root ganglia (*DRG*) have peripheral axons projecting to the heart and central axons projecting to the dorsal horn of the spinal cord. Second-order afferent neurons from the dorsal horn project to the nucleus tractus solitarius (*NTS*) of the medulla [18].

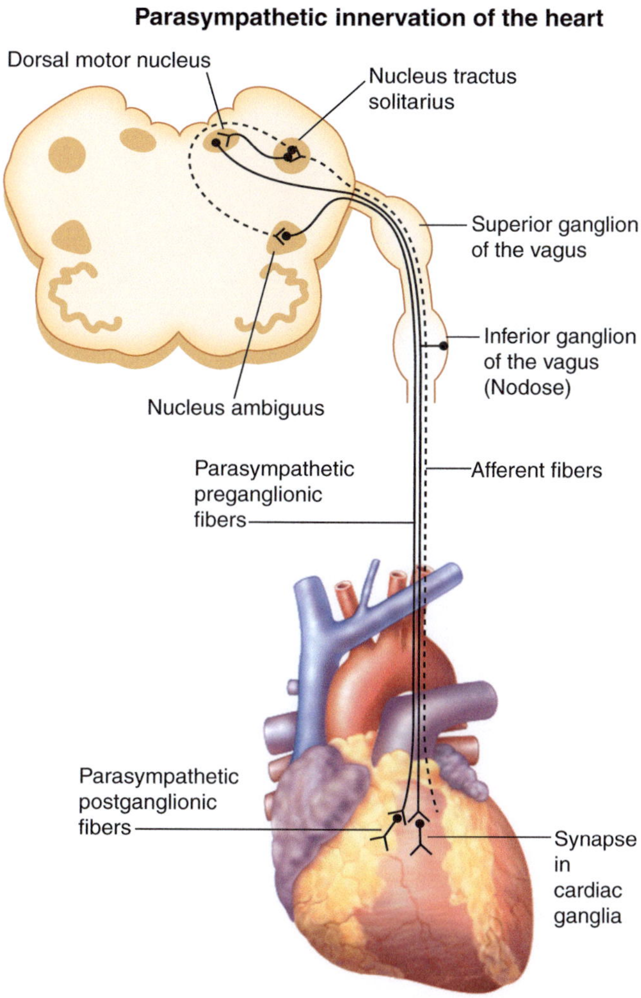

Figure 2-4. Cardiac parasympathetic innervation. The parasympathetic nervous system is the other division of the autonomic nervous system that regulates cardiac function. This diagram illustrates the path of parasympathetic nerve fibers to the heart (*solid line*). Parasympathetic preganglionic neurons innervating the heart originate in the nucleus ambiguus and dorsal motor nucleus of the medulla oblongata in the brainstem [19]. In contrast to sympathetic preganglionic neurons, parasympathetic preganglionic neurons have long axons and synapse near the target organ. Cardiac parasympathetic preganglionic neurons synapse on postganglionic neurons contained within intrinsic cardiac ganglia [13]. Postganglionic neurons from these ganglia project axons to widespread regions of the heart [20]. Although most efferent nerve fibers contained within the vagus nerve are parasympathetic, sympathetic nerve fibers also have been reported [21, 22]. Preganglionic neurons release acetylcholine, which binds to nicotinic acetylcholine receptors on postganglionic neurons. Postganglionic neurons in turn release acetylcholine, which binds to muscarinic receptors on cardiac myocytes and the coronary vasculature [19]. The vagus nerve is also an important path for sensory information from visceral organs, including the heart, to the central nervous system. In fact, approximately 80% of the fibers contained within the vagus nerve are afferent, being made up of A, B, and C fibers [23–25]. Cardiac-related bipolar neurons with cell bodies in the nodose ganglia have peripheral axons projecting to the heart and central axons projecting to the nucleus tractus solitarius of the medulla (*dashed line*) [19]. Thus, the vagus nerve contains both ascending afferent and descending efferent nerve fibers. Furthermore, as vagus nerve stimulation is evaluated as a potential therapy for a variety of chronic disorders, it is critical to understand the type of axons being activated in order to maximize the efficacy of the therapy while minimizing off-target effects (Adapted from Huang et al. [26]).

a

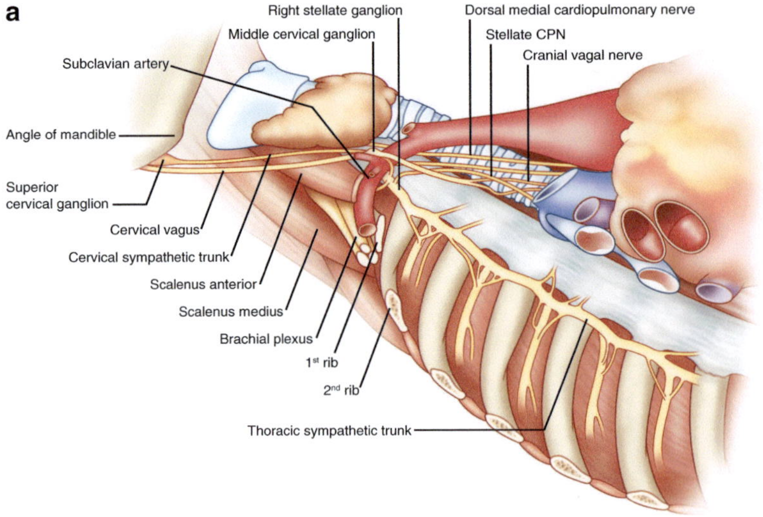

b

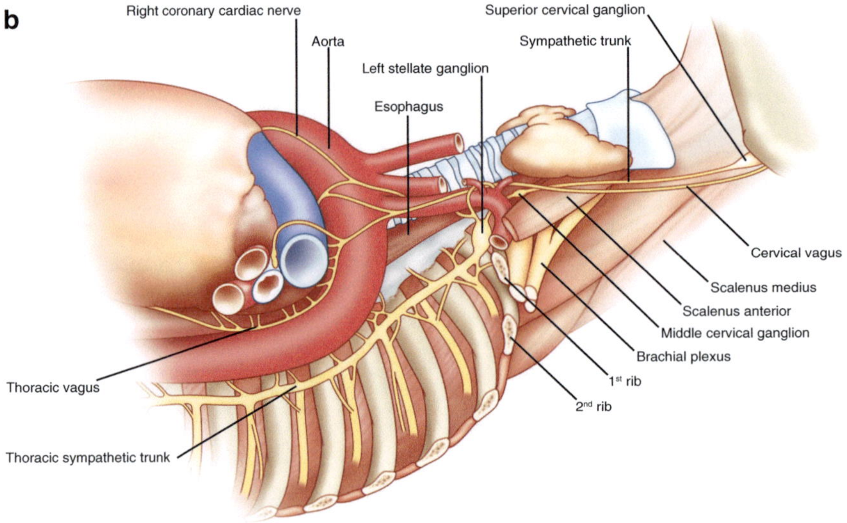

Figure 2-5. Cardiac nerves from the neck and thorax. (**a**) Right aspect of the neck and upper thorax. This view shows the course of the right sympathetic trunk, the vagus nerve, and their major branches. As the sympathetic chain proceeds cranially, the first thoracic (T1) and inferior cervical ganglia (C8) fuse, forming the stellate ganglion. Two nerves from the stellate ganglion, the ventral and dorsal ansa subclavia, course around the subclavian artery as they travel to the middle cervical ganglion. The dorsal ansa may be absent on one or both sides because of merging of the stellate and inferior portion of the middle cervical ganglia [27]. The stellate and middle cervical ganglia contain most of the postganglionic sympathetic neurons that innervate the heart. Occasional ganglia called vertebral ganglia have been identified between the middle cervical and superior cervical ganglia, which are located at the base of the skull, near the angle of the mandible. In addition to the heart, sympathetic postganglionic nerve fibers contained in the extracardiac intrathoracic ganglia innervate the esophagus, trachea, and bronchi, as well as other structures in the head and neck [13]. There are multiple cardiopulmonary nerves (CPNs) that run lateral to the trachea as they course to the base of the heart. Sympathetic CPNs have been found to arise from the stellate ganglion and cervical sympathetic trunk below the level of the cricoid cartilage [27]. Parasympathetic CPNs arise from the right vagus nerve after the recurrent laryngeal nerve branches off at the subclavian artery. (**b**) Left aspect of the neck and upper thorax. This view shows the course of the left sympathetic trunk, the vagus nerve, and their major branches. Similar to the right side, the left stellate ganglion is located at the top of the thoracic sympathetic chain as a fusion of the T1 and inferior cervical ganglia (C8). The left vagus nerve courses on the anterior aspect of the aortic arch, and the recurrent laryngeal nerve branches off and travels under the aortic arch at the ligamentum arteriosum. Parasympathetic CPNs arise from the left vagus nerve at the pulmonary hilum.

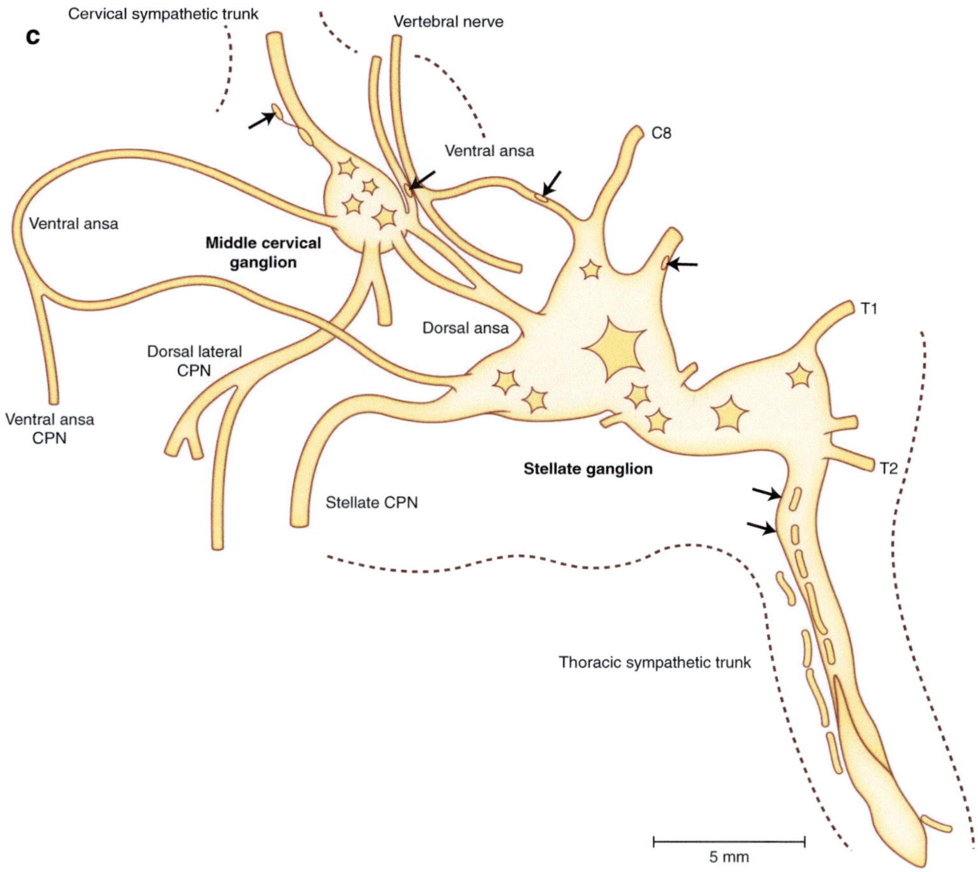

FIGURE 2-5. (**c**) Stellate and middle cervical ganglia. Axons from sympathetic postganglionic neurons contained in the stellate, as well as T2 through T4 ganglia, course through the ventral and dorsal ansa to the middle cervical ganglia as they travel to the heart. These sympathetic ganglia and nerves are covered in thick connective sheaths [27]. This is a composite drawing derived from several histologic sections of the stellate and middle cervical ganglia, along with the superior aspect of the thoracic sympathetic trunk, from human cadavers. The *arrows* indicate clusters of neuronal cell bodies, and *dashed lines* indicate the edges of connective tissue sheaths. (Adapted from Janes et al. [27]).

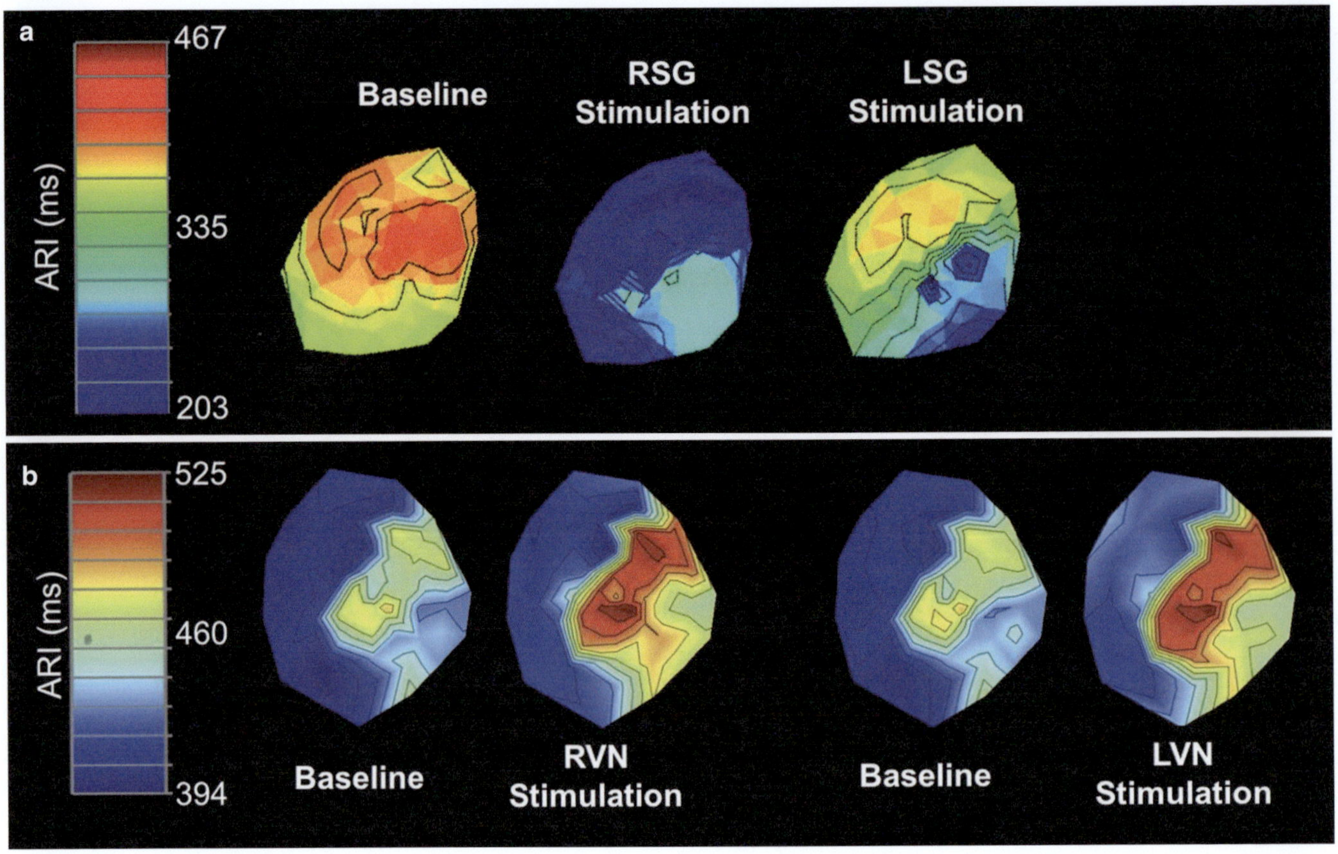

Figure 2-6. Functional innervation of the heart. (**a**) Functional sympathetic innervation. Studies recording activation recovery intervals (ARIs), a surrogate measure of local action potential duration, have been used to determine functional innervation of the heart [28]. Data from such studies have demonstrated that neural projections arising from the right (RSG) and left stellate ganglia (LSG) innervate different regions of the heart. This figure is a polar representation of the ARI from the ventricular epicardial surface at baseline and during RSG and LSG stimulation. Stimulation of the RSG caused a greater shortening of ARIs on the anterior versus the lateral or posterior walls and on the base versus the apex, whereas stimulation of the LSG caused greater shortening on the lateral and posterior walls and the apex [29]. Stimulation of both the RSG and LSG caused an increase in dispersion of repolarization [30]. Thus, each stellate ganglion exerts regional influences. (**b**) Functional parasympathetic innervation. In contrast to the regional innervation by stellate ganglia, the right (RVN) and left vagus nerves (LVN) have homogenous effects on cardiac electrical and mechanical indices [31]. This figure is a polar representation of the ARI from the ventricular epicardial surface at baseline and during RVN and LVN stimulation. No significant differences in ARI were found among the anterior, lateral, and posterior regions of the ventricles [31]. In addition, stimulation of either the RVN or LVN resulted in similar changes in heart rate, left ventricular pressure, and left ventricular contractility [31]. One possible explanation for the homogenous pattern of innervation by the vagus nerves as opposed to the stellate ganglia may be its more prominent distribution through and interactions mediated within the intrinsic cardiac nervous system (Panel **A** adapted from Vaseghi et al. [29], panel **B** from Yamakawa et al. [31]).

Cardiac Sensory Neurons

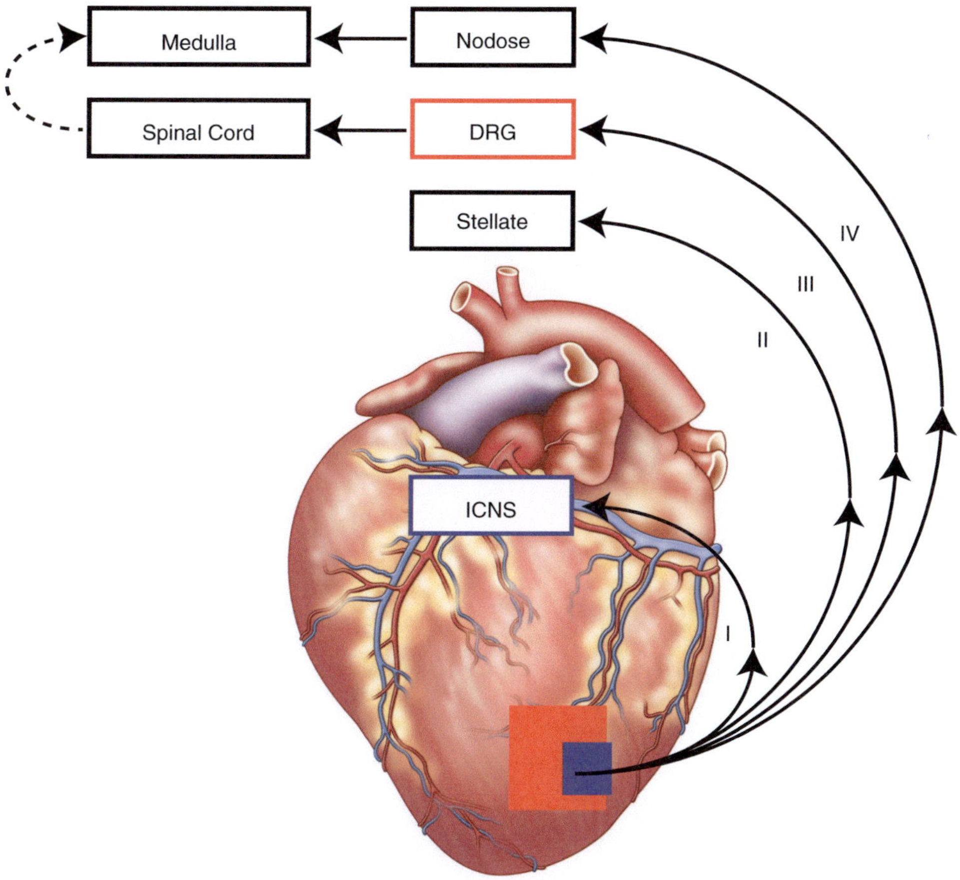

Path	SYNAPSE
I	ICNS
II	Stellate
III	Spinal cord (via DRG)
IV	Medulla (via Nodose)

Figure 2-7. University of California, Los Angeles (UCLA) classification of cardiac afferent pathways. This schematic shows the four paths through which sensory information from the heart travels to the central nervous system. Cardiac sensory (afferent) neurons are located at multiple levels of the cardiac autonomic nervous system, including intrinsic cardiac, stellate, middle cervical, mediastinal, nodose, and dorsal root ganglia (DRG) (Figs. 2.1 [12], 2.2 [1], 2.3, and 2.4 [26]) [18]. Bipolar neurons with cell bodies in the nodose ganglia have peripheral axons that project to the heart and central axons that synapse on second-order neurons contained in the nucleus tractus solitarius of the medulla [19]. Similarly, bipolar neurons with cell bodies in the DRG have peripheral axons that project to the heart and central axons that synapse on second-order neurons contained in the dorsal horn of the spinal cord [18]. Spinal cord neurons project to and interact with neurons in higher centers such as the medulla [32]. These afferent neurons transduce the local mechanical and chemical milieu of the myocardium and coronary vasculature [18]. Further, it has been shown that these neurons have multimodal transduction capabilities [2, 18]. A subpopulation of these neurons also transduce myocardial ischemia [18, 33–34], and thereby initiate a sympathoexcitatory reflex following myocardial infarction. *ICNS* intrinsic cardiac nervous system.

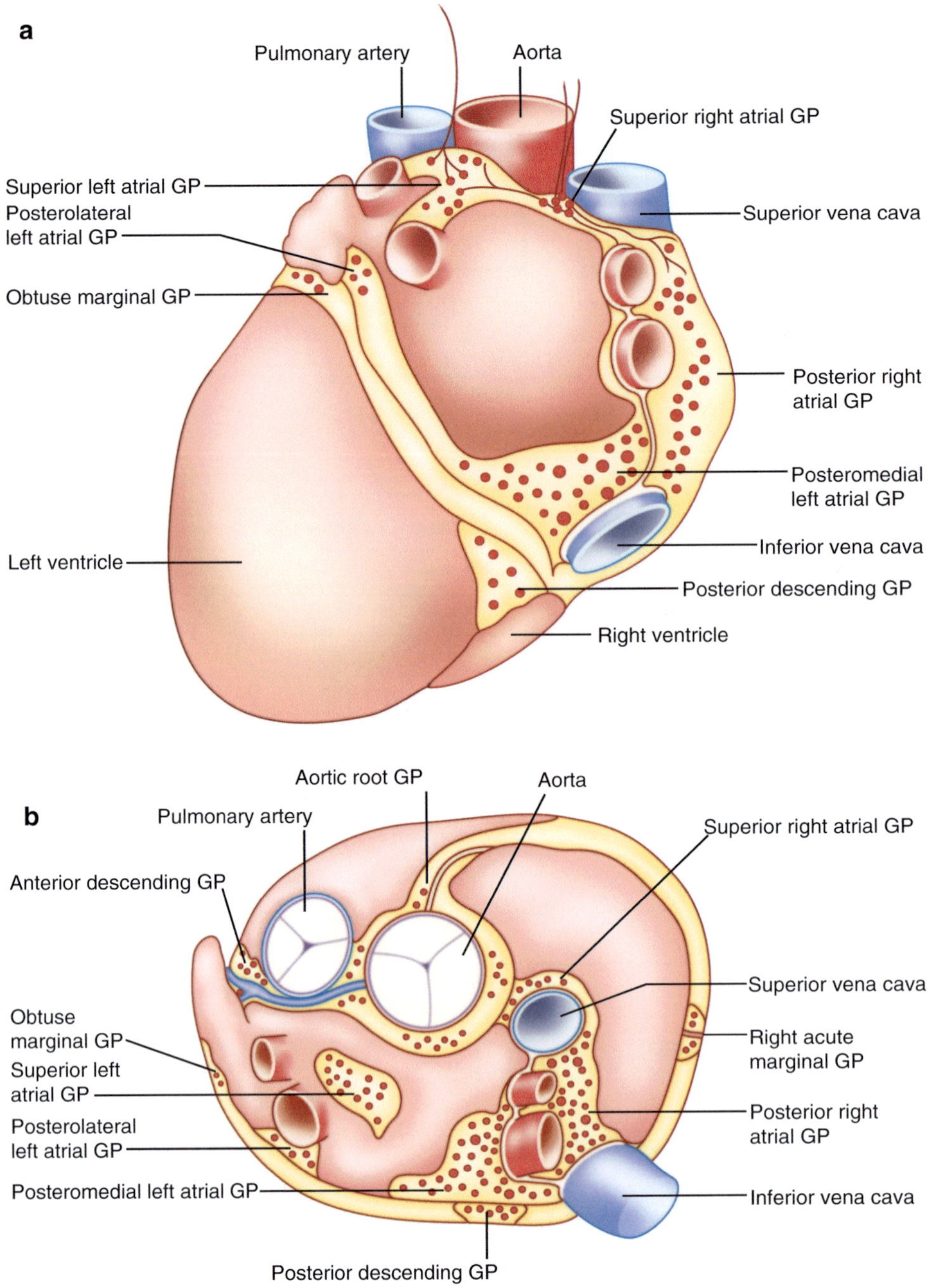

Figure 2-8. Anatomy of the intrinsic cardiac nervous system. The autonomic nervous system projects to the heart via a distributed network of ganglia and interconnecting nerves located primarily in epicardial fat—the intrinsic cardiac nervous system [2]. Contrary to prior belief, the intrinsic cardiac nervous system is not simply a motor relay station for autonomic projections to the heart [35], but instead functions in concert with higher centers to modulate regional cardiac electrical and mechanical indices on a beat-to-beat basis [2]. The intrinsic cardiac nervous system is composed of a diverse population of neurons, namely sensory and motor neurons as well as interposed local circuit neurons [2]. Hence, the intrinsic cardiac nervous system has been referred to as the "little brain on the heart" [2]. An intrinsic cardiac nervous system has been identified in multiple mammalian species [36–38]. Intrinsic cardiac neurons are located in interconnected neuronal aggregates termed ganglionated plexi (GPs) (Fig. 2.9 [37]). The number and locations of GPs vary among species [36–38]. Anatomic studies of human hearts have identified major GPs in five atrial and five ventricular regions, with the atrial GPs located on the lateral and posterior aspects of the heart and the ventricular GPs located primarily at the base of the ventricles [37]. This schematic illustrates the location of the major GPs in the human heart on the posterior (**a**) and superior surface (**b**) of the atria and ventricles. Aside from these GPs, individual neurons and smaller ganglia have been found scattered through the atrial and ventricular myocardium [37] (Adapted from Armour et al. [37]).

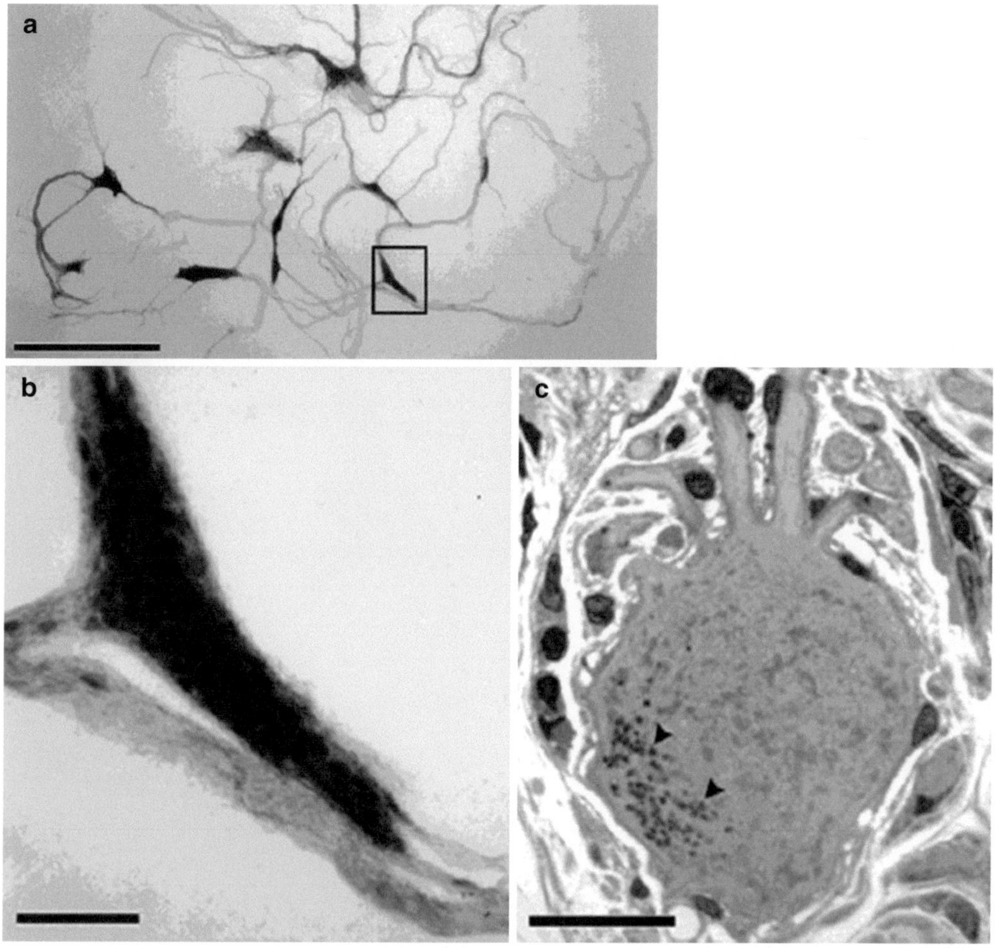

Figure 2-9. Microscopic anatomy of the intrinsic cardiac nervous system. The human intrinsic cardiac nervous system is composed of approximately 14,000 neurons that are distributed through the ganglionated plexi [37]. Neurons contained within intrinsic cardiac ganglia share histologic similarities with those from other autonomic ganglia [37]. These figures are light photomicrographs from the posteromedial left atrial ganglionated plexus of a human heart, showing ganglia, nerves, and neuronal somata. (**a**) Network of ganglia and their interconnecting nerves stained with methylene blue. (**b**) Magnified view of inset from **a** illustrating a ganglion composed of approximately 150–200 neurons. (**c**) High-magnification view of a multipolar intrinsic cardiac neuron from the ganglion. Scale bars: 2.5 mm (**a**), 250 μm (**b**), and 25 μm (**c**) (Adapted from Armour et al. [37]).

NICOTINE INJECTION	RAGP	DAGP	LAGP	IVC-ILAGP	RVGP	VSVGP	CMVGP
Heart rate effects	13 / 13	7 / 8	5 / 10	5 / 9	3 / 3	5 / 7	7 / 9
Tachycardia post-bradycardia	8 / 13	2 / 8	2 / 10	2 / 9	1 / 3	0 / 7	4 / 9
Atrial tachydysrhythmias	**0 / 13**	**2 / 8**	**1 / 10**	**0 / 9**	**0 / 3**	**0 / 7**	**3 / 9**
AV nodal block	7 / 11	3 / 6	2 / 9	1 / 7	1 / 3	0 / 5	6 / 8

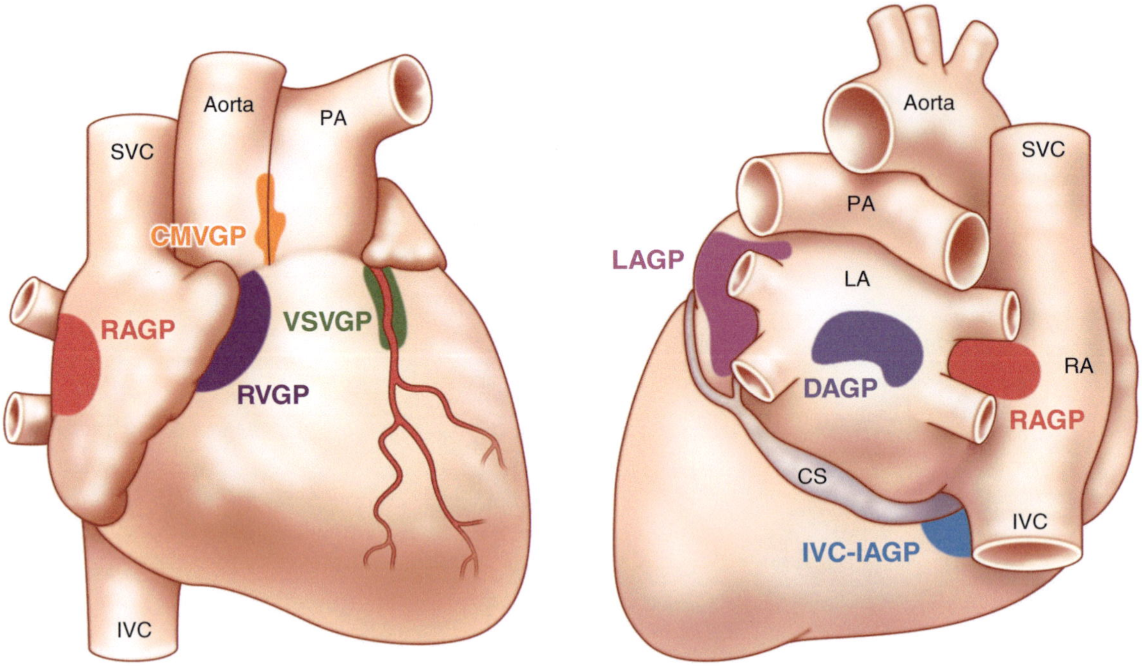

Figure 2-10. Interconnectivity of the intrinsic cardiac nervous system. The intrinsic cardiac nervous system is composed of a diverse population of neurons, namely sensory neurons, motor neurons, and interposed local circuit neurons [2]. As previously described, these neurons are located within ganglionated plexi (GPs) that are found in distinct areas of the heart. Data for this figure were obtained by administering nicotine, which activates cholinergic receptors on intrinsic cardiac neurons, directly onto the epicardial fat in which a GP was located while recording evoked cardiac responses in a canine model [20]. This figure shows that each GP exerts preferential, but not exclusive, influence over specific regions. For instance, the right atrial GP (RAGP) primarily controls sinoatrial nodal function [39]; however, ventricular GPs, such as the ventral septal ventricular GP (VSVGP), still modulate heart rate [20]. This overlap in regions of influence is mediated by local circuit neurons. In addition, the presence of local circuit neurons allows for short-loop cardio-cardiac reflexes [2]. Local circuit neurons project axons not only to neurons contained within the same intrinsic cardiac ganglion but also to those in different intrinsic cardiac ganglia, extracardiac intrathoracic ganglia, and the central nervous system [2]. Local circuit neurons also receive diverse inputs [2]. The high degree of interconnectivity among these various neuronal populations implies the presence of local information processing [2]. The constant communication among these neurons also allows for dynamic modulation of cardiac output to meet the requirements of the body on both short and long time scales [2]. *AV* atrioventricular, *CMVGP* craniomedial ventricular GP, *CS* coronary sinus, *DAGP* dorsal atrial GP, *IVC-ILA* inferior vena cava-inferior left atrial GP, *LA* left atrium, *LAGP* left atrial GP, *PA* pulmonary artery, *RA* right atrium, *RVGP* right ventricular GP, *SVC* superior vena cava (Adapted from Armour [2]).

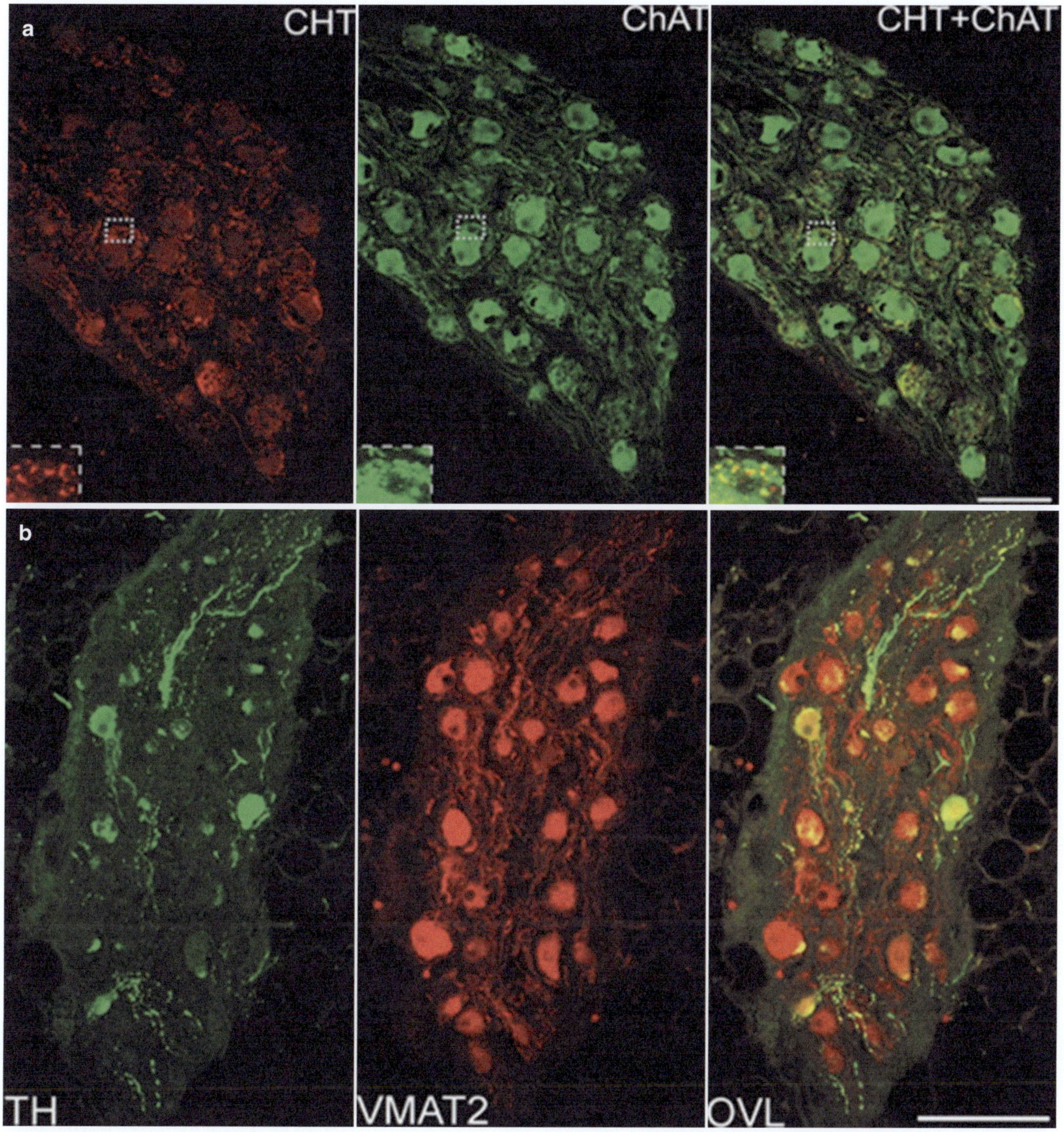

Figure 2-11. Neurotransmitter profile of the intrinsic cardiac nervous system. A variety of neurotransmitters play a role in signaling within the intrinsic cardiac nervous system [40, 41]. Immunohistochemical studies have shown that neurons in human ganglionated plexi are positive for cholinergic, noradrenergic, and nitrergic markers, among many others [41]. This confocal microscopic image of an intrinsic cardiac ganglion from a human atrial ganglionated plexus shows the presence of neurons that display a cholinergic (**a**) and noradrenergic phenotype (**b**). The ganglion in (**a**) was double-labeled with choline transporter (CHT) and choline acetyltransferase (ChAT). CHT is required for high-affinity choline uptake by cholinergic neurons, and ChAT catalyzes the synthesis of acetylcholine. The ganglion in (**b**) was double-labeled with tyrosine hydroxylase (TH) and vesicular monoamine transporter 2 (VMAT2). TH catalyzes the rate-limiting step in catecholamine synthesis, and VMAT2 facilitates the transport of norepinephrine into storage vesicles. Interestingly, there are subpopulations of neurons that display colocalization of neuronal markers, further suggesting the ability of neurons within the intrinsic cardiac nervous system to transduce multimodal signals [41]. Furthermore, this provides strong evidence of the complex neurochemical anatomy that exists within this neural network, which goes beyond the classic view of the intrinsic cardiac nervous system as a motor relay station for parasympathetic preganglionic neurons. *OVL* overlay of TH and VMAT2 images. Scale bars: 100 μm (**a**) and 150 μm (**b**) (Adapted from Hoover et al. [41]).

Cardiac ANS in Disease

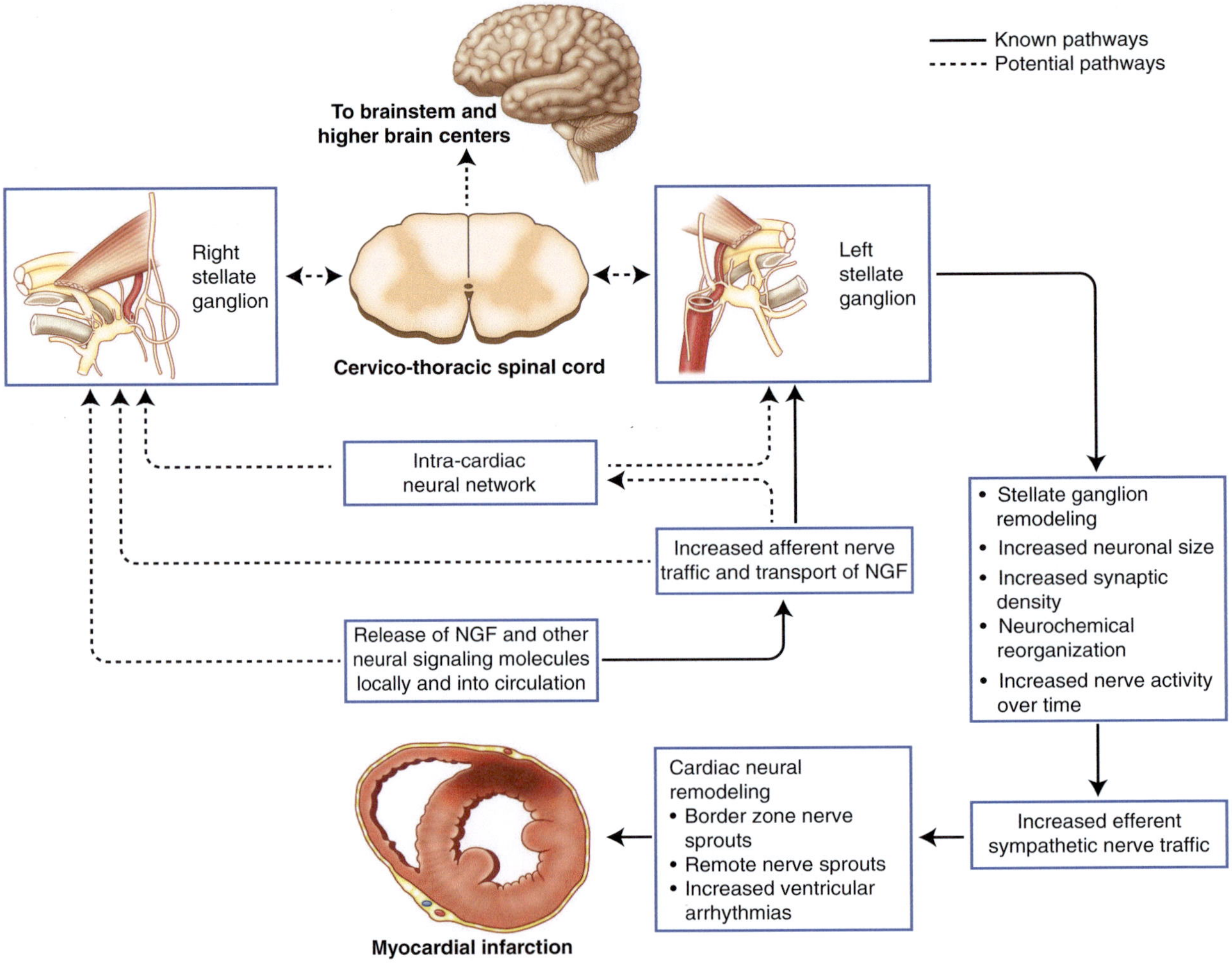

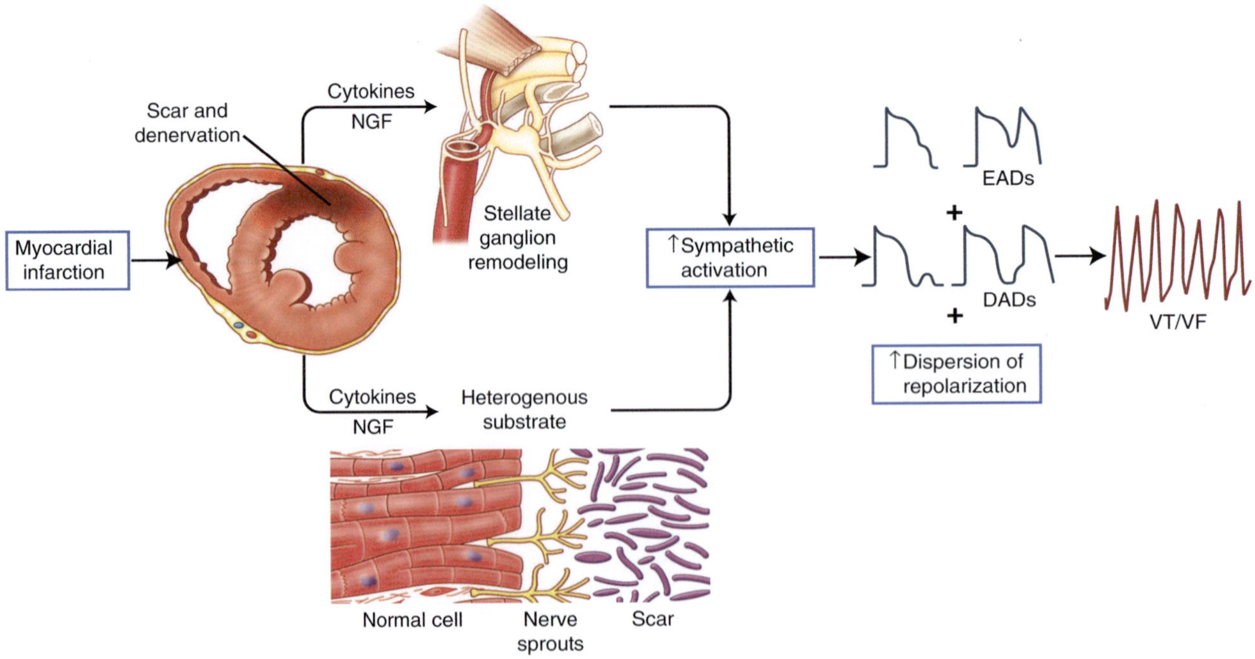

Figure 2-12. Effects of myocardial infarction on the cardiac sympathetic nervous system. Cardiac disease, such as myocardial infarction (MI), has adverse effects not only on the myocardium but also on neurons at all levels of the cardiac autonomic nervous system [1]. Nerve injury following MI causes production and release of nerve growth factor (NGF) and other neural signaling molecules, leading to myocardial nerve sprouting [42]. Further, partial denervation of the infarct scar and hyperinnervation of the scar border zone create an arrhythmogenic substrate [43, 44]. Evidence also exists suggesting that there is retrograde axonal transport of these signaling molecules to extracardiac intrathoracic ganglia, such as the stellate [42]. There are both direct and indirect effects on neurons when the coronary artery blood supply is compromised, as is the case during MI. A lack of energy substrates and an accumulation of chemicals, such as adenosine and reactive oxygen species, secondary to the local ischemia cause altered activity of cardiac sensory afferent neurons [45–47]. Aberrant and excessive activation of these afferent neurons leads to reflex sympathoexcitation [48]. Acutely, this helps maintain cardiac output; however, chronically, it leads to adaptive and maladaptive remodeling, manifested as both structural and functional changes in neurons in both intrinsic and extrinsic cardiac ganglia (Figs. 2.13 [58], 2.14 [61], 2.15 [49], and 2.16 [62]) [1]. Porcine and human stellate ganglia neurons, for example, undergo morphologic and neurochemical changes following MI, such as an increase in neuronal size, synaptic density, and neuropeptide Y expression (Fig. 2.15 [49]) [50]. Adrenergic to cholinergic phenotype transdifferentiation has also been reported in rats with congestive heart failure [51]. Together with this structural remodeling, enhanced activity of stellate ganglia neurons has been shown to precede the onset of ventricular arrhythmias after MI in canine models [52, 53]. The extent to which the spinal cord and higher centers of the central nervous system remodel with cardiac injury and disease is not as well understood. However, studies using functional magnetic resonance imaging in humans have shown abnormalities in brain areas that mediate autonomic control in heart failure, such as the hypothalamus and insular cortex [54]. The heterogeneous myocardial and neural substrate created following MI is more prone to early afterdepolarizations (EADs) and delayed afterdepolarizations (DADs), as well as increased dispersion of repolarization, which may lead to ventricular arrhythmias [55, 56]. The heightened interplay between the sympathetic nervous system and the heart underscores the therapeutic value of acute and chronic use of β-blockers after MI (Fig. 2.17) [56]. For treatment of ventricular arrhythmias resistant to medical and catheter ablation therapies, the observed remodeling of the stellate ganglia lends support to the bilateral cervicothoracic sympathetic decentralization procedure (Fig. 2.18 [10, 57]) [11]. In contrast to the increase in sympathetic drive following MI, the mechanisms underlying parasympathetic withdrawal are less well understood. *VF* ventricular fibrillation, *VT* ventricular tachycardia (Adapted from Vaseghi et al. [56] and Ajijola and Shivkumar [55]).

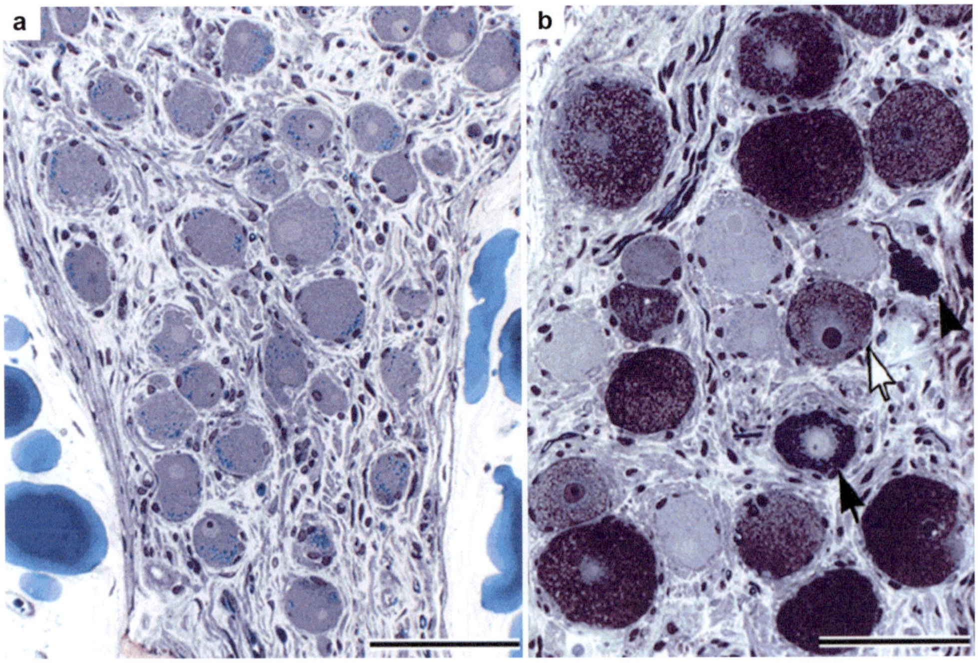

Figure 2-13. Structural remodeling of intrinsic cardiac neurons in ischemic heart disease. Intrinsic cardiac neurons undergo histologic changes in patients with ischemic heart disease [58]. Neurons have been observed to contain lamellated inclusions and vacuoles, as well as to display degenerative changes in dendrites and axons [58]. Interestingly, the inclusions seen in these neurons are similar to those in central nervous system neurons of patients with metabolic diseases, such as lysosomal storage disease [59, 60]. This is a photomicrograph of intrinsic cardiac ganglia from the posterior right atrial ganglionated plexus of two patients with ischemic heart disease stained with toluidine blue. (**a**) Neurons in this ganglion have a normal appearance, with many lipofuscin granules and a pale, eccentrically located nucleus. (**b**) In another ganglion, many neurons are enlarged and filled with dark (*black arrow*) or lucent (*white arrow*) inclusions. One neuron (*black arrowhead*) that appears to be degenerating has very darkly stained cytoplasm and is misshapen. Scale bar: 100 μm (Adapted from Hopkins et al. [58]; with permission).

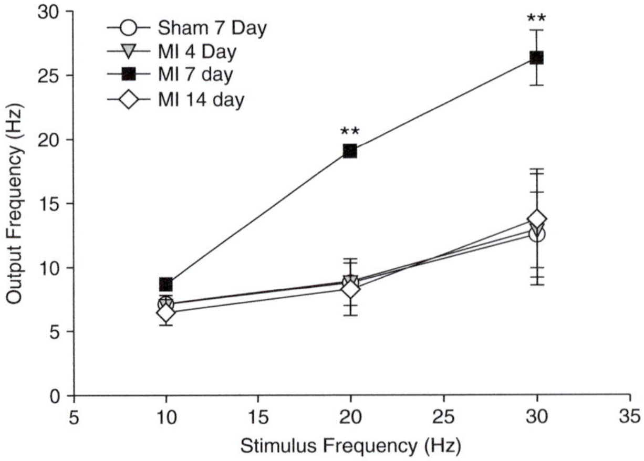

Figure 2-14. Functional remodeling of intrinsic cardiac neurons after myocardial infarction. In parallel with structural changes, intrinsic cardiac neurons also undergo functional changes. An intracellular study of intrinsic cardiac neurons from a guinea pig chronic myocardial infarction (MI) model has shown that these neurons display alterations in basal action potential frequency, synaptic efficacy, and response to neuromodulators [61]. In this study, synaptic efficacy was assessed by stimulating axons (0.1–10 V, 2 ms, 10–30 Hz) synapsing on neurons with an extracellular electrode while concurrently recording their activity with an intracellular electrode [61]. This line graph displays the output frequency of the neurons at 4, 7, and 14 days post-MI and demonstrates that their synaptic efficacy is changed during the evolution of cardiac disease [61]. Points are mean±SEM (n=6 or more cells). This is most evident in the early stages following MI, as the output frequency was significantly greater in neurons from animals 7 days post-MI at 20 and 30 Hz compared with neurons from sham animals, as well as those from animals 4 and 14 days post-MI. Taken together, the adverse structural and functional remodeling of the intrinsic cardiac nervous system—the final common pathway for autonomic modulation of cardiac function—might be a mechanism underlying many cardiac pathologies and lead to a proarrhythmic state. **$P<0.001$ by analysis of variance (Adapted from Hardwick et al. [61]).

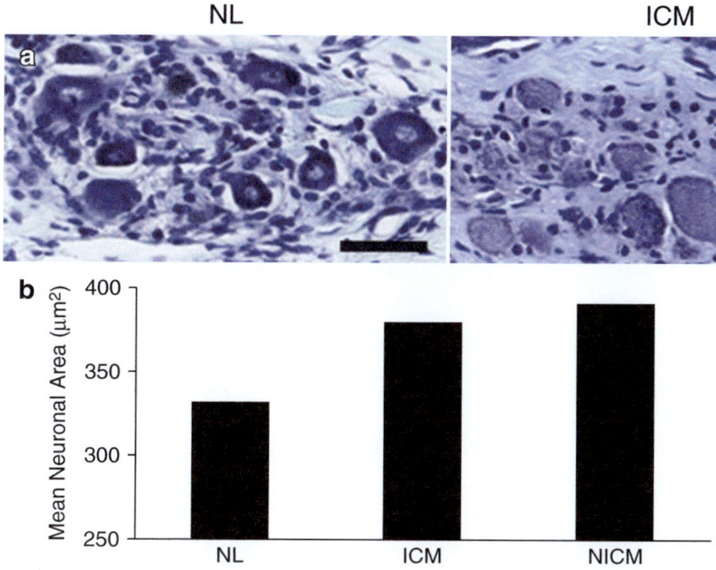

FIGURE 2-15. Structural remodeling of stellate ganglia in chronic cardiomyopathy. Similar to intrinsic cardiac neurons, neurons from the stellate ganglia undergo morphologic and neurochemical changes in both animal models and humans with ischemic heart disease [49, 50]. This figure shows enlargement of stellate ganglia neurons from humans with ischemic (ICM) and nonischemic cardiomyopathy (NICM). (**a**) Stellate ganglia neurons stained with thionin from normal (NL), ICM, and NICM hearts. Scale bar: 50 μm. (**b**) Quantification of mean stellate ganglia neuronal size from normal, ICM, and NICM hearts. In addition to neuronal enlargement, synaptic density was significantly increased in stellate ganglia from NICM compared with normal hearts [49]. These findings may be a consequence of reflex sympathoexcitation resulting from myocardial injury (Adapted from Ajijola et al. [49]).

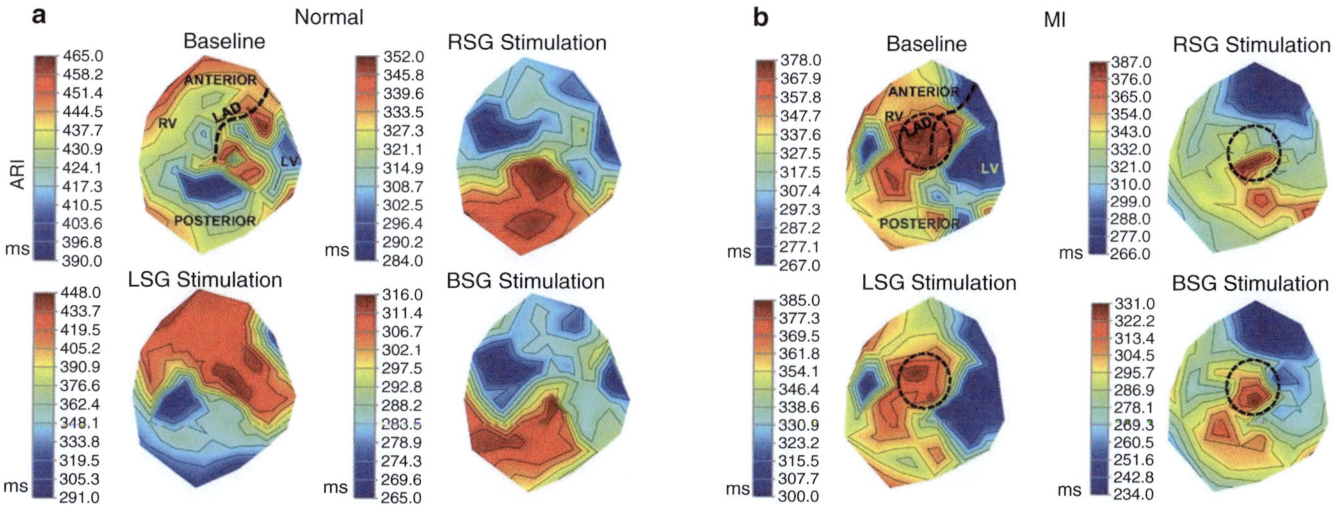

FIGURE 2-16. Functional remodeling of sympathetic innervation after myocardial infarction. These structural changes manifest as alterations in functional sympathetic innervation of the heart, as determined by measuring activation recovery intervals (ARIs) in a porcine anteroapical myocardial infarction (MI) model [62]. In control hearts, right stellate ganglion (RSG) stimulation causes greater ARI shortening on the anterior surface and left stellate ganglion (LSG) stimulation on the lateral and posterior surfaces of the heart [30]. However, this pattern is lost following MI, in addition to an increase in dispersion of repolarization and alteration in activation propagation [62]. This figure is a polar representation of ventricular epicardial ARIs in control (**a**) and MI hearts (**b**) at baseline, as well as during RSG, LSG, and bilateral stellate ganglia (BSG) stimulation. Regions of the heart are delineated in the baseline condition of the control heart, and the location of the infarct is delineated by a black circle. These data indicate that a focal MI induces global remodeling of cardiac sympathetic innervation [62]. Furthermore, the heterogeneous pattern of ARI shortening seen post-MI may create a proarrhythmic substrate. *LAD* left anterior descending coronary artery, *LV* left ventricle, *RV* right ventricle (From Ajijola et al. [62]).

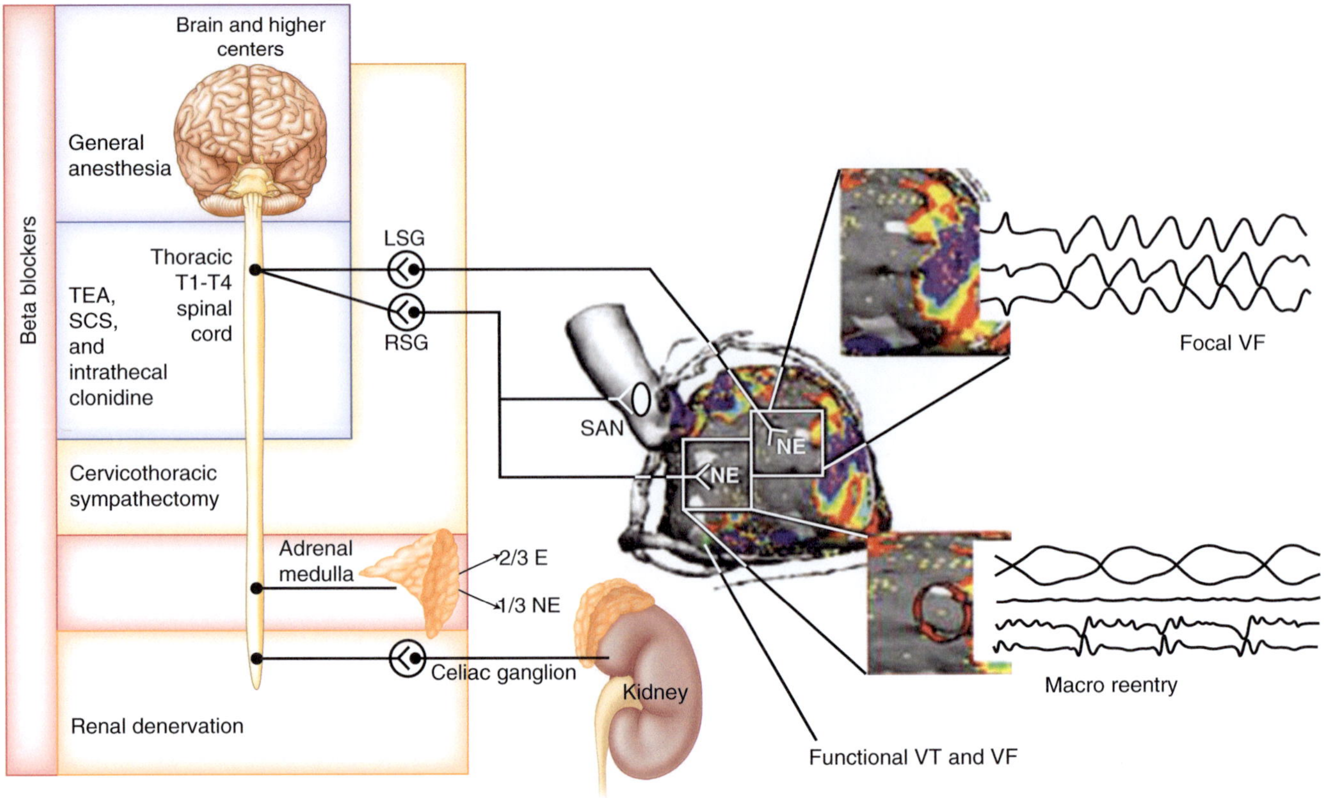

Figure 2-17. Targets of cardiac autonomic neuromodulation. This schematic depicts some aspects of the cardiac autonomic nervous system (ANS) that are being targeted via neuromodulation approaches for the treatment of cardiac diseases, especially arrhythmias and heart failure (HF). *Intrinsic cardiac nervous system*. Several mechanisms have been proposed for the pathogenesis of atrial arrhythmias, some of which involve the cardiac ANS [63]. A neural mechanism of atrial arrhythmias was first described in 1978 and has since been studied extensively [64]. Experimentally, stimulation of mediastinal nerves during the atrial refractory period has been shown to produce ectopic beats originating near the pulmonary veins and superior vena cava, which in turn may initiate atrial arrhythmias [65, 66]. It is now recognized that the cardiac ANS plays a major role in atrial arrhythmogenesis [67, 68]. The intrinsic cardiac nervous system has been proposed as a target in the treatment of atrial arrhythmias, and ganglionated plexus (GP) ablation is currently being used as an adjunctive or stand-alone treatment [69, 70]. Overall, however, GP ablation studies have yielded unclear results. The reasons for this likely are multifold. First, although each GP exerts preferential influence over specific regions of the heart, there is overlap among these regions (Fig. 2.10 [2]) [20]. This presumably ensures unperturbed neural control of cardiac function when one part of the network is compromised [2]. Second, most of these studies have relied on functionally identifying GPs to target energy delivery, on the basis of a bradycardic response to high-frequency electrical stimulation. The intrinsic cardiac nervous system is not composed solely of parasympathetic postganglionic neurons [2], and this method of identifying GPs fails to take into account the complex and heterogeneous composition of the intrinsic cardiac nervous system. Third, regeneration of neural structures may account for the return of atrial fibrillation incidence to baseline levels or worse in the long run [71]. Furthermore, there is evidence from a canine acute myocardial infarction (MI) model to suggest that ablation of atrial GPs may increase the vulnerability to ventricular arrhythmias [72]. Thus, a better understanding of the structural and functional complexity of the intrinsic cardiac nervous system is necessary before it is exploited as a therapeutic target. *Vagus nerve*. The vagus nerve is being targeted for disorders of the central nervous system (e.g., epilepsy, depression) [73], cardiovascular system (e.g., arrhythmias, HF) [8, 27], and gastrointestinal system (e.g., obesity) [74], among others. With regard to cardiac diseases, there is strong preclinical evidence supporting the use of vagus nerve stimulation (VNS) for the management of HF [8], and emerging data support its use for arrhythmias [27]. In a rat MI model of HF, VNS could attenuate adverse cardiac remodeling and improve long-term survival [75]. VNS-treated rats had reduced left ventricular remodeling, reflected by lower left ventricular end-diastolic pressures and higher left ventricular contractility [75]. The mortality rate also decreased from 50 to 14% in the treatment group [75]. In another study in a canine pacing-induced HF model, VNS-treated dogs had improved ANS control of cardiac function, indicated by increased heart rate variability, baroreflex sensitivity, and reduced plasma norepinephrine levels [76]. Plasma angiotensin II and C-reactive protein levels also were decreased in the

Figure 2-17. (continued) treatment group, suggesting that VNS may inhibit the renin–angiotensin–aldosterone system and exert an anti-inflammatory effect, respectively [76]. Based on the promising results of these preclinical studies, VNS has become the focus of three major HF clinical trials: CardioFit [77], Neural Cardiac Therapy for Heart Failure Study (NECTAR-HF) [78], and Autonomic Neural Regulation Therapy to Enhance Myocardial Function in Heart Failure (Anthem-HF) [9]. However, the results of these trials have been less clear, likely because of technical limitations in study design, including optimization of stimulation parameters. Aside from HF, VNS has a potential application in the management of arrhythmias, as it has been shown to stabilize cardiac electrical and mechanical indices [27]. In an acute canine model, VNS reversed the ventricular electrophysiologic changes induced by left stellate ganglion (LSG) stimulation, such as a decreased effective refractory period and action potential duration, as well as increased spatial dispersion of effective refractory period and maximum slope of the restitution curve [79]. Furthermore, in several animal models, VNS was shown to reduce the incidence of ventricular fibrillation and to increase the ventricular fibrillation threshold [27]. However, before this therapy moves forward clinically, a mechanistic understanding of the characteristics of the nerves being stimulated (afferent vs. efferent) and the potential impact of stimulation parameters (amplitude, frequency, pulse width, waveform, and duty cycle) is critical in order to ensure maximum efficacy while minimizing off-target effects [8]. *Spinal cord.* The spinal cord is a major convergence point for sympathetic and afferent inputs to and from the heart, respectively (Figs. 2.1 [12], 2.2 [1], 2.3, and 2.7). Thus, pharmacologic modulation (i.e., thoracic epidural anesthesia [TEA]) and electrical stimulation (i.e., spinal cord stimulation [SCS]) of the spinal cord represent another approach for the treatment of HF and arrhythmias [8, 57]. In a canine MI model of HF, SCS improved left ventricular function, reduced the incidence of ventricular arrhythmias, and slowed the progression of HF [80, 81]. Preemptive SCS reduced infarct size in a rabbit model of acute MI [82]. Similar results were found in a porcine model [83, 84]. These cardioprotective effects of SCS are thought to be the result of stabilization of reflexes at multiple levels of the cardiac ANS [8]. *Kidneys.* The activity of renal nerves may have significant effects on hemodynamic indices. Renal sympathetic nerves control renin secretion [85]. Renin causes activation of the renin–angiotensin–aldosterone system, leading to vasoconstriction as well as to sodium and water retention [86]. Aside from raising blood pressure, angiotensin II, the major hormone produced by renin–angiotensin–aldosterone system activation, has been shown to cause hypertrophy of cardiac myocytes [87]. Renal denervation is a potential treatment for arrhythmias and HF, in addition to drug-resistant hypertension [88, 89]. Because autonomic nerve fibers that innervate the kidneys run close to the renal artery [90], they can be targeted by surgical and catheter-based approaches. As previously described, MI causes denervation of the scar and hyperinnervation of the scar border and remote zones of the heart, as well as hypersensitivity to catecholamines (Figs. 2.12 [55, 56] and 2.16 [62]) [43, 44, 91]. The beneficial effects of renal denervation are thought to be through reducing afferent and autonomic efferent nerve activity. Although the results of preclinical studies and small case series of patients treated with renal denervation for ventricular arrhythmias have been encouraging, larger studies are needed [92–96]. *Other novel approaches.* Recently, novel approaches for HF management have emerged that leverage our increasing understanding of the cardiac ANS and its dysregulation in disease. For example, in a rat MI model of HF, epicardial application of resiniferatoxin, an ultrapotent agonist of transient receptor potential vanilloid 1, during MI induction attenuated adverse cardiac remodeling and improved cardiovascular dysfunction [97]. Because resiniferatoxin causes inactivation of sensory nerves, the mechanism in this study presumably is the prevention of afferent-mediated reflex sympathoexcitation. Overall, a better understanding of the cardiac ANS will allow development of rational neuromodulation therapies to manage cardiac disease. *E* epinephrine, *NE* norepinephrine, *RSG* right stellate ganglion, *SAN* sinoatrial node, *T* thoracic (Adapted from Vaseghi et al. [56]).

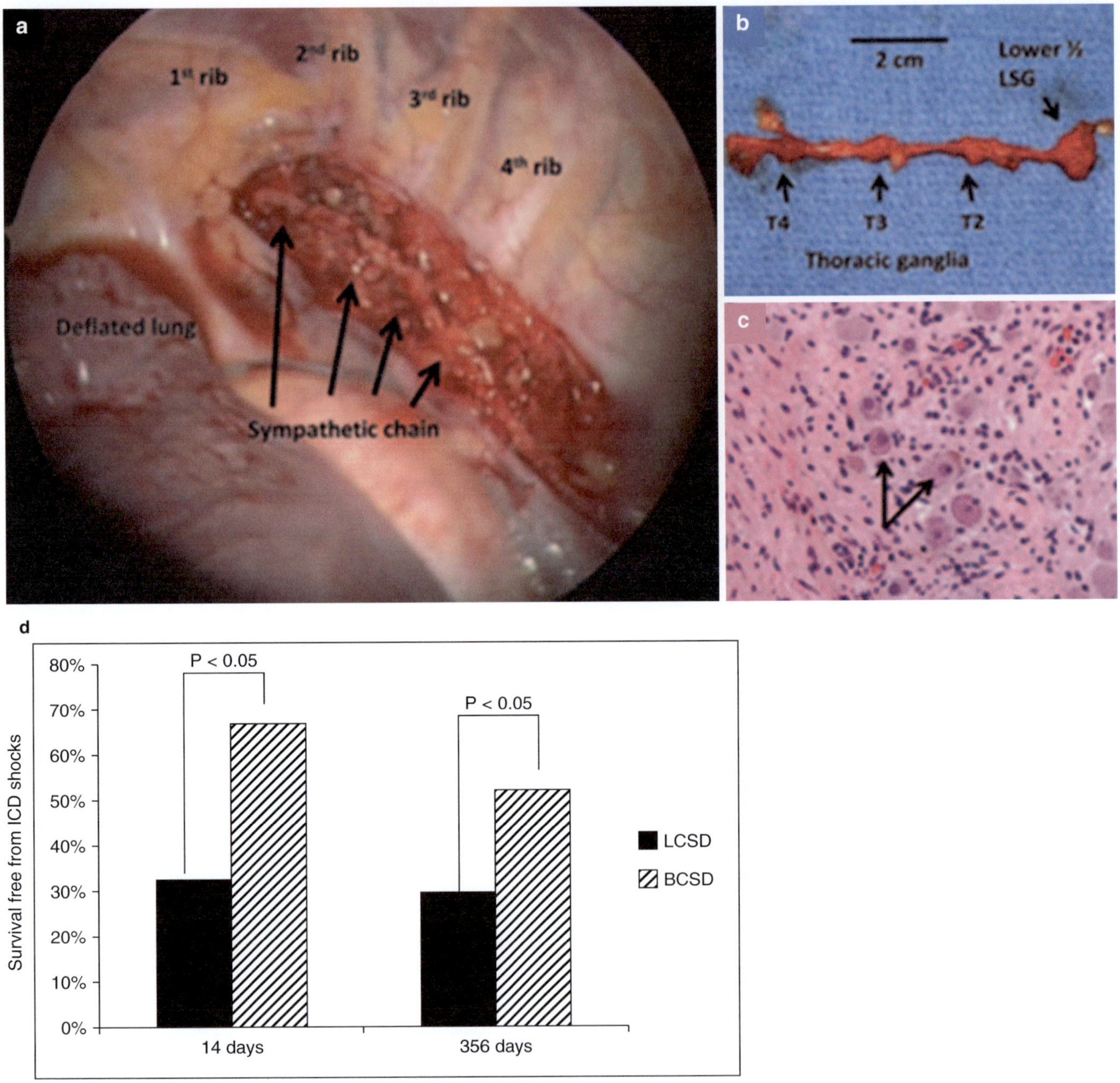

Figure 2-18. Bilateral cervicothoracic sympathetic decentralization. The remodeling observed in the stellate ganglia (Figs. 2.15 [49] and 2.16 [62], respectively) lends support to the use of bilateral cervicothoracic sympathetic decentralization (BCSD) for ventricular arrhythmias refractory to medical and catheter ablation therapy. BCSD, which consists of the removal of the lower third to half of the stellate ganglion and second (T2) through fourth thoracic (T4) ganglia bilaterally, has been shown to reduce the incidence of ventricular arrhythmias in humans [10, 11, 57]. This procedure disrupts projections from cardiac sympathetic preganglionic neurons in the intermediolateral cell column of the spinal cord to postganglionic neurons in the stellate and middle cervical ganglia, as well as some projections from the postganglionic neurons in the stellate and middle cervical ganglia to the heart. Intrathoracic reflexes remain intact after this procedure. Importantly, this procedure also disrupts one of the major paths for afferent information to the central nervous system, and may prevent afferent-mediated sympathoexcitation and conflict between central and peripheral aspects of the cardiac autonomic nervous system [1]. Furthermore, there is now evidence suggesting that patients receiving BCSD have a better prognosis, both in terms of shock-free survival and overall survival, than those receiving only left cervicothoracic sympathetic decentralization (LCSD) [10]. (**a**) Videoscopic still frame of the left sympathetic chain in the thoracic cavity before its intrathoracic resection. (**b**) Resected tissue comprising the lower half of the left stellate ganglion (LSG) to T4 ganglion. (**c**) Hematoxylin/eosin-stained section of the LSG. Ganglion cell are indicated by *arrows*. (**d**) Bar graph showing survival free from implantable cardioverter defibrillator shocks in patients receiving LCSD ($n = 14$) or BCSD ($n = 27$) at 14 and 365 days post procedure (Panels **a–c** are adapted from Bourke et al. [57], and panel **d** is adapted from Vaseghi et al. [10]).

References

1. Fukuda K, Kanazawa H, Aizawa Y, Ardell JL, Shivkumar K. Cardiac innervation and sudden cardiac death. Circ Res. 2015;116:2005–19.
2. Armour JA. Potential clinical relevance of the 'little brain' on the mammalian heart. Exp Physiol. 2008;93:165–76.
3. Gray MA, Taggart P, Sutton PM, Groves D, Holdright DR, Bradbury D, Brull D, Critchley HD. A cortical potential reflecting cardiac function. Proc Natl Acad Sci U S A. 2007;104:6818–23.
4. Oppenheimer S, Hopkins D. Suprabulbar neuronal regulation of the heart. In: Armour JA, Ardell JL, editors. Neurocardiology. New York: Oxford University Press; 1994. p. 309–42.
5. Zipes DP, Wellens HJ. Sudden cardiac death. Circulation. 1998;98:2334–51.
6. Chugh SS, Reinier K, Teodorescu C, Evanado A, Kehr E, Al Samara M, Mariani R, Gunson K, Jui J. Epidemiology of sudden cardiac death: clinical and research implications. Prog Cardiovasc Dis. 2008;51:213–28.
7. Vaseghi M, Shivkumar K. The role of the autonomic nervous system in sudden cardiac death. Prog Cardiovasc Dis. 2008;50:404–19.
8. Buckley U, Shivkumar K, Ardell JL. Autonomic regulation therapy in heart failure. Curr Heart Fail Rep. 2015;12:284–93.
9. Premchand RK, Sharma K, Mittal S, Monteiro R, Dixit S, Libbus I, DiCarlo LA, Ardell JL, Rector TS, Amurthur B, KenKnight BH, Anand IS. Autonomic regulation therapy via left or right cervical vagus nerve stimulation in patients with chronic heart failure: results of the anthem-hf trial. J Card Fail. 2014;20:808–16.
10. Vaseghi M, Gima J, Kanaan C, Ajijola OA, Marmureanu A, Mahajan A, Shivkumar K. Cardiac sympathetic denervation in patients with refractory ventricular arrhythmias or electrical storm: intermediate and long-term follow-up. Heart Rhythm. 2014;11:360–6.
11. Ajijola OA, Lellouche N, Bourke T, Tung R, Ahn S, Mahajan A, Shivkumar K. Bilateral cardiac sympathetic denervation for the management of electrical storm. J Am Coll Cardiol. 2012;59:91–2.
12. Jänig W. Sympathetic nervous system and inflammation: a conceptual view. Auton Neurosci. 2014;182:4–14.
13. Janig W. Functional anatomy of the peripheral sympathetic and parasympathetic system. In: Janig W, editor. The integrative action of the autonomic nervous system: neurobiology of homeostasis. Cambridge: Cambridge University Press; 2006. p. 13–34.
14. Palma JA, Benarroch EE. Neural control of the heart: recent concepts and clinical correlations. Neurology. 2014;83:261–71.
15. Kuntz A. The autonomic nervous system. Philadelphia: Lea & Febiger; 1934.
16. Armour JA. Activity of in situ middle cervical ganglion neurons in dogs, using extracellular recording techniques. Can J Physiol Pharmacol. 1985;63:704–16.
17. Armour JA, Janes RD. Neuronal activity recorded extracellularly from in situ canine mediastinal ganglia. Can J Physiol Pharmacol. 1988;66:119–27.
18. Armour JA, Kember G. Cardiac sensory neurons. In: Armour JA, Ardell JL, editors. Basic and clinical neurocardiology. New York: Oxford University Press; 2004. p. 79–117.
19. Waxman S. Clinical neuroanatomy. New York: McGraw Hill; 2013.
20. Cardinal R, Pagé P, Vermeulen M, Ardell JL, Armour JA. Spatially divergent cardiac responses to nicotinic stimulation of ganglionated plexus neurons in the canine heart. Auton Neurosci. 2009;145:55–62.
21. Randall WC, Priola DV, Pace JB. Responses of individucal cardiac chambers to stimulation of the cervical vagosympathetic trunk in atropinized dogs. Circ Res. 1967;20:534–44.
22. Seki A, Green HR, Lee TD, Hong L, Tan J, Vinters HV, Chen PS, Fishbein MC. Sympathetic nerve fibers in human cervical and thoracic vagus nerves. Heart Rhythm. 2014;11:1411–7.
23. Bonaz B, Picq C, Sinniger V, Mayol JF, Clarençon D. Vagus nerve stimulation: from epilepsy to the cholinergic anti-inflammatory pathway. Neurogastroenterol Motil. 2013;25:208–21.
24. Woodbury DM, Woodbury JW. Effects of vagal stimulation on experimentally induced seizures in rats. Epilepsia. 1990;31 Suppl 2:S7–19.
25. Yoo PB, Lubock NB, Hincapie JG, Ruble SB, Hamann JJ, Grill WM. High-resolution measurement of electrically-evoked vagus nerve activity in the anesthetized dog. J Neural Eng. 2013;10:026003.
26. Huang WA, Shivkumar K, Vaseghi M. Device-based autonomic modulation in arrhythmia patients: the role of vagal nerve stimulation. Curr Treat Options Cardiovasc Med. 2015;17:379.
27. Janes RD, Brandys JC, Hopkins DA, Johnstone DE, Murphy DA, Armour JA. Anatomy of human extrinsic cardiac nerves and ganglia. Am J Cardiol. 1986;57:299–309.
28. Haws CW, Lux RL. Correlation between in vivo transmembrane action potential durations and activation-recovery intervals from electrograms. Effects of interventions that alter repolarization time. Circulation. 1990;81:281–8.
29. Vaseghi M, Yamakawa K, Sinha A, So EL, Zhou W, Ajijola OA, Lux RL, Laks M, Shivkumar K, Mahajan A. Modulation of regional dispersion of repolarization and t-peak to t-end interval by the right and left stellate ganglia. Am J Physiol Heart Circ Physiol. 2013;305:H1020–30.
30. Vaseghi M, Zhou W, Shi J, Ajijola OA, Hadaya J, Shivkumar K, Mahajan A. Sympathetic innervation of the anterior left ventricular wall by the right and left stellate ganglia. Heart Rhythm. 2012;9:1303–9.
31. Yamakawa K, So EL, Rajendran PS, Hoang JD, Makkar N, Mahajan A, Shivkumar K, Vaseghi M. Electrophysiological effects of right and left vagal nerve stimulation on the ventricular myocardium. Am J Physiol Heart Circ Physiol. 2014;307(5):H722–31.
32. Armour JA. Myocardial ischaemia and the cardiac nervous system. Cardiovasc Res. 1999;41:41–54.
33. Ardell JL. Sensory transduction of the ischemic myocardium. Am J Physiol Heart Circ Physiol. 2010;299:H1753–4.
34. Hua F, Ricketts BA, Reifsteck A, Ardell JL, Williams CA. Myocardial ischemia induces the release of substance p from cardiac afferent neurons in rat thoracic spinal cord. Am J Physiol Heart Circ Physiol. 2004;286:H1654–64.
35. Langley JN. The autonomic nervous system: part I. Cambridge: W. Heffer & Sons; 1921.
36. Yuan BX, Ardell JL, Hopkins DA, Losier AM, Armour JA. Gross and microscopic anatomy of the canine intrinsic cardiac nervous system. Anat Rec. 1994;239:75–87.
37. Armour JA, Murphy DA, Yuan BX, Macdonald S, Hopkins DA. Gross and microscopic anatomy of the human intrinsic cardiac nervous system. Anat Rec. 1997;247:289–98.
38. Arora RC, Waldmann M, Hopkins DA, Armour JA. Porcine intrinsic cardiac ganglia. Anat Rec A Discov Mol Cell Evol Biol. 2003;271:249–58.
39. McGuirt AS, Schmacht DC, Ardell JL. Autonomic interactions for control of atrial rate are maintained after sa nodal parasympathectomy. Am J Physiol. 1997;272:H2525–33.

40. Hoover DB, Shepherd AV, Southerland EM, Armour JA, Ardell JL. Neurochemical diversity of afferent neurons that transduce sensory signals from dog ventricular myocardium. Auton Neurosci. 2008;141:38–45.
41. Hoover DB, Isaacs ER, Jacques F, Hoard JL, Pagé P, Armour JA. Localization of multiple neurotransmitters in surgically derived specimens of human atrial ganglia. Neuroscience. 2009;164:1170–9.
42. Zhou S, Chen LS, Miyauchi Y, Miyauchi M, Kar S, Kangavari S, Fishbein MC, Sharifi B, Chen PS. Mechanisms of cardiac nerve sprouting after myocardial infarction in dogs. Circ Res. 2004;95:76–83.
43. Cao JM, Fishbein MC, Han JB, Lai WW, Lai AC, Wu TJ, Czer L, Wolf PL, Denton TA, Shintaku IP, Chen PS, Chen LS. Relationship between regional cardiac hyperinnervation and ventricular arrhythmia. Circulation. 2000;101:1960–9.
44. Vracko R, Thorning D, Frederickson RG. Nerve fibers in human myocardial scars. Hum Pathol. 1991;22:138–46.
45. Thompson GW, Horackova M, Armour JA. Sensitivity of canine intrinsic cardiac neurons to h2o2 and hydroxyl radical. Am J Physiol. 1998;275:H1434–40.
46. Huang MH, Horackova M, Negoescu RM, Wolf S, Armour JA. Polysensory response characteristics of dorsal root ganglion neurones that may serve sensory functions during myocardial ischaemia. Cardiovasc Res. 1996;32:503–15.
47. Huang HS, Pan HL, Stahl GL, Longhurst JC. Ischemia- and reperfusion-sensitive cardiac sympathetic afferents: Influence of h2o2 and hydroxyl radicals. Am J Physiol. 1995;269:H888–901.
48. Thames MD, Kinugawa T, Dibner-Dunlap ME. Reflex sympathoexcitation by cardiac sympathetic afferents during myocardial ischemia. Role of adenosine. Circulation. 1993;87:1698–704.
49. Ajijola OA, Wisco JJ, Lambert HW, Mahajan A, Stark E, Fishbein MC, Shivkumar K. Extracardiac neural remodeling in humans with cardiomyopathy. Circ Arrhythm Electrophysiol. 2012;5:1010–116.
50. Ajijola OA, Yagishita D, Reddy NK, Yamakawa K, Vaseghi M, Downs AM, Hoover DB, Ardell JL, Shivkumar K. Remodeling of stellate ganglion neurons following spatially targeted myocardial infarction: neuropeptide and morphologic changes. Heart Rhythm. 2015;12(5):1027–35.
51. Kanazawa H, Ieda M, Kimura K, Arai T, Kawaguchi-Manabe H, Matsuhashi T, Endo J, Sano M, Kawakami T, Kimura T, Monkawa T, Hayashi M, Iwanami A, Okano H, Okada Y, Ishibashi-Ueda H, Ogawa S, Fukuda K. Heart failure causes cholinergic transdifferentiation of cardiac sympathetic nerves via gp130-signaling cytokines in rodents. J Clin Invest. 2010;120:408–21.
52. Han S, Kobayashi K, Joung B, Piccirillo G, Maruyama M, Vinters HV, March K, Lin SF, Shen C, Fishbein MC, Chen PS, Chen LS. Electroanatomic remodeling of the left stellate ganglion after myocardial infarction. J Am Coll Cardiol. 2012;59:954–61.
53. Zhou S, Jung BC, Tan AY, Trang VQ, Gholmieh G, Han SW, Lin SF, Fishbein MC, Chen PS, Chen LS. Spontaneous stellate ganglion nerve activity and ventricular arrhythmia in a canine model of sudden death. Heart Rhythm. 2008;5:131–9.
54. Woo MA, Macey PM, Keens PT, Kumar R, Fonarow GC, Hamilton MA, Harper RM. Functional abnormalities in brain areas that mediate autonomic nervous system control in advanced heart failure. J Card Fail. 2005;11:437–46.
55. Ajijola OA, Shivkumar K. Neural remodeling and myocardial infarction: the stellate ganglion as a double agent. J Am Coll Cardiol. 2012;59:962–4.
56. Vaseghi M, Ajijola O, Mahajan A, Shivkumar K. Sympathetic innervation, denervation, and cardiac arrhythmias. In: Zipes D, Jalife J, editors. Cardiac electrophysiology: from cell to bedside. Philadelphia: Saunders Elsevier; 2014. p. 409–18.
57. Bourke T, Vaseghi M, Michowitz Y, Sankhla V, Shah M, Swapna N, Boyle NG, Mahajan A, Narasimhan C, Lokhandwala Y, Shivkumar K. Neuraxial modulation for refractory ventricular arrhythmias: value of thoracic epidural anesthesia and surgical left cardiac sympathetic denervation. Circulation. 2010;121:2255–62.
58. Hopkins DA, Macdonald SE, Murphy DA, Armour JA. Pathology of intrinsic cardiac neurons from ischemic human hearts. Anat Rec. 2000;259:424–36.
59. Jv J. Cellular pathobiology. Metabolic and storage diseases. In: Electron microscopy in human medicine. New York: McGraw-Hill; 1978.
60. Lake B. Lysosomal and peroxisomal disorders. In: Adams J, Duchen L, editors. Greenfield's neuropathology. New York: Oxford University Press; 1992. p. 709–810.
61. Hardwick JC, Ryan SE, Beaumont E, Ardell JL, Southerland EM. Dynamic remodeling of the guinea pig intrinsic cardiac plexus induced by chronic myocardial infarction. Auton Neurosci. 2014;181:4–12.
62. Ajijola OA, Yagishita D, Patel KJ, Vaseghi M, Zhou W, Yamakawa K, So E, Lux RL, Mahajan A, Shivkumar K. Focal myocardial infarction induces global remodeling of cardiac sympathetic innervation: neural remodeling in a spatial context. Am J Physiol Heart Circ Physiol. 2013;305:H1031–40.
63. Wickramasinghe SR, Patel VV. Local innervation and atrial fibrillation. Circulation. 2013;128:1566–75.
64. Coumel P, Attuel P, Lavallée J, Flammang D, Leclercq JF, Slama R. [The atrial arrhythmia syndrome of vagal origin]. Arch Mal Coeur Vaiss. 1978;71:645–56.
65. Schauerte P, Scherlag BJ, Patterson E, Scherlag MA, Matsudaria K, Nakagawa H, Lazzara R, Jackman WM. Focal atrial fibrillation: experimental evidence for a pathophysiologic role of the autonomic nervous system. J Cardiovasc Electrophysiol. 2001;12:592–9.
66. Shivkumar K, Buch E, Boyle NG. Nonpharmacologic management of atrial fibrillation: role of the pulmonary veins and posterior left atrium. Heart Rhythm. 2009;6:S5–11.
67. Arora R. Recent insights into the role of the autonomic nervous system in the creation of substrate for atrial fibrillation: implications for therapies targeting the atrial autonomic nervous system. Circ Arrhythm Electrophysiol. 2012;5:850–9.
68. Ng J, Villuendas R, Cokic I, Schliamser JE, Gordon D, Koduri H, Benefield B, Simon J, Murthy SN, Lomasney JW, Wasserstrom JA, Goldberger JJ, Aistrup GL, Arora R. Autonomic remodeling in the left atrium and pulmonary veins in heart failure: creation of a dynamic substrate for atrial fibrillation. Circ Arrhythm Electrophysiol. 2011;4:388–96.
69. Katritsis DG, Giazitzoglou E, Zografos T, Pokushalov E, Po SS, Camm AJ. Rapid pulmonary vein isolation combined with autonomic ganglia modification: a randomized study. Heart Rhythm. 2011;8:672–8.
70. Nakagawa H, Scherlag BJ, Patterson E, Ikeda A, Lockwood D, Jackman WM. Pathophysiologic basis of autonomic ganglionated plexus ablation in patients with atrial fibrillation. Heart Rhythm. 2009;6:S26–34.
71. Leiria TL, Glavinovic T, Armour JA, Cardinal R, de Lima GG, Kus T. Longterm effects of cardiac mediastinal nerve cryoablation on neural inducibility of atrial fibrillation in canines. Auton Neurosci. 2011;161:68–74.
72. He B, Lu Z, He W, Wu L, Cui B, Hu X, Yu L, Huang C, Jiang H. Effects of ganglionated plexi ablation on ventricular electrophysiological properties in normal hearts and after acute myocardial ischemia. Int J Cardiol. 2013;168:86–93.
73. Groves DA, Brown VJ. Vagal nerve stimulation: a review of its applications and potential mechanisms that mediate its clinical effects. Neurosci Biobehav Rev. 2005;29:493–500.
74. Ikramuddin S, Blackstone RP, Brancatisano A, Toouli J, Shah SN, Wolfe BM, Fujioka K, Maher JW, Swain J, Que FG, Morton JM,

Leslie DB, Brancatisano R, Kow L, O'Rourke RW, Deveney C, Takata M, Miller CJ, Knudson MB, Tweden KS, Shikora SA, Sarr MG, Billington CJ. Effect of reversible intermittent intra-abdominal vagal nerve blockade on morbid obesity: the recharge randomized clinical trial. JAMA. 2014;312:915–22.

75. Li M, Zheng C, Sato T, Kawada T, Sugimachi M, Sunagawa K. Vagal nerve stimulation markedly improves long-term survival after chronic heart failure in rats. Circulation. 2004;109:120–4.
76. Zhang Y, Popovic ZB, Bibevski S, Fakhry I, Sica DA, Van Wagoner DR, Mazgalev TN. Chronic vagus nerve stimulation improves autonomic control and attenuates systemic inflammation and heart failure progression in a canine high-rate pacing model. Circ Heart Fail. 2009;2:692–9.
77. De Ferrari GM, Crijns HJ, Borggrefe M, Milasinovic G, Smid J, Zabel M, Gavazzi A, Sanzo A, Dennert R, Kuschyk J, Raspopovic S, Klein H, Swedberg K, Schwartz PJ, Investigators CMT. Chronic vagus nerve stimulation: a new and promising therapeutic approach for chronic heart failure. Eur Heart J. 2011;32:847–55.
78. Zannad F, De Ferrari GM, Tuinenburg AE, Wright D, Brugada J, Butter C, Klein H, Stolen C, Meyer S, Stein KM, Ramuzat A, Schubert B, Daum D, Neuzil P, Botman C, Castel MA, D'Onofrio A, Solomon SD, Wold N, Ruble SB. Chronic vagal stimulation for the treatment of low ejection fraction heart failure: results of the neural cardiac therapy for heart failure (nectar-hf) randomized controlled trial. Eur Heart J. 2015;36:425–33.
79. Huang J, Qian J, Yao W, Wang N, Zhang Z, Cao C, Song B. Vagus nerve stimulation reverses ventricular electrophysiological changes induced by hypersympathetic nerve activity. Exp Physiol. 2015;100:239–48.
80. Lopshire JC, Zhou X, Dusa C, Ueyama T, Rosenberger J, Courtney N, Ujhelyi M, Mullen T, Das M, Zipes DP. Spinal cord stimulation improves ventricular function and reduces ventricular arrhythmias in a canine postinfarction heart failure model. Circulation. 2009;120:286–94.
81. Issa ZF, Zhou X, Ujhelyi MR, Rosenberger J, Bhakta D, Groh WJ, Miller JM, Zipes DP. Thoracic spinal cord stimulation reduces the risk of ischemic ventricular arrhythmias in a postinfarction heart failure canine model. Circulation. 2005;111:3217–20.
82. Southerland EM, Milhorn DM, Foreman RD, Linderoth B, DeJongste MJ, Armour JA, Subramanian V, Singh M, Singh K, Ardell JL. Preemptive, but not reactive, spinal cord stimulation mitigates transient ischemia-induced myocardial infarction via cardiac adrenergic neurons. Am J Physiol Heart Circ Physiol. 2007;292:H311–7.
83. Liu Y, Yue WS, Liao SY, Zhang Y, Au KW, Shuto C, Hata C, Park E, Chen P, Siu CW, Tse HF. Thoracic spinal cord stimulation improves cardiac contractile function and myocardial oxygen consumption in a porcine model of ischemic heart failure. J Cardiovasc Electrophysiol. 2012;23:534–40.
84. Odenstedt J, Linderoth B, Bergfeldt L, Ekre O, Grip L, Mannheimer C, Andréll P. Spinal cord stimulation effects on myocardial ischemia, infarct size, ventricular arrhythmia, and noninvasive electrophysiology in a porcine ischemia-reperfusion model. Heart Rhythm. 2011;8:892–8.
85. Zanchetti AS. Neural regulation of renin release: experimental evidence and clinical implications in arterial hypertension. Circulation. 1977;56:691–8.
86. Bell-Reuss E, Trevino DL, Gottschalk CW. Effect of renal sympathetic nerve stimulation on proximal water and sodium reabsorption. J Clin Invest. 1976;57:1104–7.
87. Gray MO, Long CS, Kalinyak JE, Li HT, Karliner JS. Angiotensin II stimulates cardiac myocyte hypertrophy via paracrine release of TGF-beta 1 and endothelin-1 from fibroblasts. Cardiovasc Res. 1998;40:352–63.
88. Bradfield JS, Vaseghi M, Shivkumar K. Renal denervation for refractory ventricular arrhythmias. Trends Cardiovasc Med. 2014;24:206–13.
89. Bhatt DL, Kandzari DE, O'Neill WW, D'Agostino R, Flack JM, Katzen BT, Leon MB, Liu M, Mauri L, Negoita M, Cohen SA, Oparil S, Rocha-Singh K, Townsend RR, Bakris GL. Investigators SH-. A controlled trial of renal denervation for resistant hypertension. N Engl J Med. 2014;370:1393–401.
90. Atherton DS, Deep NL, Mendelsohn FO. Micro-anatomy of the renal sympathetic nervous system: a human postmortem histologic study. Clin Anat. 2012;25:628–33.
91. Kammerling JJ, Green FJ, Watanabe AM, Inoue H, Barber MJ, Henry DP, Zipes DP. Denervation supersensitivity of refractoriness in noninfarcted areas apical to transmural myocardial infarction. Circulation. 1987;76:383–93.
92. Linz D, Wirth K, Ukena C, Mahfoud F, Pöss J, Linz B, Böhm M, Neuberger HR. Renal denervation suppresses ventricular arrhythmias during acute ventricular ischemia in pigs. Heart Rhythm. 2013;10:1525–30.
93. Ukena C, Bauer A, Mahfoud F, Schreieck J, Neuberger HR, Eick C, Sobotka PA, Gawaz M, Böhm M. Renal sympathetic denervation for treatment of electrical storm: first-in-man experience. Clin Res Cardiol. 2012;101:63–7.
94. Tsioufis C, Papademetriou V, Tsiachris D, Dimitriadis K, Kasiakogias A, Kordalis A, Antonakis V, Kefala A, Thomopoulos C, Kallikazaros I, Lau EO, Stefanadis C. Drug-resistant hypertensive patients responding to multielectrode renal denervation exhibit improved heart rate dynamics and reduced arrhythmia burden. J Hum Hypertens. 2014;28:587–93.
95. Remo BF, Preminger M, Bradfield J, Mittal S, Boyle N, Gupta A, Shivkumar K, Steinberg JS, Dickfeld T. Safety and efficacy of renal denervation as a novel treatment of ventricular tachycardia storm in patients with cardiomyopathy. Heart Rhythm. 2014;11:541–6.
96. Hoffmann BA, Steven D, Willems S, Sydow K. Renal sympathetic denervation as an adjunct to catheter ablation for the treatment of ventricular electrical storm in the setting of acute myocardial infarction. J Cardiovasc Electrophysiol. 2013;24:E21.
97. Wang HJ, Wang W, Cornish KG, Rozanski GJ, Zucker IH. Cardiac sympathetic afferent denervation attenuates cardiac remodeling and improves cardiovascular dysfunction in rats with heart failure. Hypertension. 2014;64:745–55.
98. Armour JA, Kember G. Cardiac sensory neurons. In: Armour JA, Ardell JL, editors. Basic and clinical neurocardiology. New York:Oxford University Press; 2004. p. 79–117.

3 Chemistry and Biology of Radiotracers Designed to Target Changes in the Myocardial Sympathetic and Parasympathetic Nervous Systems as a Function of Disease or Treatment

William C. Eckelman and Vasken Dilsizian

The parasympathetic nervous system (PSNS) uses chiefly acetylcholine (ACh) as its neurotransmitter, although peptides (such as cholecystokinin) may act on the PSNS as a neurotransmitter. The ACh acts on two types of receptors, the muscarinic and nicotinic cholinergic receptors. Most transmissions occur in two stages: When stimulated, the preganglionic nerve releases ACh at the ganglion, which acts on nicotinic receptors of postganglionic neurons. The postganglionic nerve then releases ACh to stimulate the muscarinic receptors of the target organ.

The (ortho-) sympathetic nervous system (SNS) is one of three major parts of the autonomic nervous system (the others being the enteric and parasympathetic systems). The sympathetic nervous system originates in the spinal cord and its main function is to activate the physiological changes that occur during the fight or flight response. This component of the autonomic nervous system utilizes and activates the release of norepinephrine (NE) in the reaction. Its general action is to mobilize the body's nervous system fight-or-flight response. It is, however, constantly active at a basic level to maintain homeostasis.

V. Dilsizian, J. Narula (eds.), *Atlas of Cardiac Innervation*, DOI 10.1007/978-3-319-45800-7_3

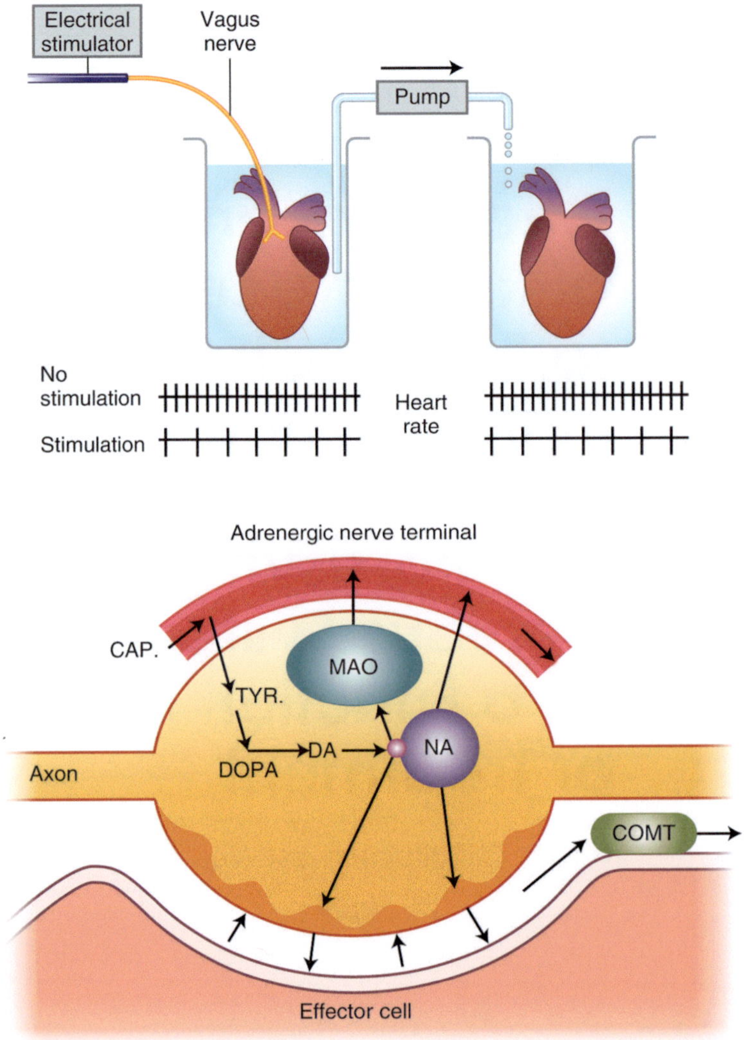

Figure 3-1. Although Otto Loewi discovered chemical transmission of nerve impulses using acetylcholine [1], it was von Euler who discovered in 1946 that the true agent of sympathetic transmission is noradrenaline, also know as NE [2]. That led to the differentiation of adrenergic and cholinergic neurons and synapses. On left above is Otto Loewi's experiment where he took fluid from one frog heart which had been stimulated, and applied it to another. The result was slowing of the second heart, which showed that synaptic signaling used chemical messengers. On the right above is von Euler's description of the adrenergic nerve terminal based on his experiments [3] (Taken from his Nobel Award presentation on 12/1/1970).

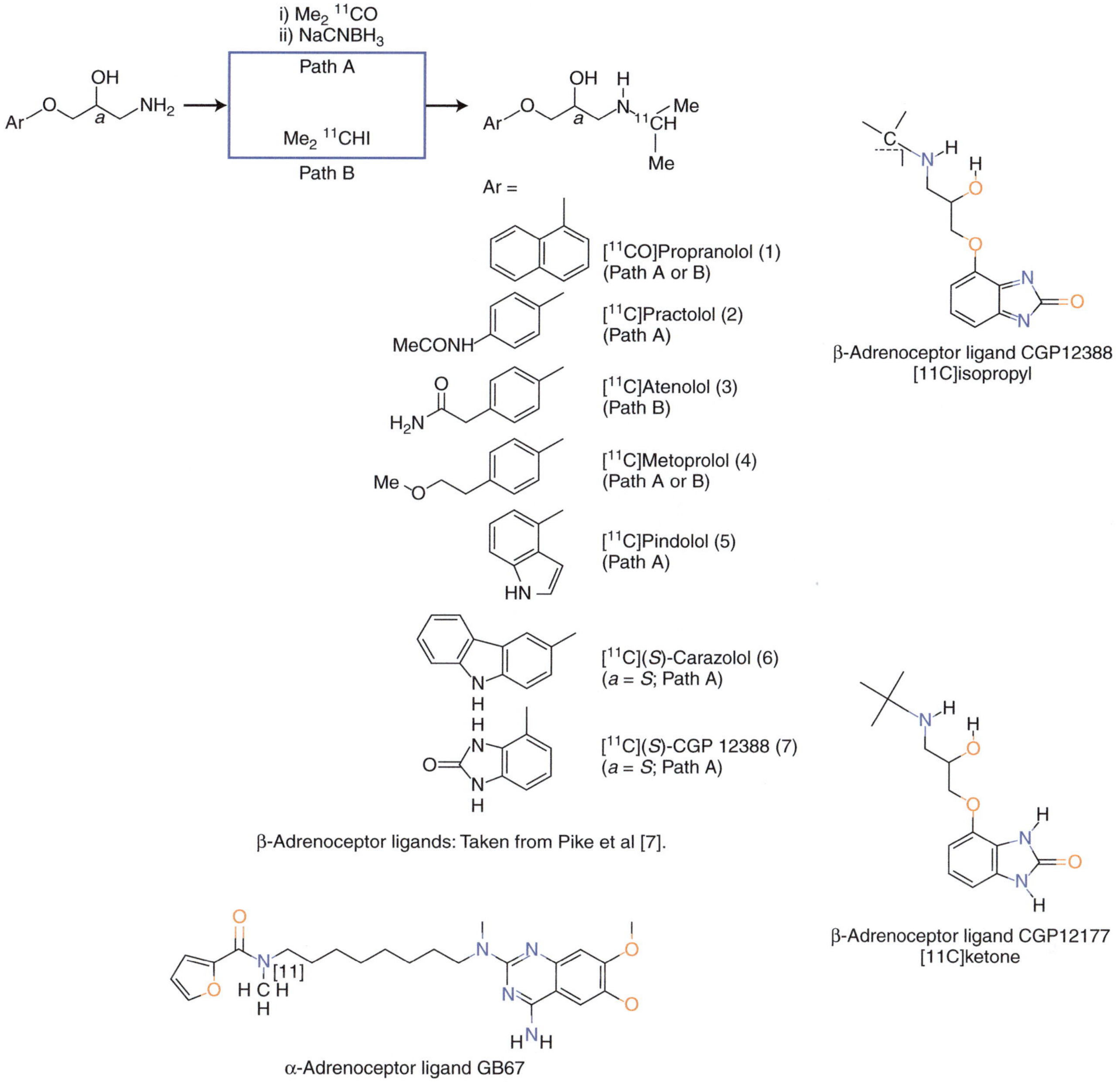

Figure 3-2. Positron emission tomography (PET) imaging of receptors in the sympathetic and the parasympathetic systems of heart and lung has been carried out for three systems, the alpha and beta adrenoceptors (BAR) and the muscarinic acetylcholine receptors (mAChR). For the alpha-adrenoceptor, only [^{11}C]GB67 (N2-[6-[(4-amino-6,7-dimethoxy-2-quinazolinyl)(methyl)amino]hexyl]-N2-[^{11}C]methyl-2-furamide hydrochloride) has been developed. Its potential for application in patients needs to be assessed [4, 5]. The mAChR radioligand [^{11}C]MQNB (N-[^{11}C]methylquinuclidinyl benzilate) was the highest affinity radiotracer for the mAChR straightforward chemistry using the N-[^{11}C]methylation approach [6]. The early BAR radioligands were based on the first drugs for that receptor, i.e., propranolol, practolol, atenolol, metoprolol, etc. [7] and upper left structures. In general, drugs seldom lead to ideal radiotracers given their weaker affinities and higher log P [8]. The most promising BAR radioligands are: [^{11}C]CGP12177: S-(3′-t-butylamino-2′-hydroxypropoxy)-benzimidazol-2-[^{11}C]one [9, 10] and [^{11}C]CGP12388: (S)-4-(3-(2′-[^{11}C]isopropylamino)-2-hydroxypropoxy)-2H-benzimidazol-2-one [11] and qualitatively in lung [^{11}C]VC002: N-[11C]-methyl-piperidin-4-yl-2-cyclohexyl-2-hydroxy-2-phenylacetate [5]. [^{11}C]-S-CGP 12177 had high specific uptake in the heart and lungs (both tissues have high density BAR). This was a success by the accepted technical design criteria, except for the challenging synthesis. A synthesis to introduce the C-11 in the last step led to [^{11}C]CGP12388, also a high affinity radioligand [9–11]. However, the uptake was rapid with minimal efflux indicating that the concentration in the heart and lung was influenced by flow. Therefore an approach to obtain the B_{max} using at least two contractions of radioligand was proposed based on the Scatchard equation, $B/F = B_{max}/K_i - B/K_i$ where the second term is considered negligible if the bound radioligand is <5% of the B_{max} [12]. In summary, for both the beta-adrenergic and the muscarinic systems, potent radioligands have been prepared and evaluated in patients. For both it has been possible to measure receptor densities quantitatively in human heart, but not by the single scan technique that is used routinely in the clinic (Taken from Pike et al. [7]).

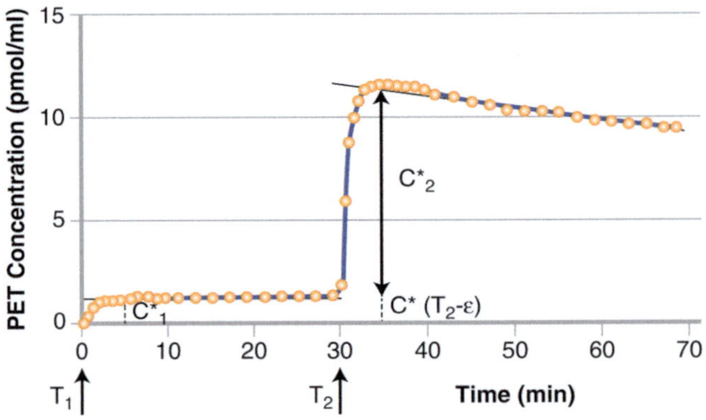

Figure 3-3. The approach for the two injection/ two scan technique to estimate β-adrenergic receptor density using a graphic method. The experimental protocol includes two injections with doses D1* and D2* at times T1 and T2, respectively. The graphic method is based on measurement of 2 plateau levels at end of distribution phase (C1* and C2*). From the analytical data using the specific activity of 29,415 MBq/μmol with D1* = 3.09 nmol and D2* = 22.19 nmol and using a vascular fraction of 40%, receptor concentration was estimated at 18.6 pmol/mL. As demonstrated, the clinical implementation of this requires acquisition of a time-activity curve and at least two images, one at the NCA level and one at ~50% saturation. This approach is complicated and the target density (B_{max}) is difficult to validate using ex vivo data and therefore only a few studies have been pursued by other groups in the routine clinic [13]. It appears that the initial biodistribution of beta adrenergic binding radioligands is heavily weighted by flow. In addition, the target density (B_{max}) is not high compared to the affinity constant. The metrics derived from mathematical analysis using the two injection system using the most easily synthesized beta adrenoceptor ligand (CGP 12388) yielded B_{max} values of 9.74 ± 1.80 nM and a K_d of 0.58 ± 0.22 nM. This yields a $B_{max}/K_d = 17$, which a rule of thumb from in vitro studies of the maximum bound to free ratio to be expected in vivo, One other ramification of this ratio is that a high ratio will be beneficial as the field moves to imaging abnormal tissue that is smaller than twice the instrument resolution [27].

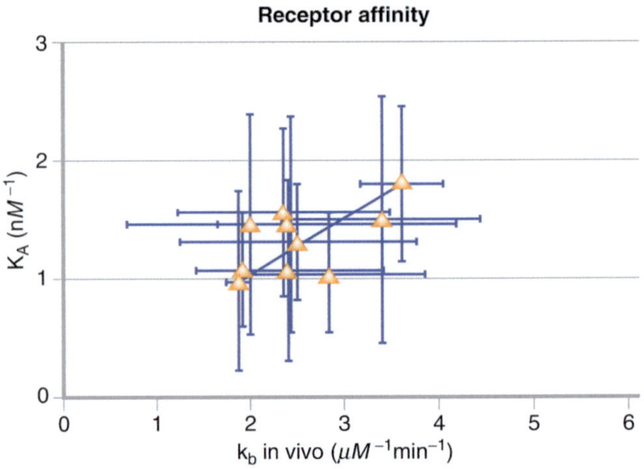

Figure 3-4. Model parameter k_b and an independent measurement of 99mTc-NGA-HBP affinity, K_A, were highly correlated. The correlation was determined by weighted linear regression. Approaches to measuring receptor density for receptor binding radiotracers whose early distribution is heavily weighted by flow and the parent compound toxicity is low. The best example of this is the validation of in vivo receptor measurements via in vitro radioassay: Technetium-99m-Galactosyl-Neoglycoalbumin as Prototype Model [14]. The authors point out various stages of validation:

The ligand should not produce a physiologic effect

The localization in vivo should be receptor mediated

An alteration in biodistribution should reflect a change in disease or disease treatment

A pharmacokinetic method that allows quantitation of changes in receptor density should be developed and validated

Kinetic sensitivity of the analysis with respect to published changes in receptor density as a function of disease should be verified

Receptor density in tissue obtained from images should agree with that measured ex vivo

The key factor is sensitivity to changes in receptor density. Based on in vitro data developed from the original radioimmunoassays, a saturation of ~50% will yield maximal change in binding as a function of receptor density changes.

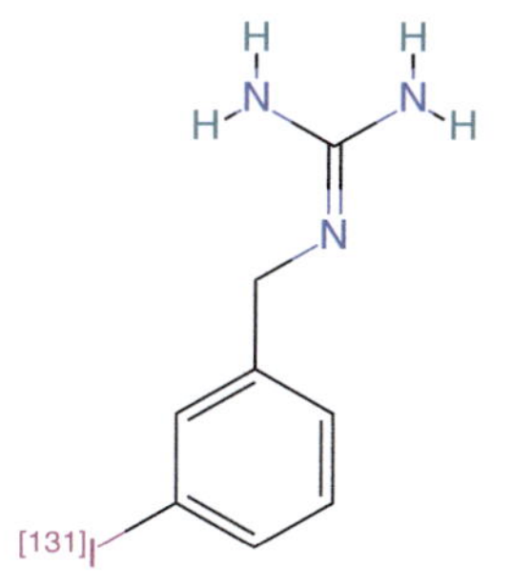

[$^{123/131}$I]MIBG

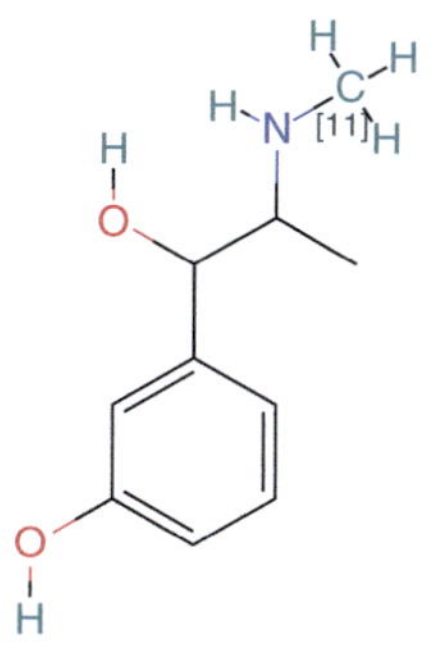

[^{11}C]*meta*-hydroxyephedrine or [^{11}C]mHED

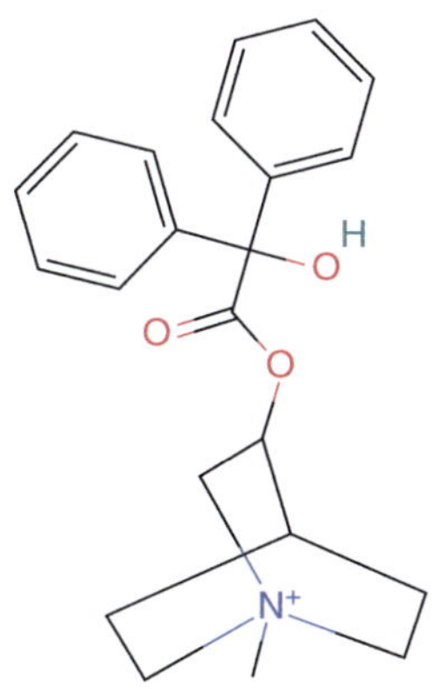

N-[^{11}C]methyl quinuclidinyl RS benzylate

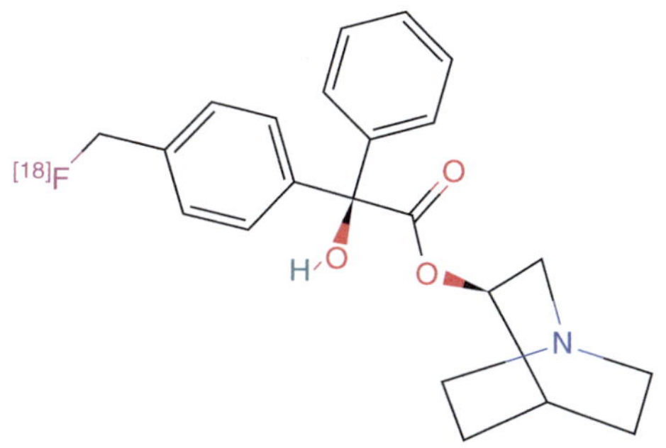

Quinuclidinyl 4-[^{18}F]fluoromethylbenzilate

Figure 3-5. Chemistry: Compared to N-methylation using C-11 methyl iodide or methyl triflate, preparing the precursor for radiofluorination or radioiodination is complicated. N-[^{11}C] methyl quinuclidinyl benzoate was prepared using this method [16, 17]. The original method to produce radiolabeled QNB inserted the C-11 in the benzylic acid. This was achieved by carbonation of the benzophenone dianion followed by ester formation with 3-quinuclidinol [18–20]. Both were validated as specifically targeting the muscarinic receptor but the MQNB was used more often given the straightforward chemistry. The C-11 synthesis can also be complicated if the C-11 is not inserted in the final chemical step. For the two beta adrenoceptor ligands [^{11}C]CGP12177 and [^{11}C]CGP12388, the former is a complicated synthesis starting with C-11 phosgene followed by a multistep synthesis whereas the latter is a more straightforward radiolabeling of the isopropyl group via a reductive alkylation using [^{11}C]acetone of the corresponding (S)-desisopropyl compound [9–11]. The complicated synthesis for [^{11}C]CGP12177 prevented a detailed clinical study. Quinuclidinyl 4-[^{18}F]fluoromethyl-benzilate was also developed and validated as binding to the muscarinic receptors and could be imaged in the monkey myocardium, but showed uptake in bone [21]. [^{123}I]MIBG was originally synthesized by an exchange method using the non radioactive MIBG. Later, the trialkyl tin precursor was used to increase the specific activity. A procedure using a solid phase resin containing the covalently bound stannylbenzyl-guanidine precursor has the potential to produce the highest specific activity [22]. This is important given the potential side effects of carrier MIBG (Taken from PubChem [15]).

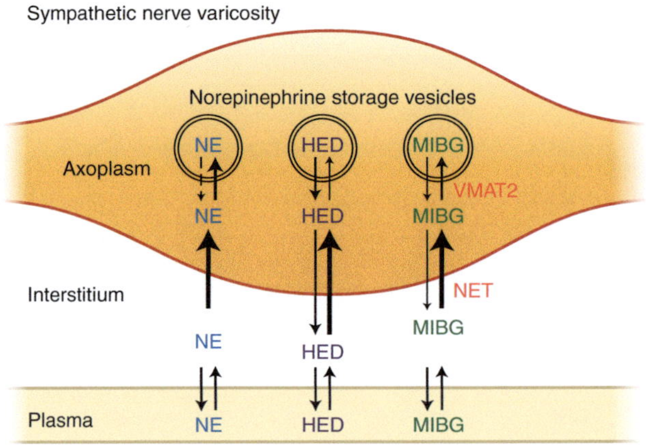

FIGURE 3-6. Schematic illustration of the uptake of norepinephrine (NE), [^{11}C]meta-hydroxyephedrine (HED), and meta[^{123}I] iodobenzylguanidine (MIBG) into cardiac sympathetic nerve varicosities. After extraction from plasma, HED and MIBG are transported into sympathetic nerve terminal axons by the norepinephrine transporter (NET). Once in the neuronal axoplasm, they are subsequently transported into NE storage vesicles by the second isoform of the vesicular monoamine transporter (VMAT2). Because the radiotracers targeting receptors, enyzmes, and transporters of the sympathetic and parasympathetic nervous system are small molecules, the radionuclides used were chosen to introduce the minimal perturbation to the parent drug candidate from C-11, which replaced a stable carbon and therefore did not alter the biochemistry, to F-18 and I-123 that produced changes in the biochemistry. The C-11 radioligands had the biochemical properties of the parent compound, often a well-characterized drug candidate. The F-18 and I-123 analogs showed similarities in the biochemistry compared to the parent drug candidate, but validation studies were needed to elucidate the key biochemical parameters. This requires extensive effort using in vitro and in in vivo models. For example, the biochemistry of [^{18}F]Fludeoxyglucose and [^{18}F]Fluorothymidine are similar to that of deoxyglucose and thymidine, but there are key differences and the biochemistry of fluorothymidine is more unlike that of thymidine than fluorodeoxyglucose is from deoxyglucose (and glucose) [24] (Taken from Raffel [23]).

NET Substrate	Acronym	Structure	K_1 (μM)	K_m (μM)	V_{max} (pmol/min/mg protein)	V_{max}/K_m (μl/min/mg protein)
[^{3}H]-(−)-norepinephrine	NE	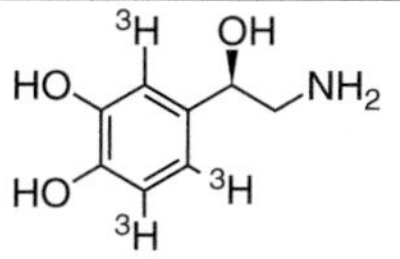	63.9±2.3	0.28±0.03	5.83±0.49	21.3±2.4
[^{3}H]dopamine	DA	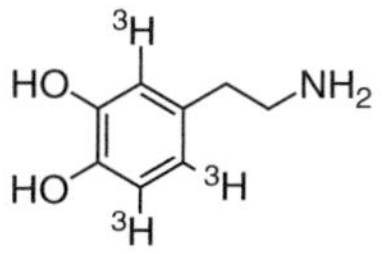	8.1±0.5	0.24±0.04	2.91±0.47	12.2±1.8
[^{11}C]-(−)-epinephrine	EPI	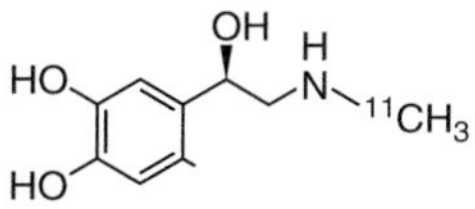	68.4±7.6	3.16±0.78	6.09±1.04	2.0±0.2
[^{11}C]-(−)-*metn*-hydroxyephedrine	HED	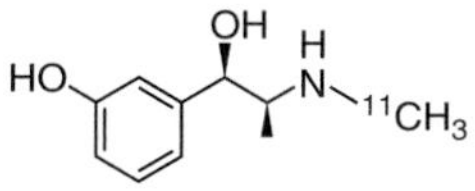	43.2±1.8	0.48±0.08	5.43±0.71	11.4±1.3
[^{11}C]*metn*-hydroxyphenethylguanidine	MHPG	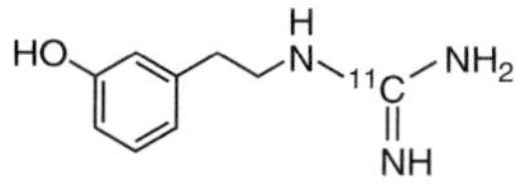	4.9±0.5	0.73±0.20	7.83±1.73	11.2±2.8
[^{11}C]*para*-hydroxyphenethylguanidine	PHPG	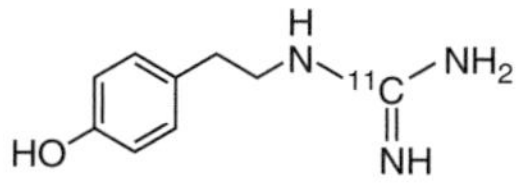	1.9±0.2	0.52±0.06	3.31±0.40	6.4±1.1
(−)-N-[^{11}C]*guanyl*-metn-octopamine	GMO	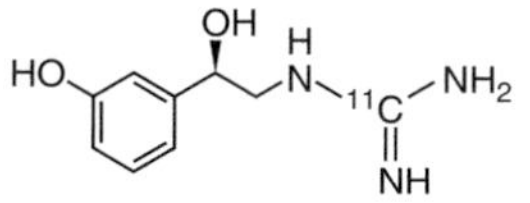	20.3±2.5	4.43±0.31	5.57±0.30	1.3±0.1
[^{11}C]4-fluoro-*metn*-hydroxyphenethylguanidine	4F-MHPG	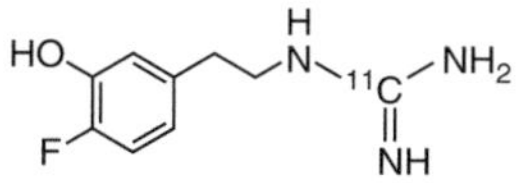	5.6±0.5	2.57±0.35	7.46±0.64	3.0±0.5
[^{11}C]6-fluoro-*metn*-hydroxyphenethylguanidine	6F-MHPG	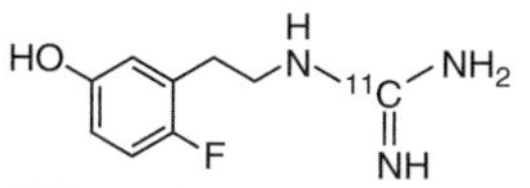	17.7±0.5	2.86±0.43	4.06±0.66	1.4±0.3

Figure 3-7. NET substrates have been more completely validated for measuring the kinetics of various key biochemical steps. The goal is a diagnostic test per se, but also increasing the understanding of the underlying mechanisms of autonomic dysfunction and its contribution to the manifestation and progression of cardiac diseases. The search continues for a radioligand whose distribution is not primarily affected by flow or by endogenous NE, but rather sensitive to moderate levels of cardiac denervation. One recent attempt is to find a radiotracer that has a lower extraction than MIBG or HED. The new lead compound is 4-[^{18}F]fluoro-m-hydroxyphenethyl-guanidine (4-[^{18}F]F-MHPG) [26]. The compound was originally compared to NE and HED using the Michaelis-Menten enzyme analysis. The analysis in the current study was analyzed using a compartment model (net uptake K_i=0.341 mL/min/g) and the Patlak analysis (K_p=0.302 mL/min/g). The radio tracer, 4-[18 F] FMHPG, has a weaker Km with about the same maximum velocity, which was the design goal. It is worth noting that the K_i from Fig. 3.7 measures the inhibition of these ligands in the micromolar range. If the goal were to inhibit the transporter (as it is in the brain) then these affinity constants would have to be in the nanomolar range [28]. For substrates, the main concern is the competition with endogenous NE and therefore one design goal is to develop a substrate that binds with an affinity less than that of NE, which is 63.9 μM in this assay (Taken from Raffel et al. [25]).

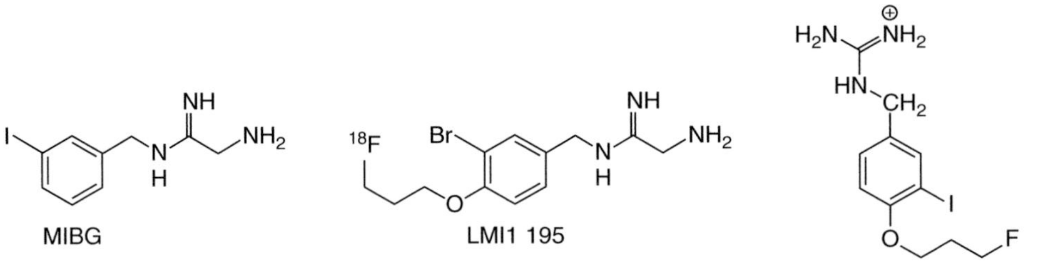

Figure 3-8. MIBG, radioiodinated using I-123, is approved for visualization of myocardial sympathetic innervation in certain heart failure patients and therefore is the gold standard for other radiotracers seeking the same indication. LMI1195 (named FBOBBG by Vaidyanathan et al. [30]) is in Phase III studies. FPOIBG can be radiolabeled with either I-123 or F-18. Recently another analog of mIBG, radiolabeled with F-18 has been evaluated, namely N-[3-bromo-4-(3-[^{18}F]fluoro-propoxy)-benzyl]-guanidine (LMI1195). The affinity constants of LMI1195 are similar to those found for NE and the uptake in the heart is similar to meta[^{123}I]IBG, but the heart to liver and lung are significantly higher for LMI1195 compared to mIBG. Desipramine (1 mg/kg), a selective NET inhibitor, blocked LMI1195 heart uptake by 82% whereas only 53% of meta[^{123}I]IBG was blocked in rabbits [29]. In sympathetically denervated rabbits, LMI1195 showed minimal heart uptake compared to the control rabbits, but Flurpiridaz F-18, a myocardial perfusion marker, showed no difference in myocardial uptake compared to a normal rabbit. This latter study was repeated by the same group using the phenol model whereas the earlier study used chemical denervation with 6-hydroxydopamine and found the same defect with MLI1195 at delayed times after denervation [29]. In the isolated perfused rabbit heart, the extraction fraction was 44.4, 28.2 and 21.5% at flow rates at 2, 4, and 8 mL/min/g, which may account for the differences between LMI1195 and a perfusion agent in the denervated rabbit myocardium [29].

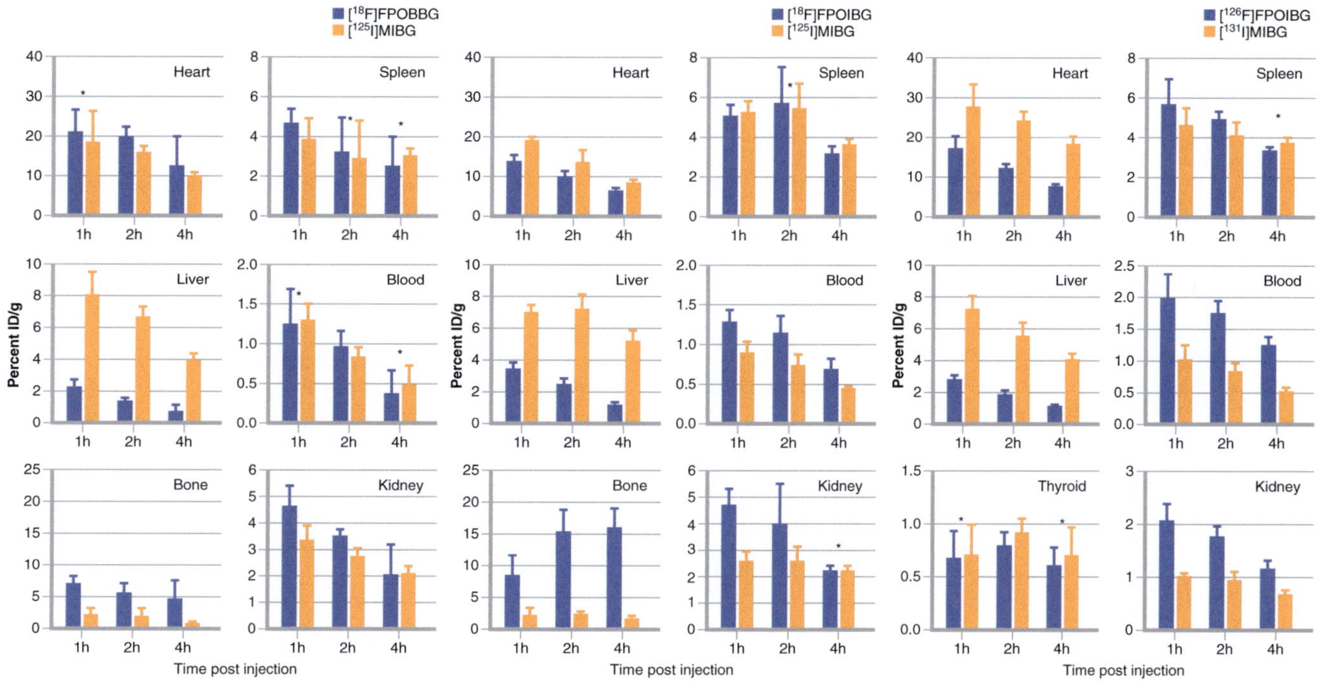

FIGURE 3-9. Vaidyanathan et al. reported on a similar series of compounds and compared those to ML1195 [30]. In these experiments, the affinity constants for the three compounds from competitive inhibition experiments using UVW-NAT cells for MIBG, FPOBBG, and FPOIBG were 1.5±1.1, 11.0±2.9, and 20.0±0.1 μM respectively. Defluorination was evident in both FPOBBG (MLI1195) and FPOIBG. MLI1195 had the highest heart/liver ratios.The basis for developing a radiotracer should be an unmet clinical need. This is not limited to other imaging procedures, but rather an evaluation of all diagnostic tests presently in use. The Rationale of an unmet need for radiolabeled adrenoceptor antagonists is based on post mortem studies, which showed that the numbers of human cardiac adrenoceptors (ARs) are associated with various diseases, such as myocardial ischemia, congestive heart failure, cardiomyopathy and hypertension. "There is a clear need for capability to assess human cardiac ARs directly in vivo, so that their distribution, concentration and occupancy by endogenous ligand or drugs can be monitored throughout the progress of specific diseases and their treatments. This would have the potential to give new insights into the involvement of the sympathetic nervous system (SNS) in the aetiology of myocardial disease" [31]. Caldwell and Link point out that measuring perfusion in the heart when the tracer is fixed at a density for a long enough period to image the distribution has been shown to be useful in patient management. However, the many rapid changes in the biochemical pathways in, for example, heart failure, a single static image at an arbitrary time may need add relevant information [32]. However, given the efficient extraction of the radioligands by the alpha and beta adrenoreceptor and by NET for NE metabolism, the measurement for the adrenoceptors requires the use of a two dose injection [16–20] and for NE metabolism requires monitoring the efflux from the myocardium [33–35]. Monitoring radioactivity and converting it to biochemical parameters in both these situations is a major challenge. Given the technical challenges in developing and validation new radiotracers for the adrenoceptors and the NE system that are sensitive to small biochemical changes, the emphasis should be on defining the unmet need for a targeted imaging agent and therefore the patient impact [36, 37].
Caldwell and Link point out that measuring perfusion in the heart when the tracer is fixed at a density for a long enough period to image the distribution has been shown to be useful in patient management. However, the many rapid changes in the biochemical pathways in, for example, heart failure, a single static image at an arbitrary time may need add relevant information [32]. However, given the efficient extraction of the radioligands by the alpha and beta adrenoreceptor and by NET for NE metabolism, the measurement for the adrenoceptors requires the use of a two dose injection [16–20] and for NE metabolism requires monitoring the efflux from the myocardium [33–35]. Monitoring radioactivity and converting it to biochemical parameters in both these situations is a major challenge. Given the technical challenges in developing and validation new radiotracers for the adrenoceptors and the NE system that are sensitive to small biochemical changes, the emphasis should be on defining the unmet need for a targeted imaging agent and therefore the patient impact [36, 37].

References

1. Zimmer H-G. Otto Loewi and the chemical transmission of vagus stimulation in the heart. Clin Cardiol. 2006;29:135–6.
2. Von Euler US. Some aspects of the clinical physiology of noradrenaline. Scand J Clin Lab Invest. 1952;4:254–62.
3. von Euler US. Adrenergic neurotransmitter functions. Science. 1971;173:202–6.
4. Riemann B, Schäfers M, Law MP, Wichter T, Schober O. Radioligands for imaging myocardial alpha- and beta-adrenoceptors. Nuklearmedizin. 2003;42:4–9.
5. Elsinga PH, van Waarde A, Vaalburg W. Receptor imaging in the thorax with PET. Eur J Pharmacol. 2004;499:1–13.
6. Mazière M, Comar D, Godot JM, Collard P, Cepeda C, Naquet R. In vivo characterization of myocardium muscarinic receptors by positron emission tomography. Life Sci. 1981;29:2391–7.
7. Pike VW, Law MP, Osman S, Davenport RJ, Rimoldi O, Giardinà D, Camici PG. Selection, design and evaluation of new radioligands for PET studies of cardiac adrenoceptors. Pharm Acta Helv. 2000;74(2–3):191–200.
8. Moran NC. The development of beta adrenergic blocking drugs: a retrospective and prospective evaluation. Ann N Y Acad Sci. 1967;139:649–60.
9. Nanoff C, Freissmuth M, Schüz W. Naunyn schmiedebergs. Arch Pharmacol. 1987;336:519.
10. Brady F, Luthra SK, Tochon-Danguy HJ, et al. Asymmetric synthesis of a precursor for the automated radiosynthesis of S-(3′-t-butylamino-2′-hydroxypropoxy)-benzimidazol-2-[11C] one (S-[11C]CGP 12177) as a preferred radioligand for beta-adrenergic receptors. Int J Rad Appl Instrum A. 1991;42: 621–8.
11. Elsinga PH, van Waarde A, Jaeggi KA, Schreiber G, Heldoorn M, Vaalburg W. Synthesis and evaluation of (S)-4-(3-(2′-[11C] isopropylamino)-2-hydroxypropoxy) -2H-benzimidazol –2-one ((S)-[11C]CGP 12388) and (S)-4-(3-((1′-[18 F]-fluoroisopropyl) amino)-2-hydroxypropoxy) -2H- benzimidazol-2-one ((S)-[18 F] fluoro-CGP 12388) for visualization of beta-adrenoceptors with positron emission tomography positron. J Med Chem. 1997;40:3829–35.
12. Delforge J, Mesangeau D, Dolle F, Merlet P, Loc'h C, Bottlaender M, et al. In vivo quantification and parametric images of the cardiac-adrenergic receptor density. J Nucl Med. 2002;43:215–26.
13. Tsukamoto T, Morita K, Naya M, et al. Decreased myocardial b-adrenergic receptor density in relation to increased sympathetic tone in patients with nonischemic cardiomyopathy. J Nucl Med. 2007;48:1777–82.
14. Kudo M, Vera DR, Trudeau WL, Stadalnik RC. Validation of in vivo receptor measurements via in vitro radioassay: technetium-99 m-galactosyl-neoglycoalbumin as prototype model. J Nucl Med. 1991;32(6):1177–82.
15. National Center for Biotechnology Information. PubChem BioAssay Database. http://pubchem.ncbi.nlm.nih.gov/. Accessed 07/07/2015.
16. Mazière M, Comar D, Godot JM. In vivo characterization of myocardium muscarinic receptors by positron emission tomography. Life Sci. 1981;7(29):2391–7.
17. Syrota A, Comar D, Paillotin G, et al. Muscarinic cholinergic receptor in the human heart evidenced under physiological conditions by positron emission tomography. Proc Natl Acad Sci U S A. 1985;82:584–8.
18. Mazzadi AN, Pineau J, Costes N, Le Bars D, Bonnefoi F, Croisille P, Porcher R, Chevalier P. Muscarinic receptor upregulation in patients with myocardial infarction: a new paradigm. Circ Cardiovasc Imaging. 2009;2:365–72.
19. Prenant C, Barre L, Crouzel C. Synthesis of [11C]QNB. Lab Comp Pharm. 1989;27:1257.
20. Varastet M, Brouillet E, Chavoix C, et al. In vivo visualization of central muscarinic receptors using [11C]quinuclidinyl benzilate and positron emission tomography in baboons. Eur J Pharmacol. 1992;213(2):275–84.
21. Eckelman WC. Design criteria for targeted molecules: Muscarinic cholinergic systems biology. In: Welch MJ, Eckelman WC, editors. Targeted molecular imaging. Boca Raton: CRC Press, Taylor & Francis Group; 2012. p. 388–215.
22. Barrett JA, Joyal JL, Hillier SM, Maresca KP, Femia FJ, Kronauge JF, Boyd M, Mairs RJ, Babich JW. Comparison of high-specific-activity ultratrace 123/131I-MIBG and carrier-added 123/131I-MIBG on efficacy, pharmacokinetics, and tissue distribution. Cancer Biother Radiopharm. 2010;25:299–308.
23. Raffel DM. Targeting norepinephrine transporters in cardiac sympathetic nerve terminals. In: Welch MJ, Eckelman WC, editors. Targeted molecular. Imaging. Boca Raton: Taylor & Francis Group, LLC. ISBN: 978-1-4398-4195-2; 2012. pp 305–18.
24. Krohn KA, Mankoff DA, Muzi M, Link JM, Spence AM. True tracers: comparing FDG with glucose and FLT with thymidine. Nucl Med Biol. 2005;32:663–71.
25. Raffel DM, Chen W, Jung YW, Jang KS, Gu G, Cozzi NV. Radiotracers for cardiac sympathetic innervation: transport kinetics and binding affinities for the human norepinephrine transporter. Nucl Med Biol. 2013;40:331–7.
26. Jang KS, Jung YW, Gu G, Koeppe RA, Sherman PS, Quesada CA, Raffel DM. 4-[18 F]Fluoro-m-hydroxyphenethylguanidine: a radiopharmaceutical for quantifying regional cardiac sympathetic nerve density with positron emission tomography. J Med Chem. 2013;56:7312–23.
27. Eckelman WC, Jones AG, Duatti A, Reba RC. Progress using Tc-99 m radiopharmaceuticals for measuring high capacity sites and low density sites. Drug Discov Today. 2013;18:984–91.
28. Eckelman WC. Choosing a target for targeted radionuclide therapy using biomarkers to personalize treatment. J Diagn Imaging Ther. 2014;1:103–9.
29. Werner RA, Rischpler C, Onthank D, et al. Retention kinetics of the 18 F-labeled sympathetic nerve PET tracer LMI1195: comparison with 11C-hydroxyephedrine and 123I-MIBG. J Nucl Med. 2015;56:1429–33.
30. Vaidyanathan G, McDougald D, Koumarianou E, Choi J, Hens M, Zalutsky MR. Synthesis and evaluation of 4-[18 F]fluoropropoxy-3-iodobenzylguanidine n[18 F]FPOIBG): A novel 18 F-labeled analogue of MIBG. Nucl Med Biol. 2015;42(8):673–84.
31. Olshansky B, Sabbah HN, Hauptman PJ, Colucci WS. Parasympathetic nervous system and heart failure: pathophysiology and potential implications for therapy. Circulation. 2008;118:863–71.
32. Caldwell JH and Link JM. Imaging Left Ventricular Muscarinic Receptor Heterogeneity. A Tool to Evaluate Inividuals at Risk for Sudden Death? Circ Cardiovasc Imaging. 2009;2(5):353–5
33. DeGrado TR, Hutchins GD, Toorongian SA, Wieland DM, Schwaiger M. Myocardial kinetics of carbon-11-meta-hydroxyephedrine: retention mechanisms and effects of norepinephrine. J Nucl Med. 1993;34:1287–93.
34. Glowniak JV. Cardiac studies with metaiodobenzylguanidine: a critique of methods and interpretation of results. J Nucl Med. 1995;36:2133–7.
35. Caldwell JH, Kroll K, Li Z, Seymour K, Link JM, Krohn KA. Quantitation of presynaptic cardiac sympathetic function with carbon-11 -meta-hydroxyephedrine. J Nucl Med. 1998;39:1327–34.
36. Eckelman WC, Lau CY, Neumann RD. Perspective, the one most responsive to change. Nucl Med Biol. 2014;41:297–8.
37. Eckelman WC, Mankoff DA. Choosing a single target as a biomarker or therapeutic using radioactive probes. Nucl Med Biol. 2015;42:421–5.

4

Neuronal Imaging in Heart Failure

Arnold F. Jacobson and Jagat Narula

Introduction

Radionuclide imaging provides the capability to noninvasively monitor important physiologic functions. Nuclear imaging may be used to identify the condition of an organ or one of its functional elements at a single point in time or serially over a short or long interval, thereby permitting assessment of the effects of therapy or documentation of disease progression. Because most radiopharmaceuticals have benign adverse event profiles and deliver low radiation doses to the patient, they may be used periodically as deemed clinically appropriate to provide valuable physiologic information to the treating clinician.

The single-photon emitting radiopharmaceutical iodine-123 metaiodobenzylguanidine (^{123}I-MIBG), an analogue of norepinephrine (NE), has been used widely for more than 20 years to facilitate assessment of cardiac sympathetic neuronal function in patients with heart failure (HF) [1–3]. Quantitative measurement of myocardial ^{123}I-MIBG uptake is performed readily by using both planar and single-photon emission CT (SPECT) imaging techniques [4–6]. Reduced myocardial ^{123}I-MIBG uptake is common in HF patients, and there is a strong association between the severity of global and regional abnormalities and the likelihood of adverse outcomes, such as ventricular arrhythmias and cardiac and all-cause mortality [7–11]. ^{123}I-MIBG imaging also can identify recovery of sympathetic nerve function as a result of medical or device therapy for HF, as well as early evidence of reinnervation in transplanted hearts [12–19]. Comparison of the extent of ^{123}I-MIBG tomographic defects in relation to myocardial perfusion assessed with thallium- or technetium-labeled tracers offers insights into susceptibility to unstable arrhythmias associated with sudden cardiac death (SCD) and the need for implanted defibrillators (ICDs) [20–24]. The potential for use of ^{123}I-MIBG imaging as a cost-effective noninvasive means to individualize HF treatments to optimize patient outcomes is largely untapped [2].

Physiology and Pharmacokinetics

MIBG is a structural and functional analogue of NE, but it possesses only weak sympathomimetic effects and is a poor ligand for adrenergic receptors [25–27]. MIBG is taken up by the NE transporter (NET), with a higher affinity than NE ($K_m = 0.31$ μM and 1.8 μM, respectively) but with a similar capacity. MIBG also may enter cells via non–NET-dependent uptake activity [28, 29]. MIBG is not metabolized by either monoamine oxidase (MAO) or catechol-O-methyltransferase (COMT) [30, 31]. Slightly less than 1% of an intravenously injected dose of MIBG localizes to the myocardium [32].

V. Dilsizian, J. Narula (eds.), *Atlas of Cardiac Innervation*, DOI 10.1007/978-3-319-45800-7_4

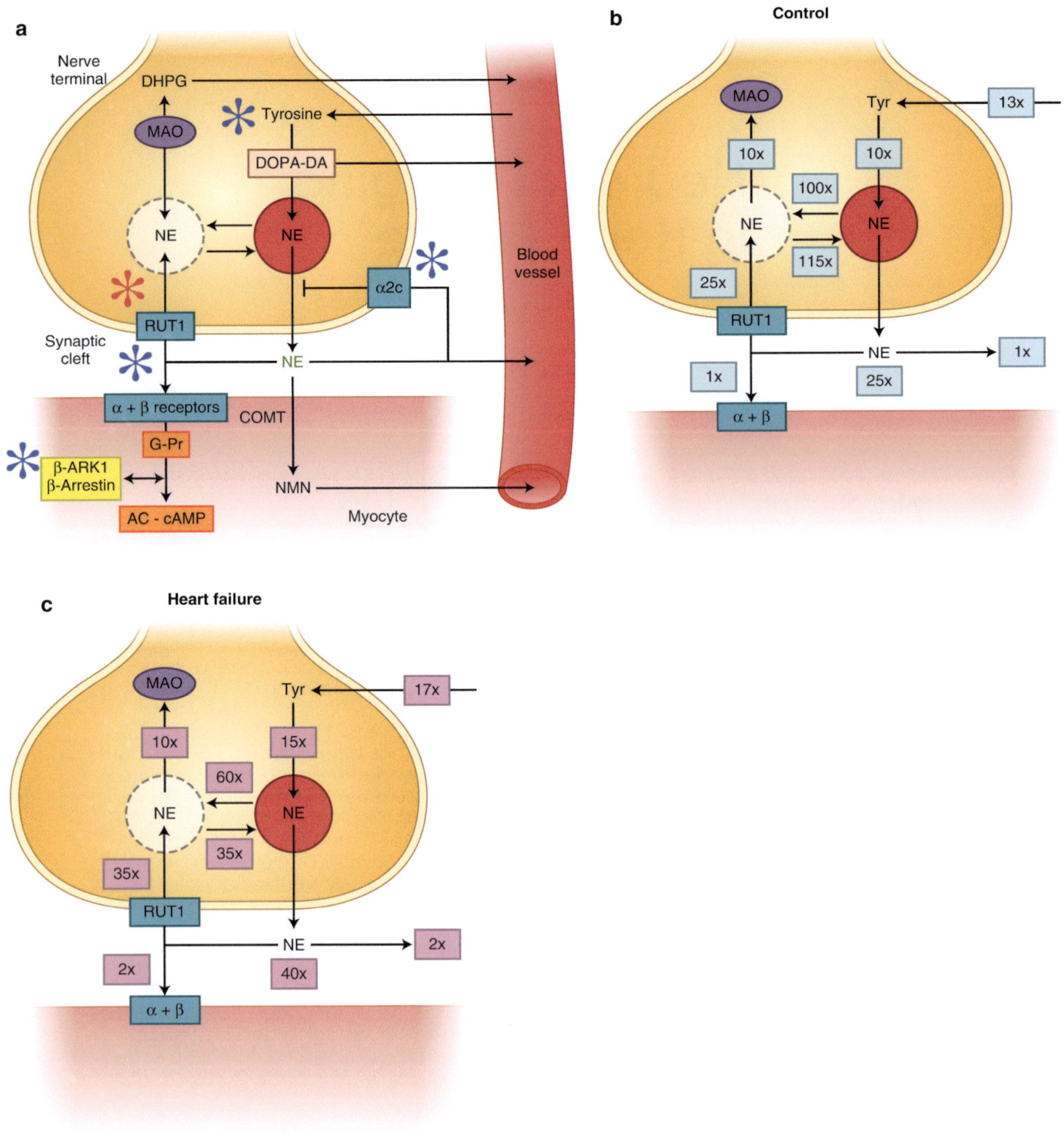

Figure 4-1. (**a**) Norepinephrine (*NE*) cascade from synthesis to vesicular storage, release into synaptic cleft, reuptake, and partial inactivation. (**b**, **c**) The processes of synthesis, vesicular–axoplasmic exchange, metabolism, release, neuronal and extraneuronal uptake, spillover, and turnover of NE for sympathetic nerves of the normal (**b**) and failing (**c**) human heart at rest. Both NE release and uptake are increased in the failing heart; the efficiency of the NE uptake is reduced such that cardiac spillover of NE is increased disproportionately more than neuronal uptake. As such, cardiac NE stores are 50% lower in HF. Numbers with each arrow represent the rates of each process in a hundredth of actual picomoles per minute value (100 pg or 1× is the normal amount of NE spilled into the circulation, and representation as 1/100th of values makes it easier to understand the relative changes in the NE cascade). *AC* adenyl cyclase, *cAMP* cyclic adenosine monophosphate, *COMT* catechol-O-methyltransferase; *DA* dopamine, *DHPG* dihydroxyphenylglycol, *DOPA* dihydroxyphalanine, *NE* norepinephrine, *NMN* normetanephrine, *MAO*, monoamineoxidase, *RUT1* reuptake 1 (Adapted from Narula and Sarkar [33]).

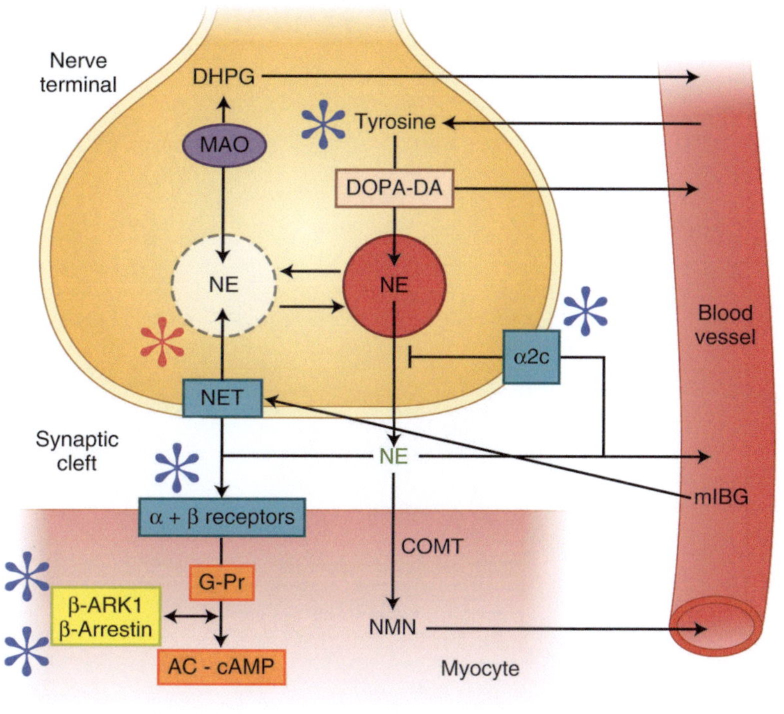

Figure 4-2. Representation of postganglionic presynaptic sympathetic neuron, synapse, and postsynaptic myocyte. MIBG enters the synapse and is taken up into the neuron by the NET and stored in NE vesicles. With each cycle of neuronal stimulation and release of NE, a small amount of MIBG reenters the synapse and diffuses back into the vascular system, where it is transported to and excreted by the kidneys unchanged. In HF patients, increased sympathetic outflow [34] and a decrease in the number and function of NET sites [35] result in more rapid clearance of neuronal MIBG, usually quantified by the parameter "washout" in terms of the percentage reduction in MIBG activity between early (15-min) and late (4-h) images. High levels of washout (>40–50%) are associated with an increase in adverse events, such as HF progression and cardiac death [5].

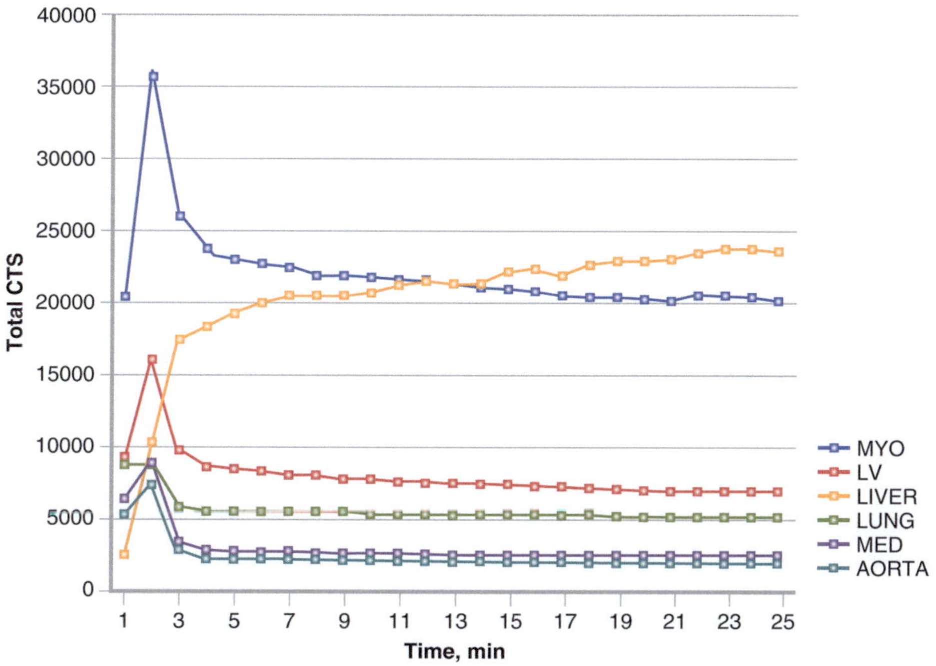

Figure 4-3. Time–activity curves from dynamic MIBG acquisition from the anterior chest of a 69-year-old patient with New York Heart Association (NYHA) class III HF. The MYO curve (*blue*) represents counts (CTS) in the whole heart, whereas the LV curve (*red*) reflects the myocardial region of interest (ROI), excluding the left ventricular cavity. Both MYO and LV curves reach a relative plateau by minute 4, reflecting first-pass extraction of MIBG, and then show a slow decrease in counts thereafter as a manifestation of washout. Washout typically is quantified in terms of relative decrease in myocardial activity between the 15-min (early) and 4-h (late) postinjection images, with a normal range of 10–20%. Note that liver counts increase continuously throughout this period, reflecting the high proportion of MIBG that accumulates in this organ (typically about 30% of the injected activity) [36]. *MED* mediastinum (Image courtesy of A. Jacobson).

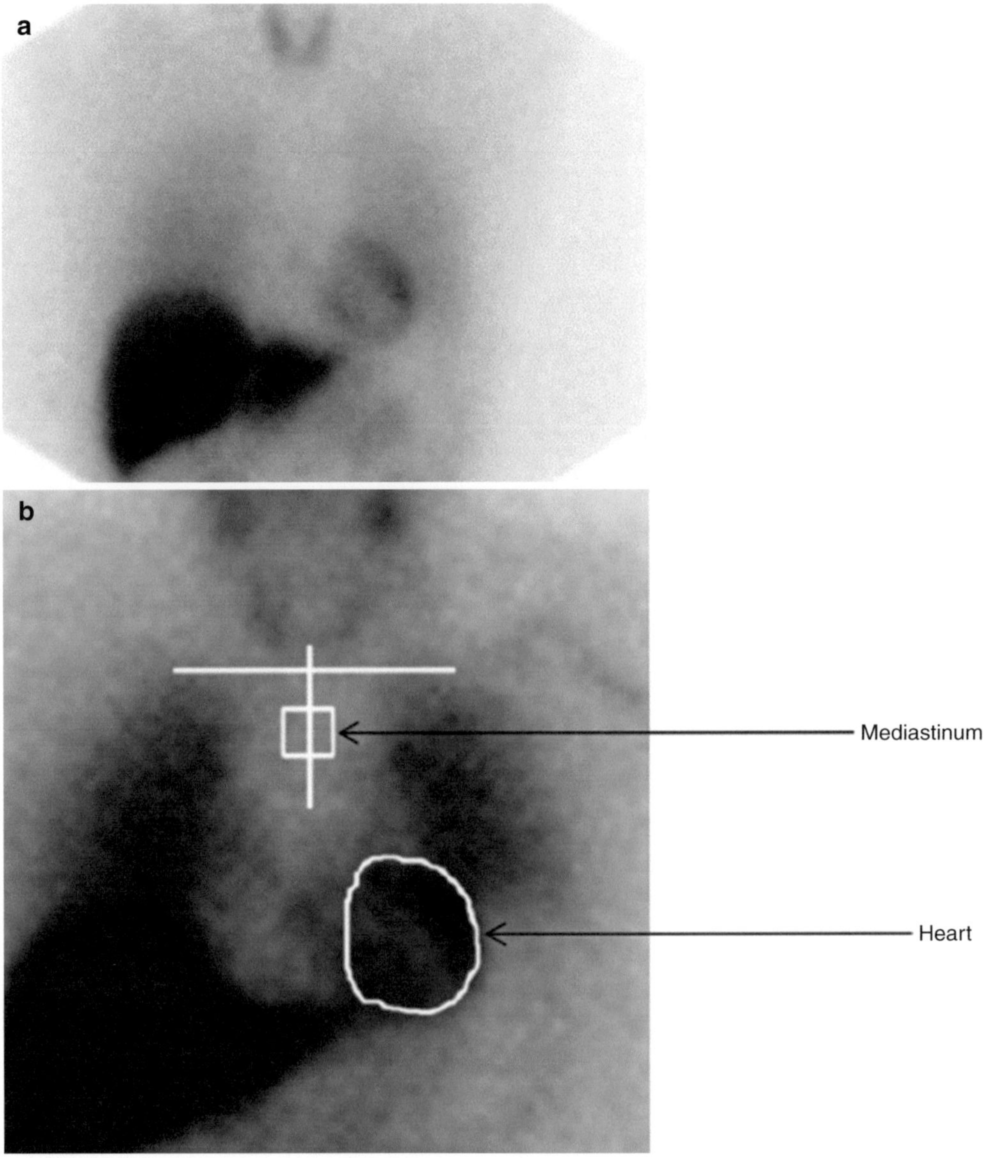

Figure 4-4. MIBG images and quantitation of uptake on planar views. Images are commonly acquired shortly (15–20 min) after MIBG administration ("early") and repeated after 3–4 h ("late"). (**a**) In a normal heart, both early and late images show uniform myocardial uptake of MIBG, with clear delineation from the surrounding lung and mediastinum. There is always intense liver uptake, as this organ accumulates about 30% of the injected dose. (**b**) Quantitation of myocardial uptake usually is done in terms of the heart/mediastinum (H/M) ratio of counts/pixel values; a typical method for drawing ROIs on planar anterior thorax images is illustrated here. Normal H/M values primarily depend on the type of collimator used on the nuclear camera [37]; for late images, these ratios typically are in the 1.8–2.2 range for the low-energy high-resolution collimators widely used in the United States and Europe [38] and 2.4–2.8 for the low–medium and medium energy collimators more commonly used in Japan [5]. (**c**), Washout rate (WR) reflects the change in myocardial activity between early and late images. The normal washout rate typically is in the 10–20% range, whereas HF patients commonly have rates as high as 30–50% [8]. Both low late H/M ratios and high washout rates are associated with poor outcomes in HF patients [9]. (**a** and **b** from AdreView package insert; images courtesy of GE Healthcare. **c** from Yamada et al. [8]; with permission).

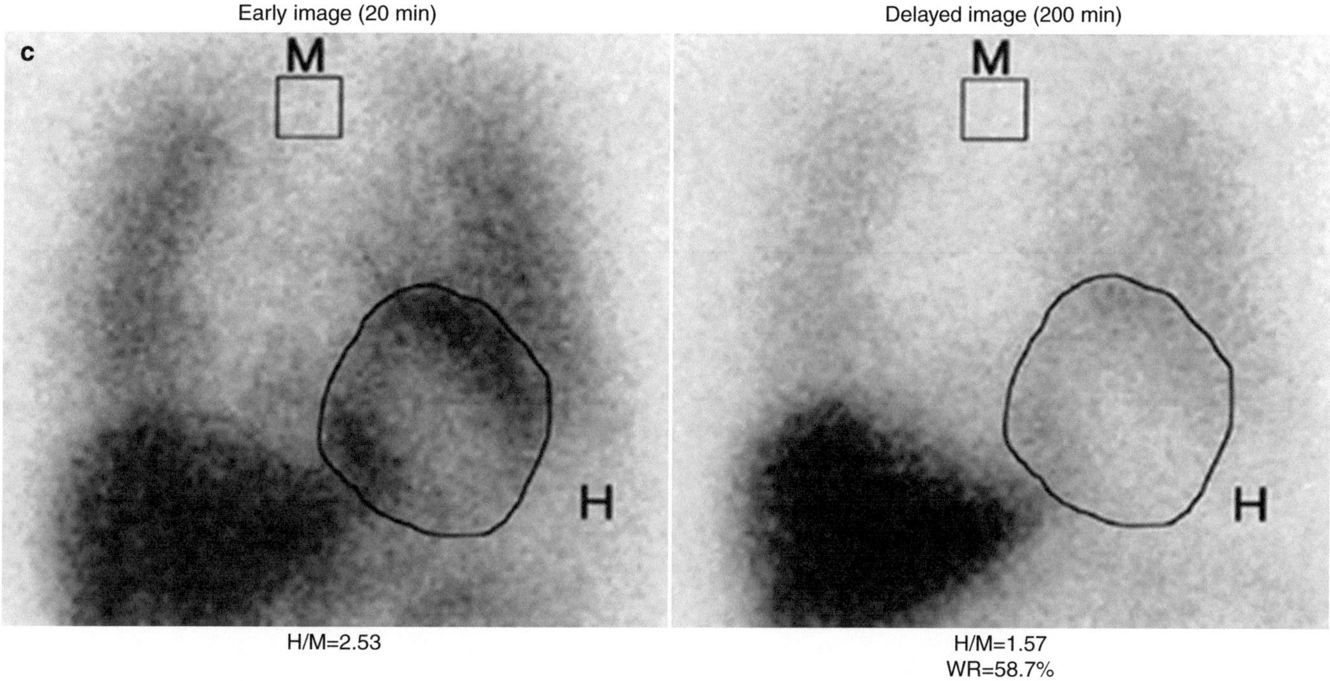

Figure 4-4. (continued)

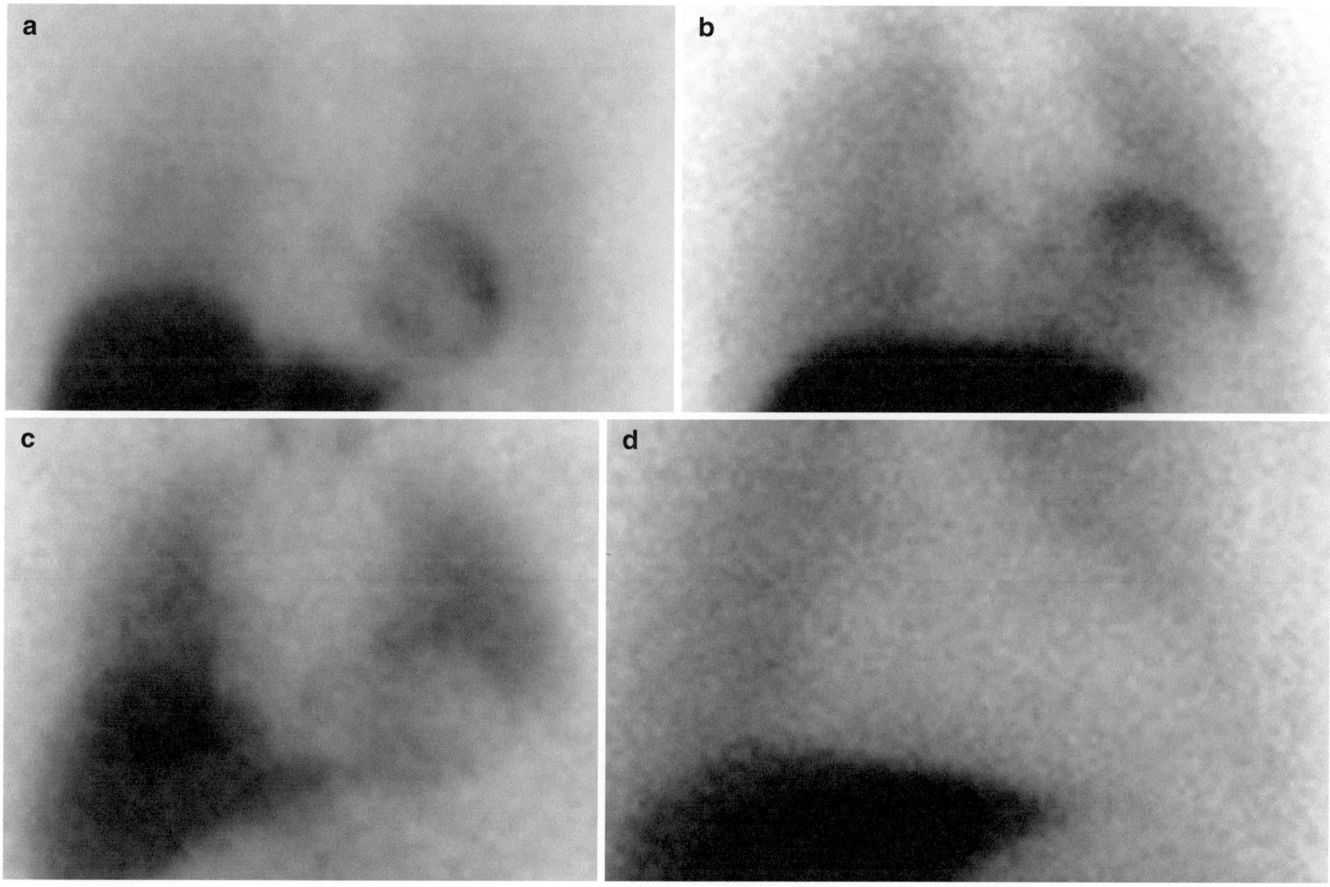

Figure 4-5. Spectrum of 4-h delayed planar MIBG images of the anterior chest. (**a**) This image, from a patient without heart disease, shows uniform uptake and a normal H/M ratio (2.4). (**b**) This image, from a patient with NYHA class II nonischemic cardiomyopathy, shows relatively preserved uptake with an H/M ratio of 1.8. (**c**, **d**), These images are from HF patients with moderate and severe reduction in MIBG cardiac uptake; H/M ratios are 1.3 and 1.0, respectively. HF patients with poor cardiac uptake of MIBG are at increased risk for adverse cardiac outcomes [38].

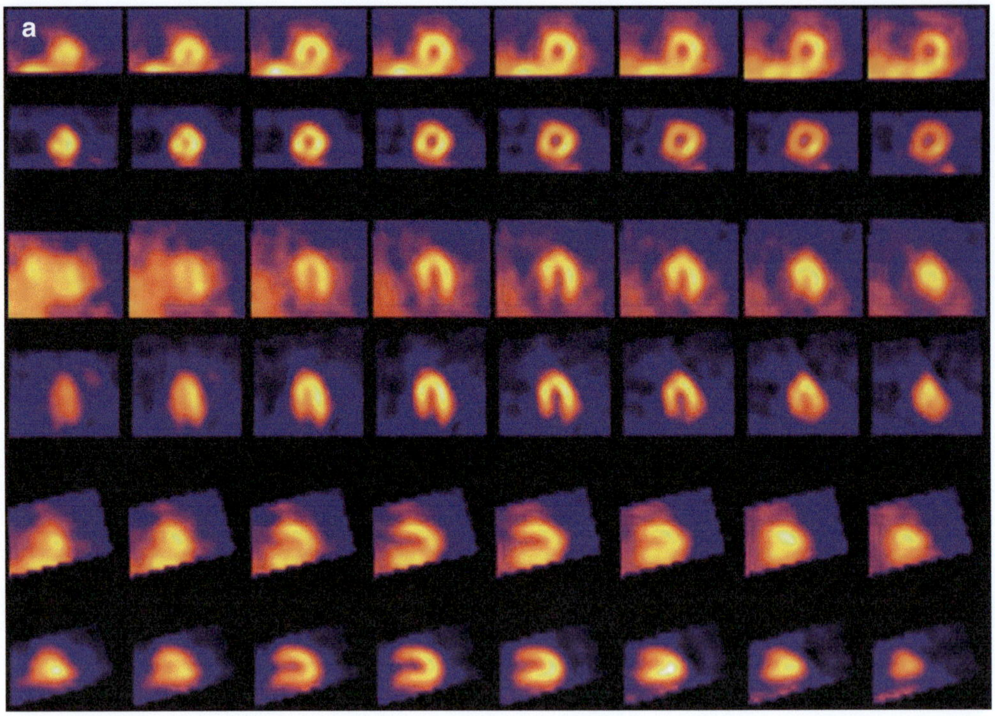

Figure 4-6. MIBG and technetium-99m (^{99m}Tc)-tetrofosmin SPECT in a patient without heart disease (**a**) and in a patient with ischemic HF (**b**). Each display alternates between rows of MIBG and myocardial perfusion imaging (MPI) slices. There is uniform uptake in all myocardial walls of the normal patient. The HF patient has a perfusion defect in the basal inferolateral wall (*white arrow*), consistent with a prior myocardial infarction (MI). The associated innervation defect is much larger, involving most of the surrounding inferior and lateral walls and apex (*blue arrows*). This pattern of innervation/perfusion mismatch—that is, abnormal innervation in a region with preserved perfusion—is common in patients with MI and has been associated with increased susceptibility to ventricular arrhythmic events [22, 39].

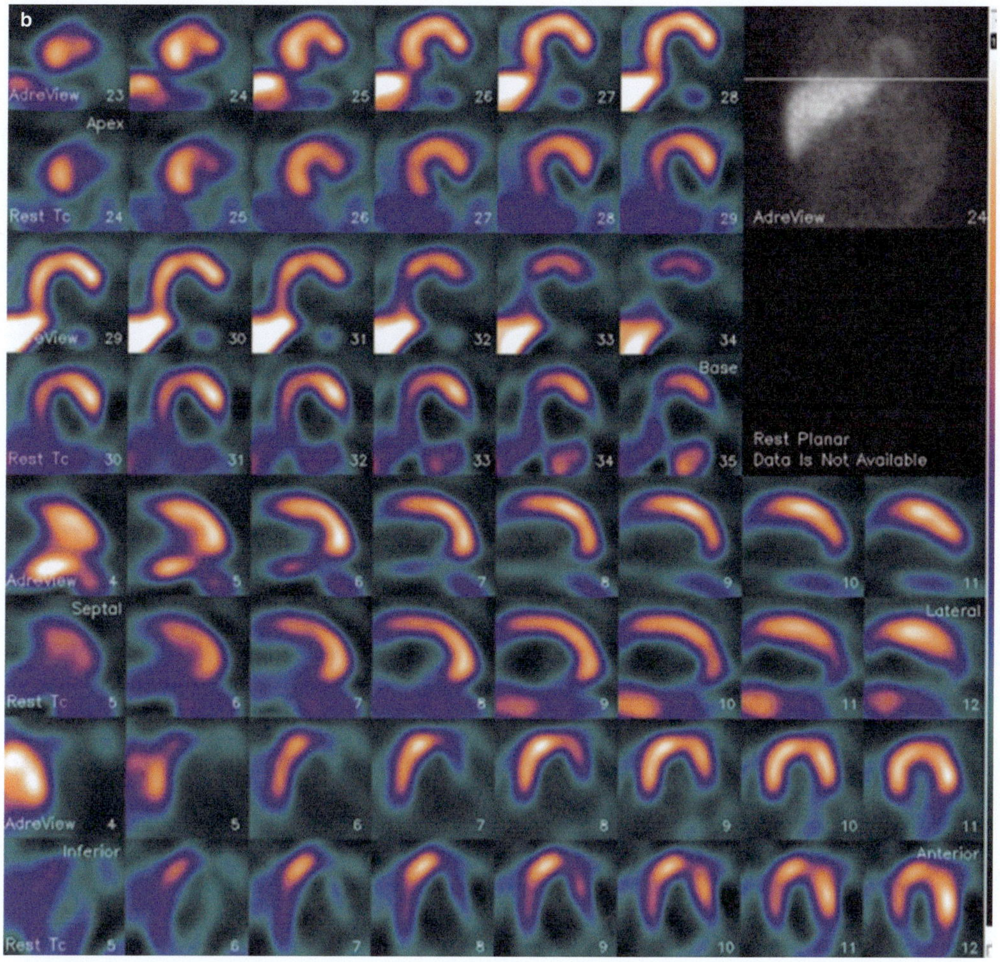

Figure 4-6. (continued)

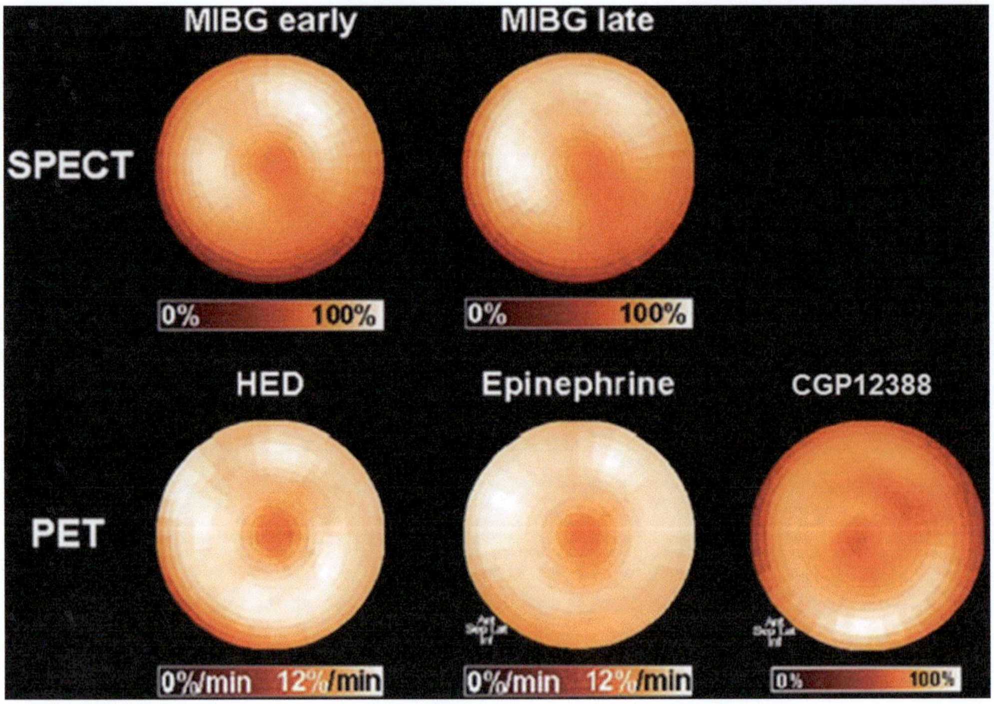

FIGURE 4-7. Polar maps of myocardial distribution (center–apex to periphery–base) of MIBG from early (15 min post injection) and late (4 h post injection) SPECT images of the normal heart for comparison with those of selected carbon-11 (^{11}C)-labeled positron emission tomography (*PET*) tracers also used to assess functional status of the sympathetic nervous system. The mechanism of neuronal uptake for hydroxyephedrine (HED) and epinephrine is the same as that for MIBG, with the NET responsible for transferring the compounds into the neuronal cytoplasm. CGP12388 binds to postsynaptic β-receptors, providing a means to assess the distribution and density of these adrenergic receptors. Distribution patterns for all five image sets are equivalently uniform, confirming that all tracers are interrogating attributes of the same physiologic system [40].

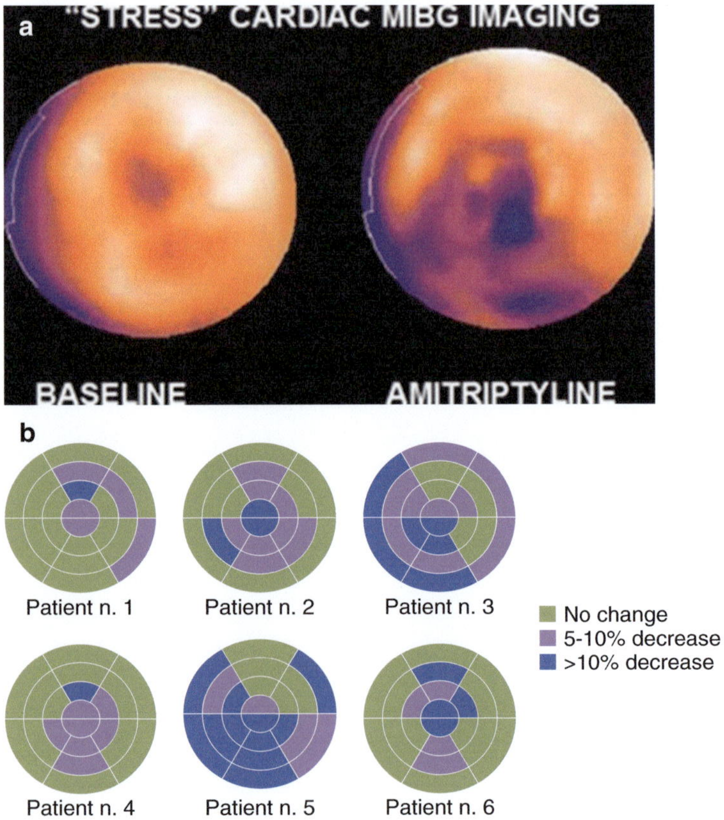

FIGURE 4-8. MIBG imaging in conjunction with the NET inhibitor amitriptyline as a means to stress the neuronal system to uncover covert dysfunction. (**a**) MIBG polar maps from SPECT studies performed at rest and after administration of amitriptyline show induction of a severe regional decrease in tracer uptake in the inferior, septal, and apical walls after pharmacologic stress. (**b**) Individual change in regional distribution of cardiac MIBG uptake based on a polar map (20-segment model) in six patients demonstrates the variable effect of amitriptyline, with patients 3 and 5 showing substantially greater reduction in uptake than the other four patients. This might reflect a greater susceptibility to worsening neuronal dysfunction with cardiac stress (ischemic, psychological, etc.) that might place the patient at increased risk for morbidity and mortality [41] (**a** from Estorch et al. [41]; **b** adapted from Estorch et al. [41]).

Planar MIBG Imaging for Prognostic Assessment

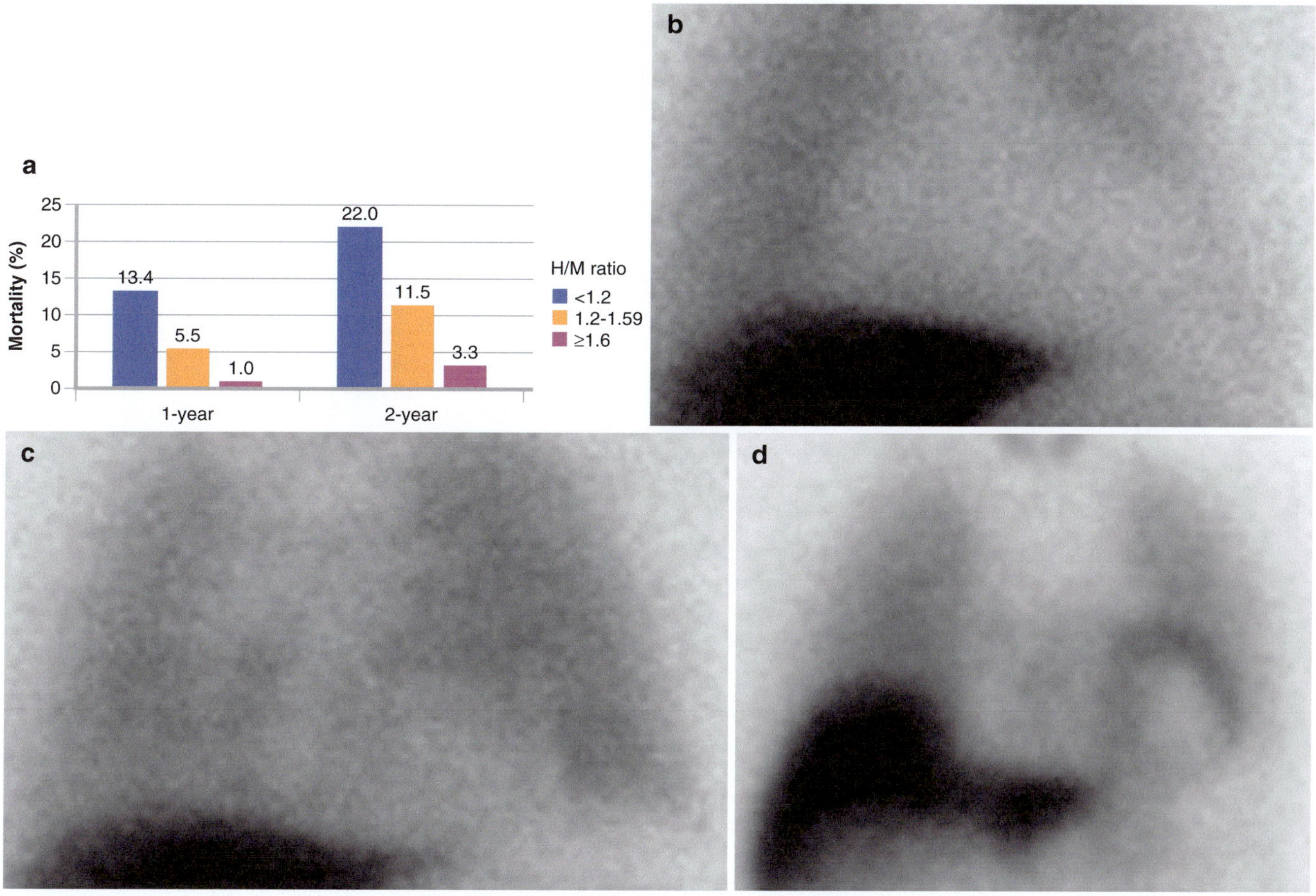

Figure 4-9. (**a**) One- and 2-year all-cause mortality rates for the 961 HF subjects in the ADMIRE-HFX (AdreView Myocardial Imaging for Risk Evaluation in Heart Failure Extension) study. For the 10% of subjects with the lowest H/M ratios ($H/M < 1.20$, $n = 92$), mortality rates were 13 and 7 times greater, respectively, than for the 20% of subjects with $H/M \geq 1.60$ ($n = 201$). (**b–d**) The clinical consequence of this difference in innervation status is illustrated in these scans from three NYHA class II male patients in the trial: (**b**) a 65-year-old with a left ventricular ejection fraction (LVEF) 25% and an H/M of 0.96 (outcome: death from HF progression at 8 months); (**c**), a 51-year-old with an LVEF of 33% and an H/M of 1.38 (outcome: SCD at 8 months); and (**d**), a 64-year-old with an LVEF of 30% and an H/M of 1.67 (outcome: survival to 2 years with no events) (Bar graph adapted from AdreView Package insert; images courtesy of GE Healthcare).

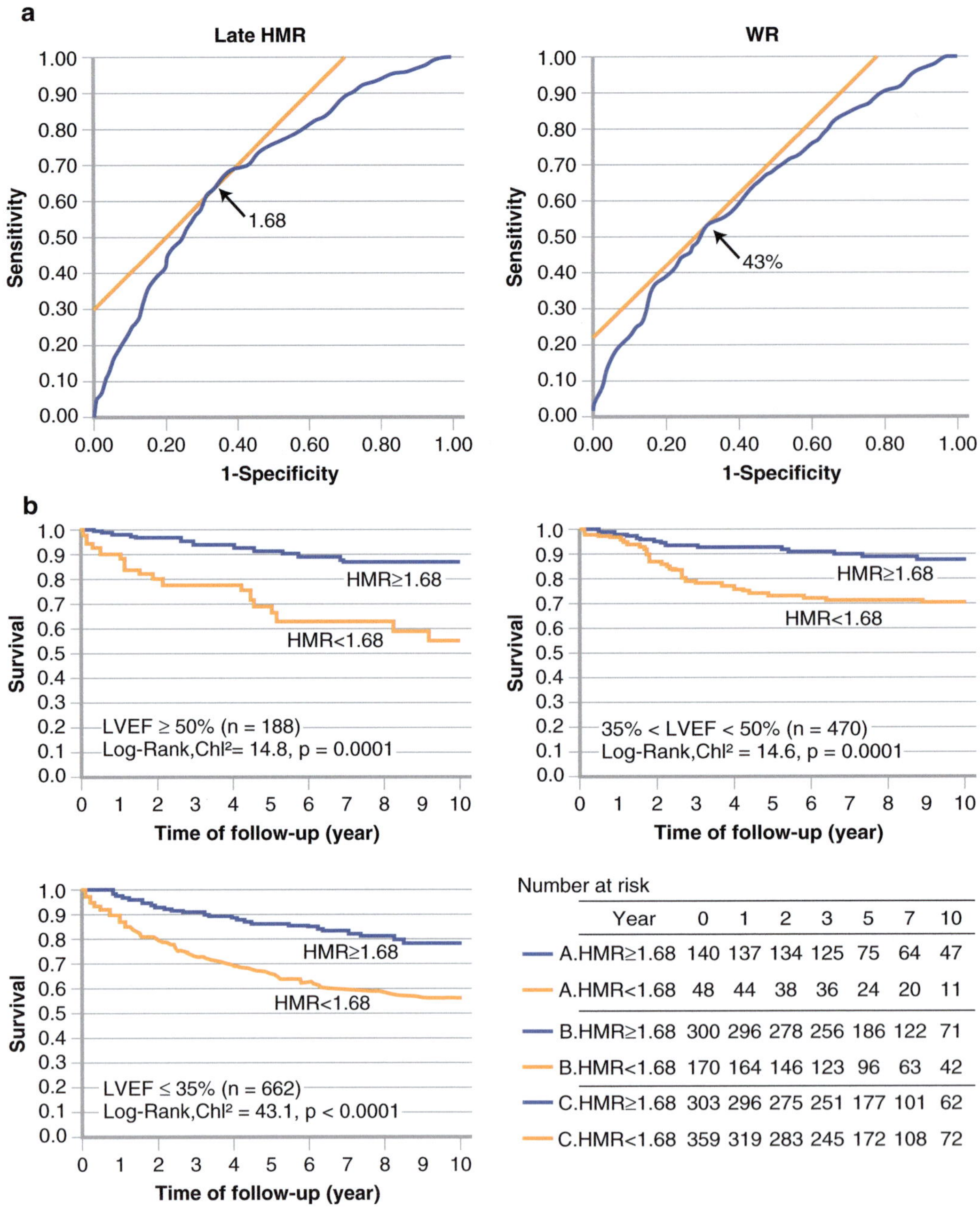

Year	0	1	2	3	5	7	10
A.HMR≥1.68	140	137	134	125	75	64	47
A.HMR<1.68	48	44	38	36	24	20	11
B.HMR≥1.68	300	296	278	256	186	122	71
B.HMR<1.68	170	164	146	123	96	63	42
C.HMR≥1.68	303	296	275	251	177	101	62
C.HMR<1.68	359	319	283	245	172	108	72

Figure 4-10. The largest amount of data on MIBG imaging in HF has been collected in Japan. (**a**) Based on data from 1322 NYHA I to IV HF patients followed up for a median of 5.6 years after planar MIBG imaging [10], the optimal values for distinguishing patients with a higher risk of all-cause mortality from those with a lower one were an H/M ratio (HMR) of 1.68 and a washout rate of 43%. (**b**) These discriminators were independent of LVEF, as shown here, confirming previous observations that cardiac neuronal imaging provides information different from that obtained by measuring ventricular systolic function [42]. As such, MIBG may be used to evaluate prognosis in HF patients who have either reduced or preserved systolic function.

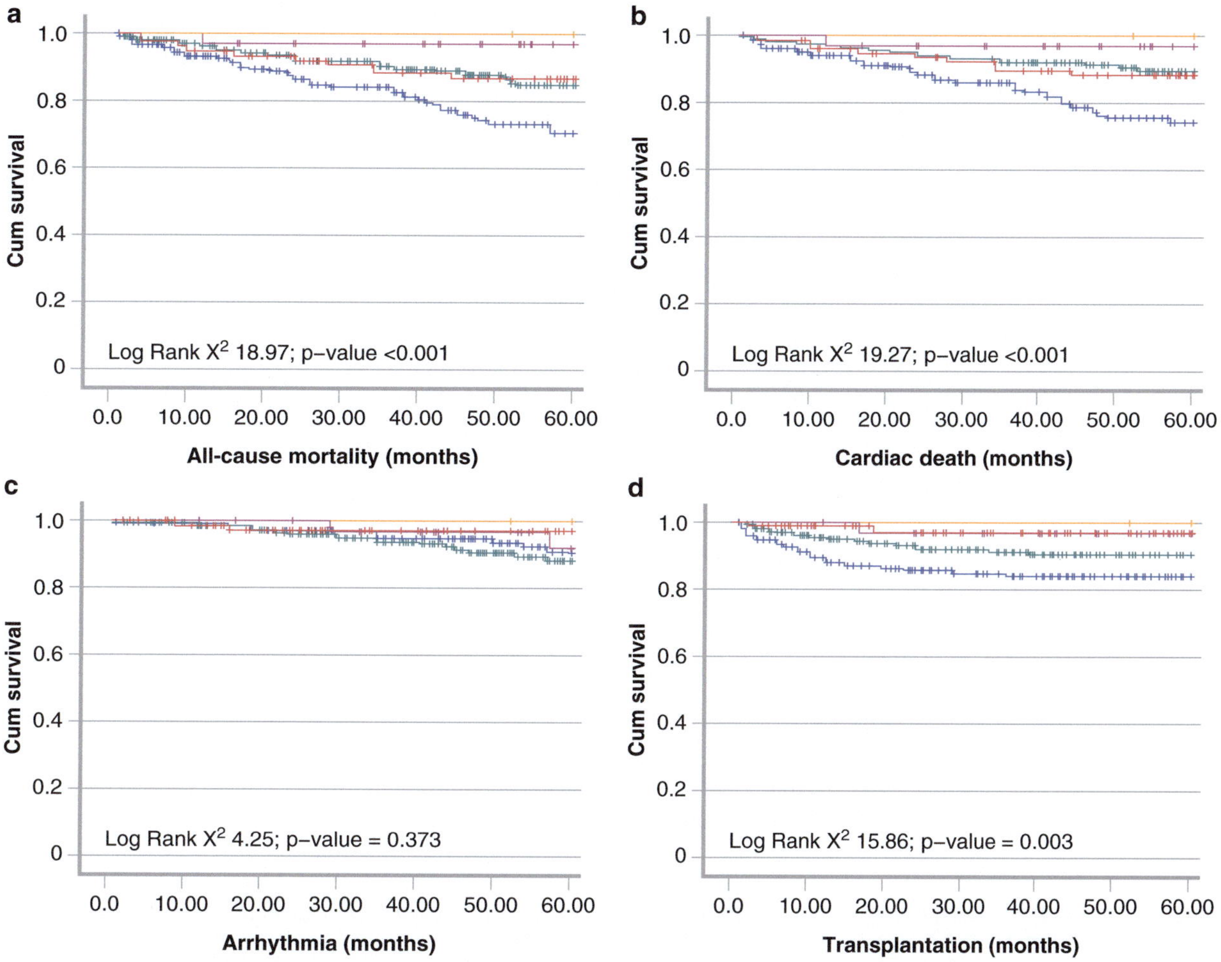

Figure 4-11. Event-free survival analyses from a European meta-analysis of 636 HF patients studied with planar MIBG imaging. Shown are curves for all-cause mortality (**a**), cardiac mortality (**b**), arrhythmic events (resuscitated cardiac arrest, appropriate ICD discharge, or sustained ventricular tachycardia longer than 30 s and heart rate >100 bpm) (**c**), and cardiac transplantation (**d**). During a maximum follow-up of 60 months (mean 36 mo), there were 83 deaths (67 cardiac), 33 arrhythmic events, and 56 cardiac transplantations. H/M first quintile (*blue line*) was ≤1.32, second to fourth quintiles (*green, beige, and purple lines respectively*) were 1.33–1.97, and fifth quintile (*horizontal yellow line at 1.0*) was ≥1.98. For all end points, decreasing late H/M was associated with increased event risk, but for arrhythmic events, the differences among quintiles were not statistically significant. This reflects the nonlinear relationship between arrhythmic events and cardiac MIBG uptake, as presented in further detail in Fig. 4.12 [11].

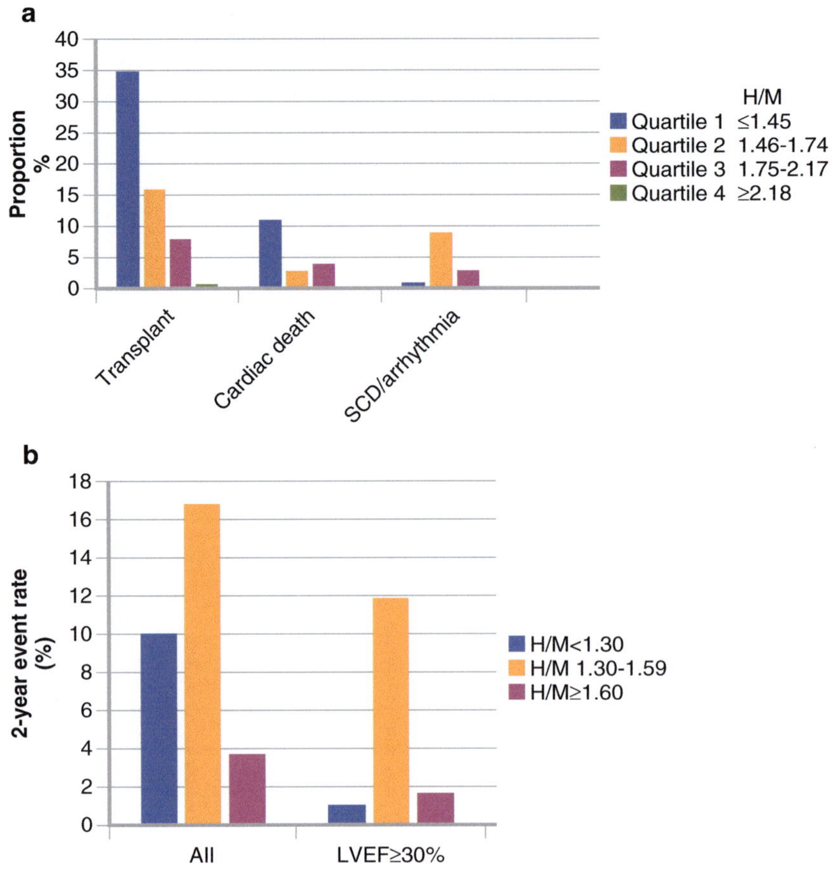

Figure 4-12. Occurrence of arrhythmic events in relation to H/M ratio on planar MIBG imaging. (**a**) Data from a European retrospective study with 290 HF patients. (**b**) Data from 961 HF patients in the prospective ADMIRE-HF study. In the European study, the highest event proportions for cardiac transplant and cardiac death were in patients with H/M ratios in the lowest quartile (≤1.45), whereas the lowest proportions were for those in the highest H/M ratio quartile (≥2.18) [43]. In contrast, the highest proportion of arrhythmic events was among patients in the second quartile (1.46–1.74), representing those with only mild–moderate neuronal dysfunction. This observation was confirmed in the 2-year results from ADMIRE-HF, in which the highest arrhythmic event rate (nonfatal and fatal) was in subjects with an H/M between 1.30 and 1.59 [44]; 1.30 was the lower limit of normal for control subjects in the trial, and 1.60 was the prospectively defined threshold for preserved cardiac innervation. The event rate difference among H/M ratio groups was particularly dramatic among the 471 subjects with LVEF above the median value of 29%. This suggests that in HF patients with less severe left ventricular (LV) dysfunction, cardiac neuronal abnormalities of moderate severity play an important role in the occurrence of unstable ventricular rhythms.

MIBG SPECT for Arrhythmic Risk Assessment

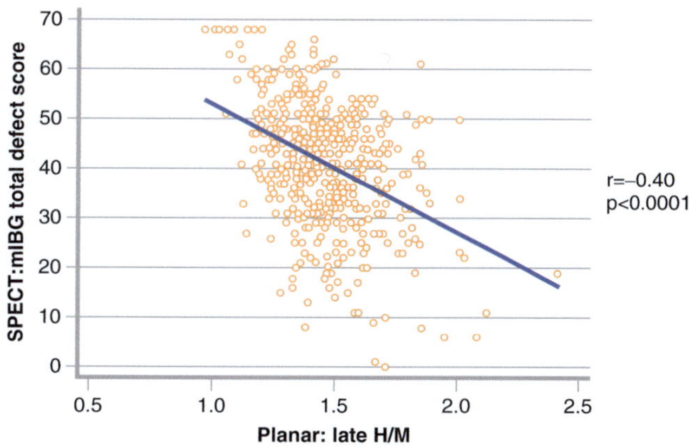

Figure 4-13. Relationship between planar and SPECT MIBG results in patients with ischemic HF ($n=471$). The graph shows the results of late H/M ratio on planar images compared with summed defect score determined by visual assessment of SPECT images using a 17-segment model (0–4 score, maximum 68). There is moderate correlation between the values. However, there is a wide distribution of SPECT scores for patients with H/M ratios <2.0, reflecting the relative insensitivity of the two-dimensional planar technique for detecting potentially significant regional neuronal abnormalities, especially in the posterolateral wall and toward the base of the heart. These results suggest that planar and SPECT MIBG imaging methods provide complementary information and should both be performed when feasible [45].

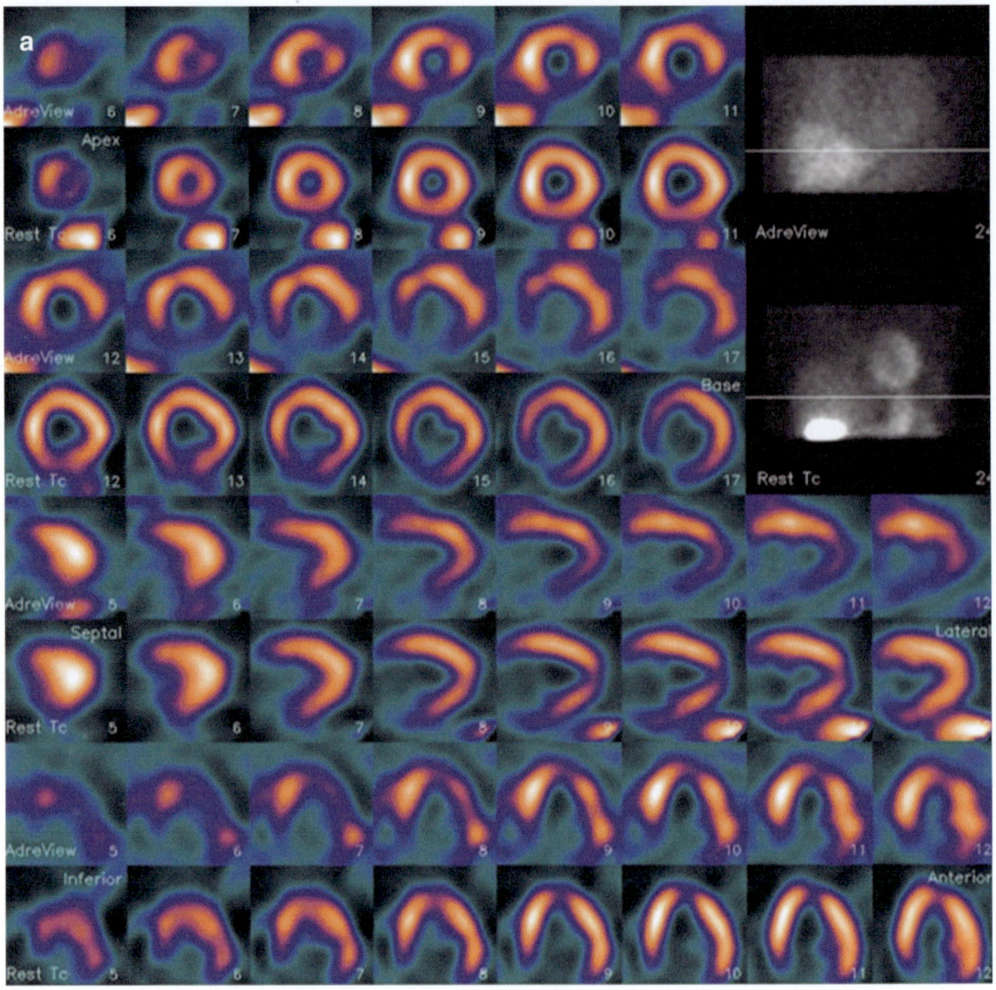

Figure 4-14. SPECT studies with MIBG (rows 1, 3, 5, and 7) and rest ^{99m}Tc-tetrofosmin (rows 2, 4, 6, and 8) in two patients with ischemic HF. MIBG defect scores are based on visual assessment using a standard 17-segment model (score 0–4, maximum 68). (**a**) This patient has moderate cavity dilatation on MPI, but uptake is nearly normal except for a small area at the base of the inferior septum. There is a larger abnormality in the inferior wall on the MIBG images, representing an area of innervation/perfusion mismatch (MIBG defect score, 14). (**b**) This patient has a large matched defect in the inferior and inferolateral walls on both MIBG and tetrofosmin images (MIBG defect score, 22). Based on the results of several studies, the risk for arrhythmic events is increased for HF patients with large innervation defects on MIBG SPECT imaging [45, 46]. The ^{123}I-MIBG/perfusion mismatch score hazard ratio (HR) is 1.06 (95% confidence interval [CI], 1.02–1.09), $P<0.01$ on univariate Cox analysis and 1.01 (95% CI, 0.97–1.06), $P=0.5$ on multivariate Cox analysis (Images courtesy of GE Healthcare).

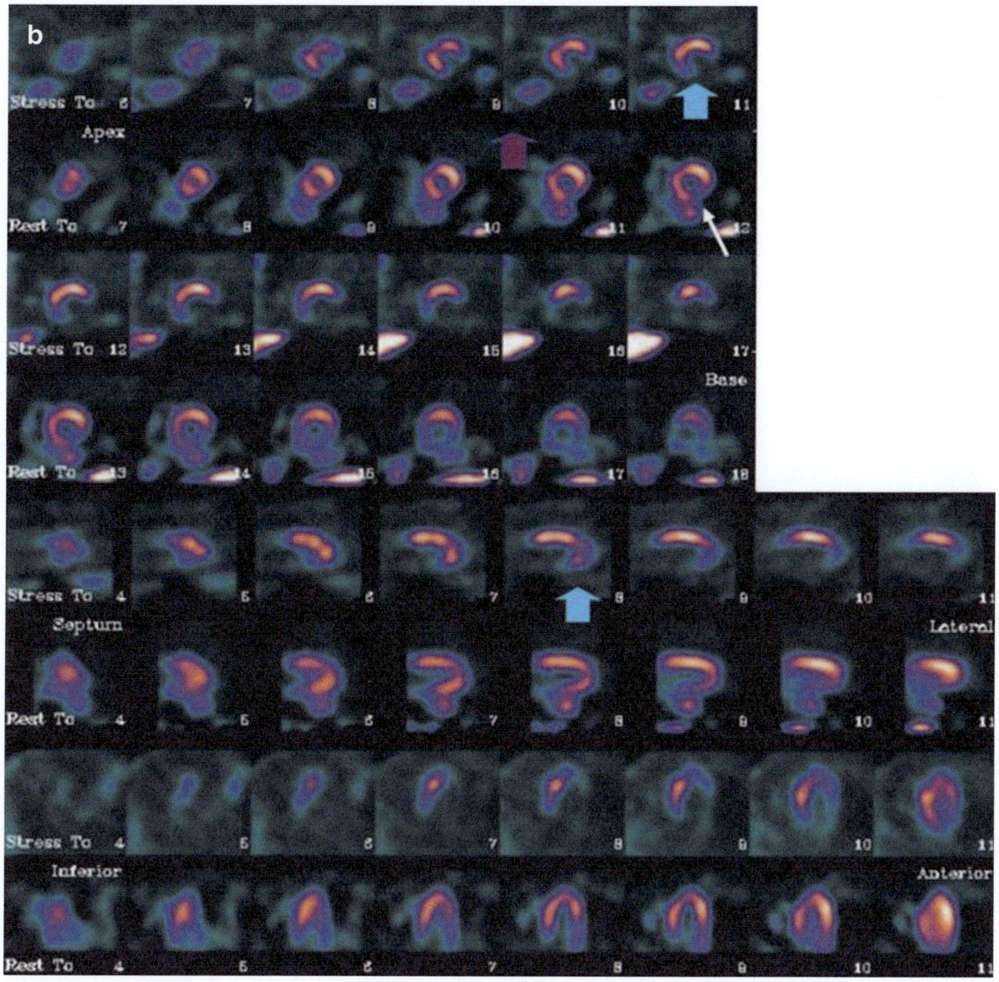

Figure 4-14. (continued)

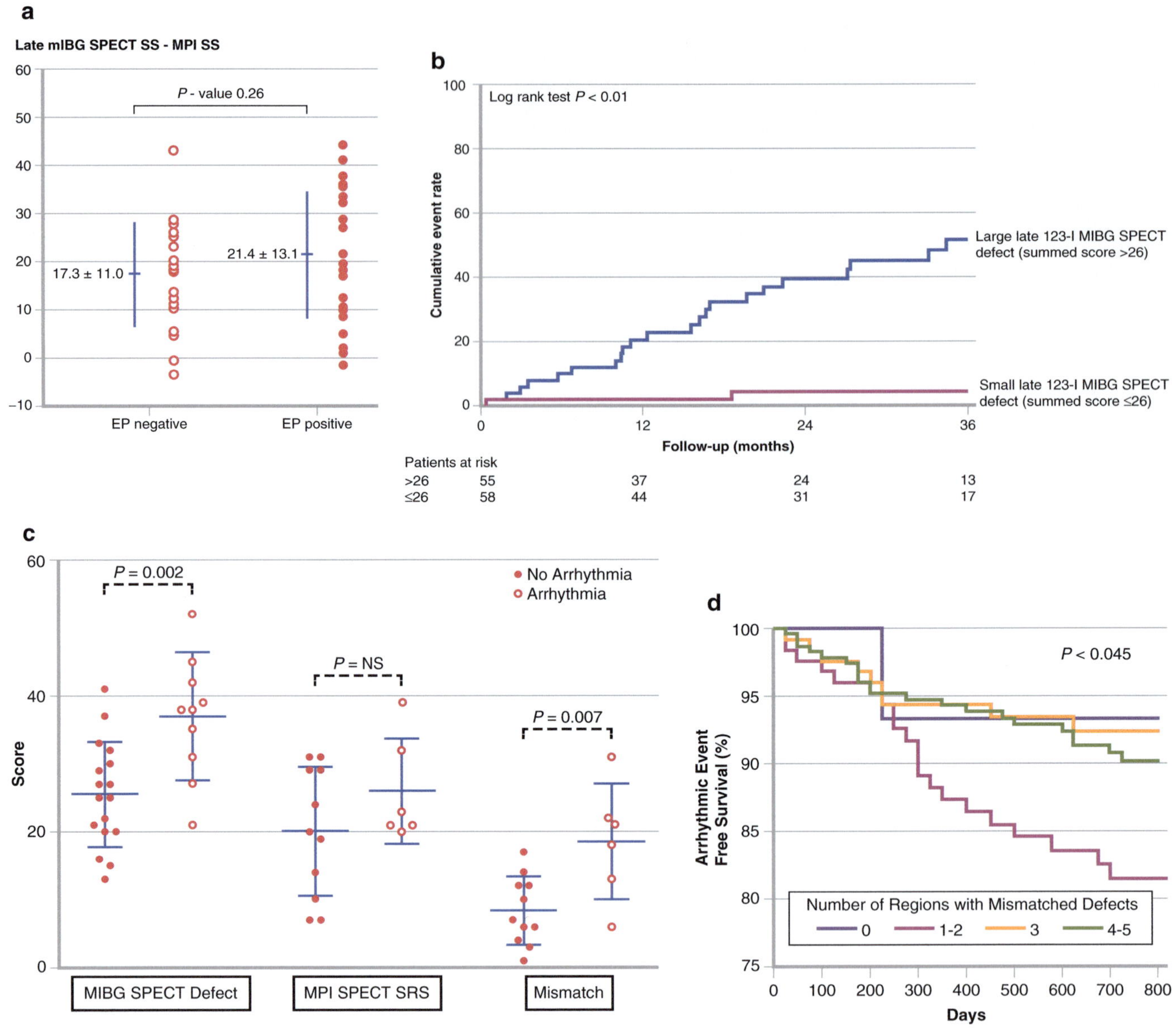

FIGURE 4-15. Analyses examining the prognostic significance of mismatch between MIBG and MPI SPECT for the occurrence of arrhythmic events. Although numerous studies have examined the significance of innervation/perfusion mismatch, results based on visual scoring of SPECT scans occasionally have been contradictory. (**a**) In a study in 50 patients with ischemic heart disease referred for electrophysiologic (EP) testing, mismatch score did not predict the inducibility of sustained ventricular tachycardia [24]. *SS* summed score. (**b**) In a study with 116 HF patients referred for ICD placement, mismatch score predicted subsequent ICD shocks on univariate but not multivariate Cox analysis [46]. (**c**) A small study of 27 HF patients referred for ICD placement showed the significance of mismatch scores as a predictor of ICD activations during a mean follow-up of 16 months [39]. *NS* not significant, *SRS* summed rest score. (**d**) A recent informed reread of 500 MIBG and tetrofosmin SPECT studies from ischemic HF patients in ADMIRE-HF found that those with innervation/perfusion mismatches in one or two wall regions (of anterior, septum, inferior, lateral, and apex) had a 2-year arrhythmic event rate two times higher than patients with either less or greater abnormalities [45]. In all four studies cited, MIBG SPECT defect score was a significant predictor of subsequent arrhythmic events. In aggregate, these and other studies have confirmed that medium to large innervation defects on MIBG SPECT studies (typically involving 20–50% of the myocardium) are associated with an increased risk for arrhythmias. Although the precise role of MPI SPECT as an adjunctive technique remains to be elucidated, interpretation of location and severity of MIBG defects on visual reads is facilitated by the availability of correlative perfusion SPECT images.

Risk Assessment with MIBG Imaging in Conjunction with Other Clinical Measurements and Multivariate Models

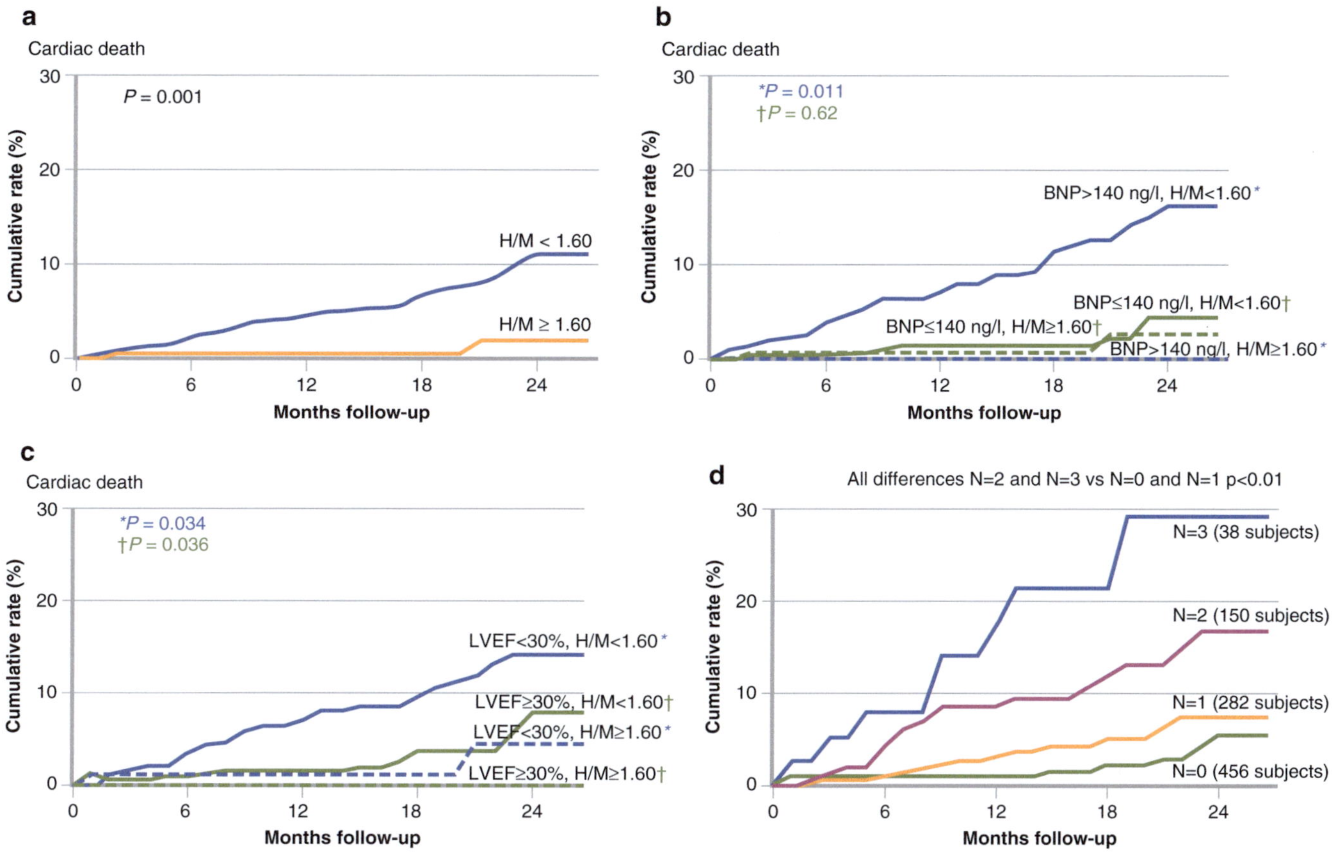

Figure 4-16. Use of MIBG imaging combined with B-type natriuretic peptide (BNP) and LVEF. In ADMIRE-HF, a planar H/M ratio of 1.60 was prospectively defined as the lower limit of preserved neuronal uptake. (**a**) Considering the end point of cardiac death, this threshold identified patients at low absolute risk, with only two events (among 201 patients) over a median follow-up of 17 months. (**b**, **c**), Using the median values of BNP (140 ng/L) and LVEF (29%) as further discriminators, the highest event rates clearly were found among those with high BNP and low LVEF. (**d**) Cumulative event curves for cardiac death, categorized in terms of the presence of parameter values in the most abnormal quartile. In relation to the most abnormal quartiles of BNP (>310 ng/L), LVEF (≤23%), and H/M (≤1.30), there was a significant difference between subjects with zero or one such value and those with two or three values. Cardiac death during 2 years was about six times more likely in a patient with the highest risk values of LVEF, BNP, and H/M compared with a patient with no such values. The multivariate event model developed from the ADMIRE-HF study included four variables: H/M ratio, LVEF, NYHA functional class, and BNP [38].

Figure 4-17. Influence of LVEF on the predictive value of MIBG imaging in HF patients. Although in ADMIRE-HF the inclusion of NYHA class II/III patients required on-site determination of LVEF≤35%, echocardiograms also were submitted to a core laboratory for independent determination of LVEF. The latter LVEF data, which included 386 participants with values >35.0%, were used in analyses of the prognostic significance of the dichotomous division of patients based on a planar H/M ratio <1.60 versus ≥1.60 [47]. Based on the end point of death or arrhythmic event, event rates for patients with a low H/M ratio were more than two times higher at all levels of LVEF examined. These results are consistent with other analyses showing MIBG uptake as independent of LVEF in predicting adverse cardiac outcomes, even among patients with normal or only mildly reduced systolic function [10]. *HR* hazard ratio.

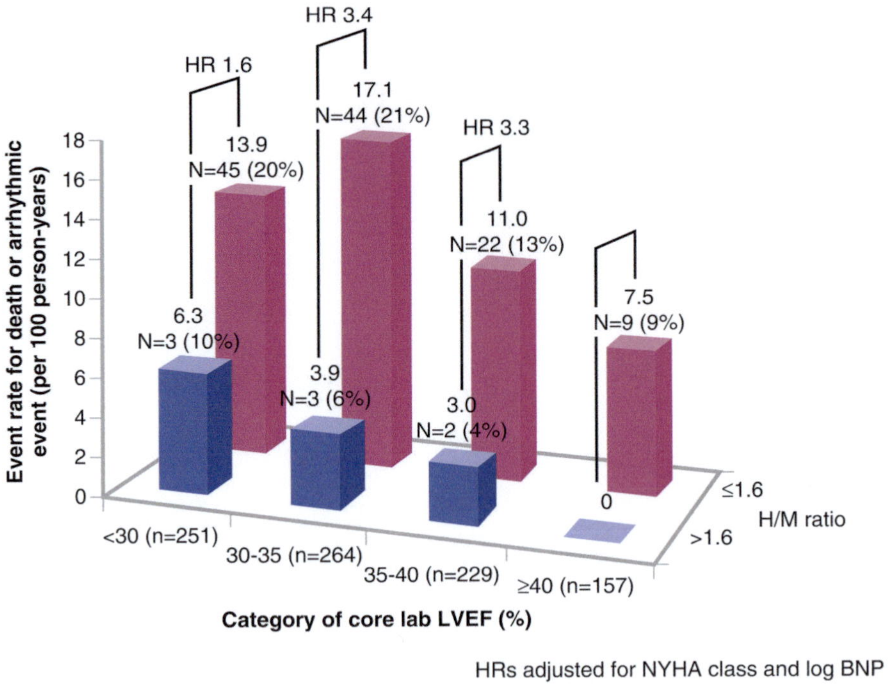

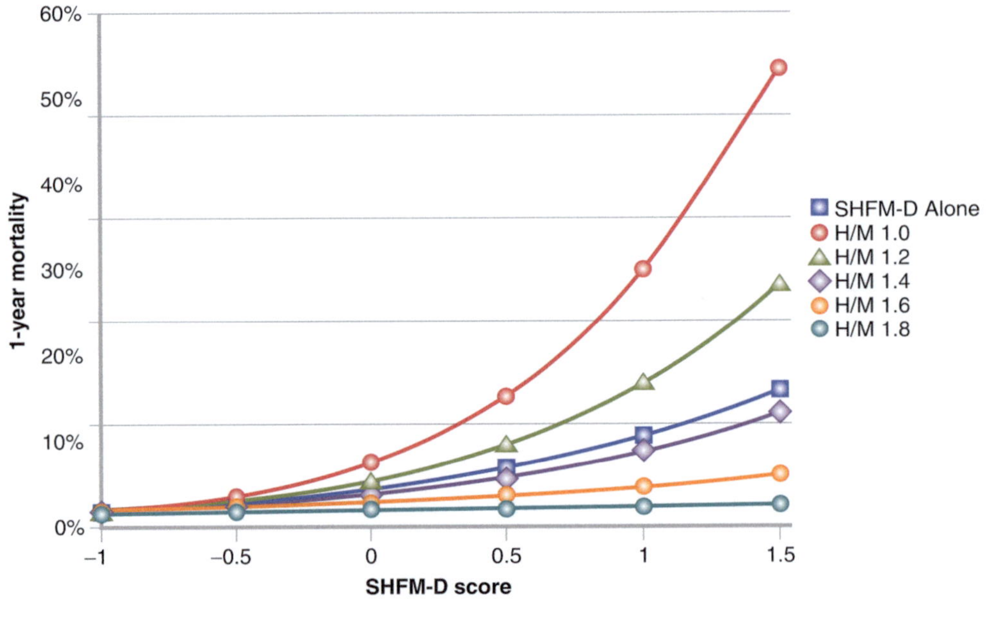

Figure 4-18. Effect of adding MIBG imaging results to a multivariate clinical risk model for predicting 1-year all-cause mortality. Mortality estimates for the ADMIRE-HF population using the multivariate Seattle Heart Failure Model, version D (SHFM-D) [48] are represented by the blue line with squares. Addition of the planar H/M ratio at five different levels (1.0, 1.2, 1.4, 1.6, and 1.8) is represented by the other lines in the graph [49]. Whereas an H/M ratio of 1.4 produces little change in the risk estimate, as the H/M value decreases, risk rises substantially. For an SHFM-D score of 1, equivalent to a 1-year mortality rate of about 10%, an HF patient with an H/M of 1.0 has a predicted mortality rate three times higher. Conversely, an H/M of 1.8 is associated with a greater than three times reduction in risk. Analyses of the source data using risk models developed from four large prospective trials (EFFECT, Care-HF, MADIT-II, and PACE) produced similar results, with the addition of H/M ratio to each model providing improved HF risk assessment [50].

Considerations for Clinical Use of MIBG Imaging in HF Patients

Table 4-1. Change in cardiac MIBG Uptake after Initiation of New Pharmacotherapy.

Study	Population	Medication/ intervention	Therapy category	Patients, n	Interscan interval, mo	Mean baseline HMR	Mean follow-up HMR	% Change in HMR
Kasama et al. (2005) [16]	HF	Perindopril	ACE inhibitor	20	6	1.62	1.76	8.6
Kasama et al. (2003) [14]	DCM	Spironolactone	Aldosterone inhibitor	15	6	1.64	1.86	13.4
Kasama et al. (2003) [15]	HF	Valsartan	ARB	16	6	1.66	1.81	9
Toyama et al. (2008) [51]	DCM	Carvedilol	β-Blocker	15	12	1.64	1.86	13.4
Cha et al. (2008) [18]	HF	CRT	CRT	12	6	1.8	2.1	16.7
Drakos et al. (2010) [19]	NYHA IV	LVAD	LVAD	12	3	1.25	1.43	14.4

Shown are the results from a representative sample of studies examining changes in H/M ratio (HMR) after initiation of new heart failure (HF) therapy. Each study involved a baseline MIBG examination before initiation of a new therapy followed by a repeat imaging procedure a minimum of 3 months later. For interscan intervals ranging from 3 to 12 months in these six studies, the mean improvement in HMR ranged from 8.6 to 16.7% for medications—angiotensin-converting enzyme (ACE) inhibitors, angiotensin II receptor blockers (ARBs), β-blockers, and aldosterone antagonists—and device interventions—cardiac resynchronization therapy (CRT) and left ventricular assist device (LVAD) implantation. In total, more than 40 such therapy-response studies using all major current HF therapies have been published in the past 20 years, 90% of which show statistically significant improvement in MIBG cardiac uptake as a result of the initiation of new medical or device therapies. These results establish that MIBG imaging can document the positive effects of therapies that affect the activity of the renin–angiotensin–aldosterone system (RAAS). As such, this imaging modality may be used to evaluate the effectiveness of new RAAS therapies and potentially identify nonresponders earlier than other diagnostic methods. *DCM* dilated cardiomyopathy, *NYHA IV* New York Heart Association class IV

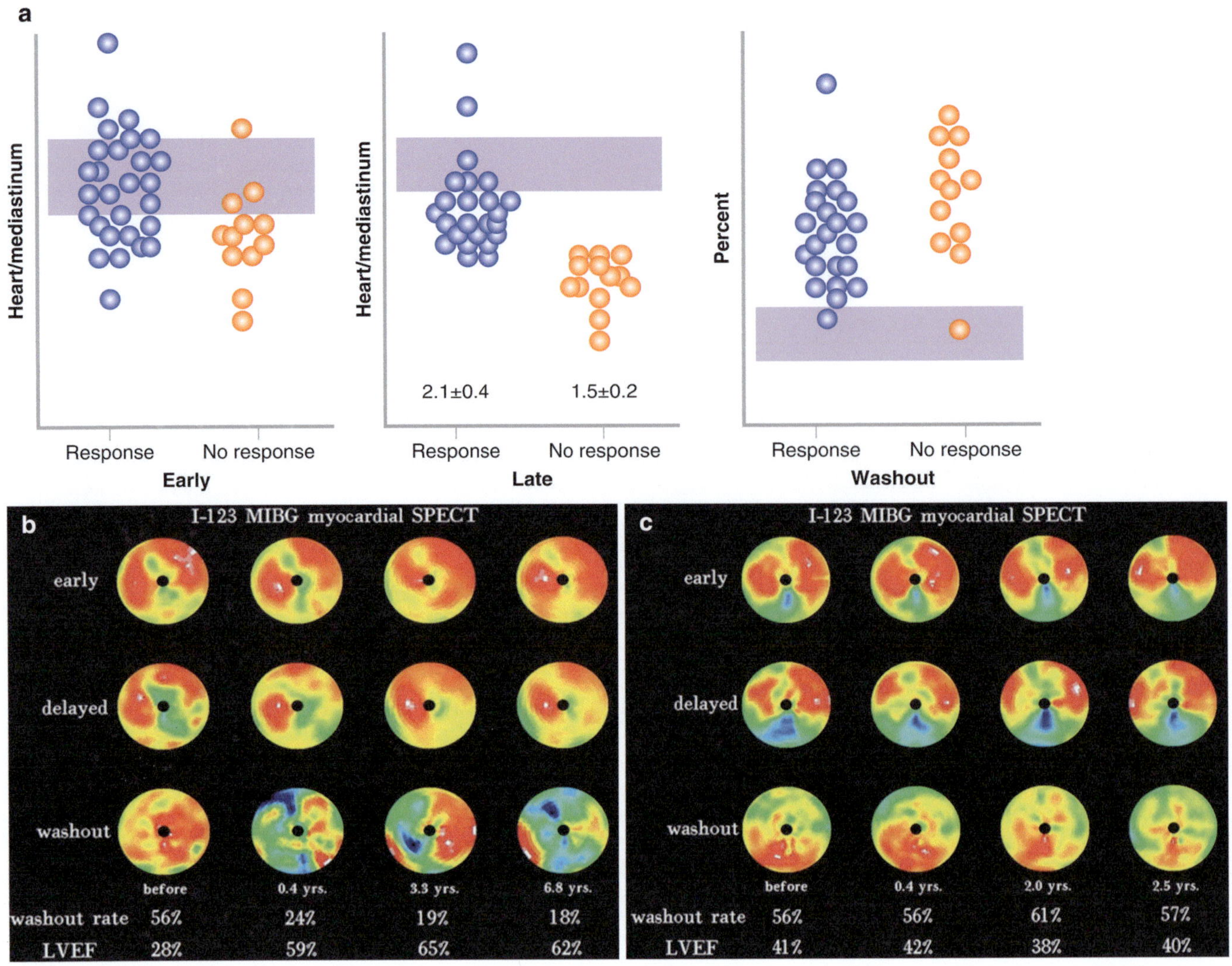

Figure 4.19. Serial cardiac MIBG imaging in HF patients treated with β-Blockers. (**a**) Results from a series of 45 patients with dilated cardiomyopathy (NYHA III or IV) who underwent imaging before starting bisoprolol therapy. After 8 months, 30 patients were determined to have had a clinical response to the treatment. A late H/M ratio >1.7 (mean for nine controls, 2.6; *blue* bar represents mean ± standard deviation) discriminated responders from nonresponders with a 91% sensitivity and 92% specificity [52]. (**b**, **c**), Representative SPECT bullseye plots from HF patients in another study who underwent multiple sequential MIBG SPECT studies following initiation of β-blocker therapy with metoprolol, carvedilol, or nipradilol. (**b**) Among patients who showed clinical improvement, an improvement also was observed in cardiac neuronal function, as reflected by MIBG uptake. (**c**) Nonresponders showed no change in imaging findings following initiation of β-blocker therapy [53] (**b**, **c** from Yamazaki et al. [53]; with permission).

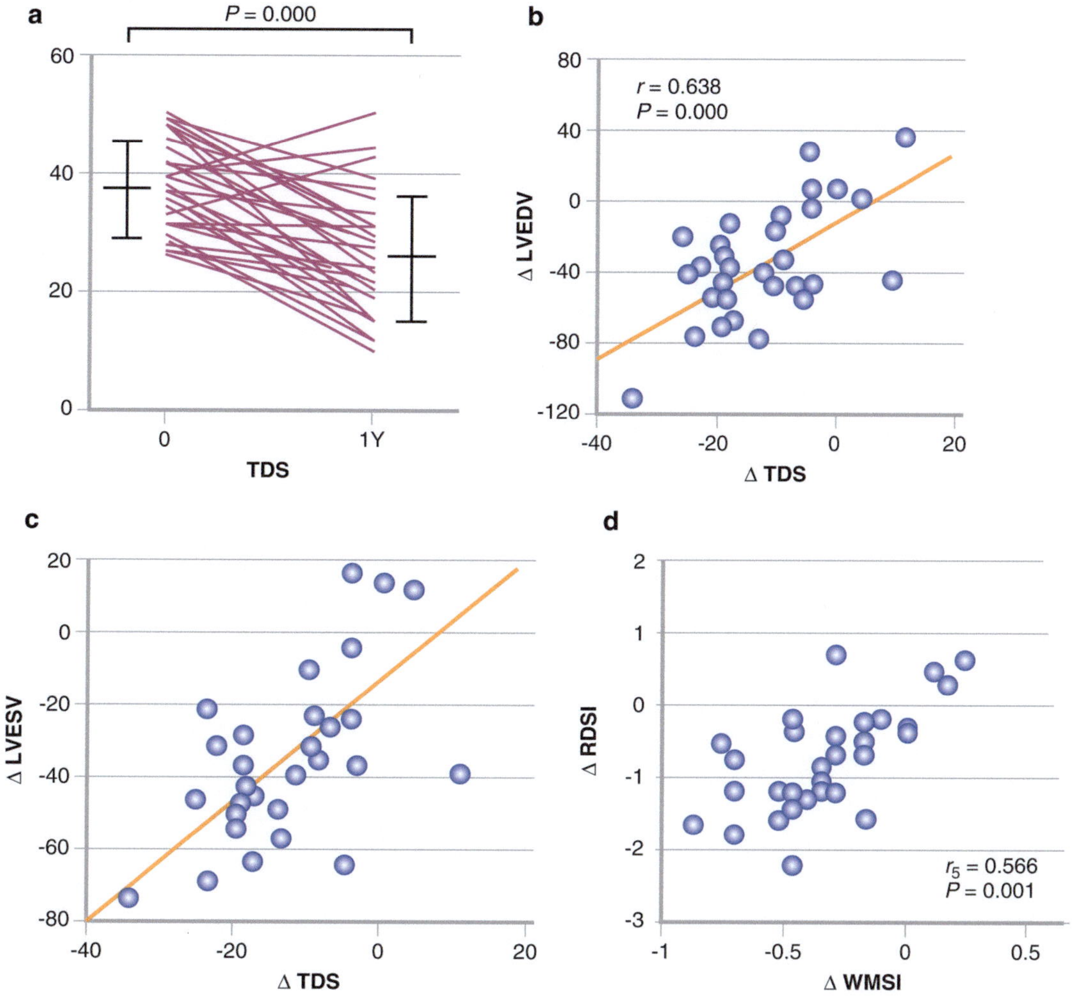

Figure 4-20. Utility of MIBG SPECT for evaluating the effect of HF therapy on ventricular remodeling. (**a**) In a study of 30 patients with dilated cardiomyopathy who underwent MIBG SPECT and echocardiography before beginning carvedilol therapy and again approximately 12 months later, an interval significant decrease was observed in the 17-segment total defect score (*TDS*) in most of the patients [54]. With regard to the change in TDS (*ΔTDS*), there were strong correlations with changes in (**b**) LV end-diastolic volume (*LVEDV*) and (**c**) end-systolic volume (*LVESV*). (**d**) Good correlation also was found between the changes in the average segmental MIBG defect score (regional defect score index [*RDSI*]) and a similarly calculated wall motion score index (*WMSI*) on echocardiography. Improvement and worsening of segmental MIBG uptake on SPECT are associated with the morphologic changes that occur secondary to LV remodeling in HF patients. MIBG SPECT provides functional information that may be used to assess the physiologic effects of HF therapies.

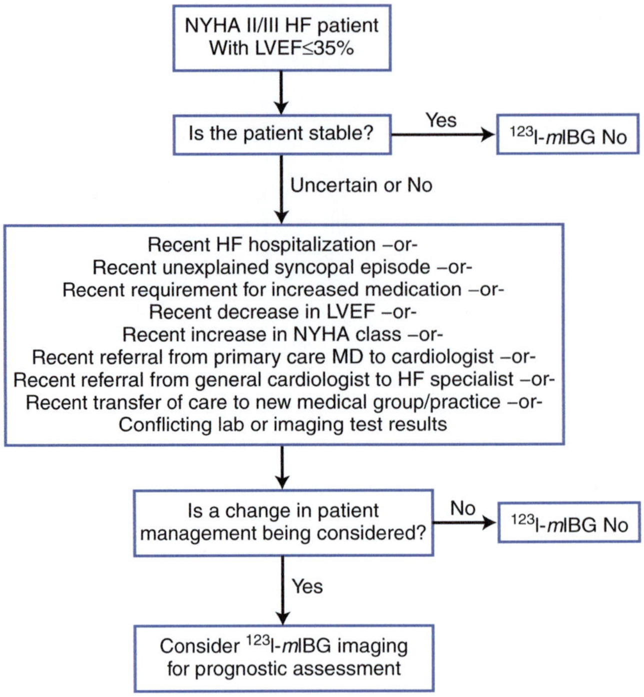

Figure 4-21. Proposed flow chart to help the clinician determine whether to use MIBG cardiac neuronal imaging in an HF patient with significant LV dysfunction. Information on cardiac neuronal status may be of value in decision making regarding patients with only borderline indications for guideline-based therapies or for whom the benefits of such therapies might be outweighed by their risks. Numeric estimation of mortality probability using MIBG imaging in conjunction with clinical risk models provides an individualized means to judge the most appropriate approach to future clinical management.

References

1. Travin M. Cardiac autonomic imaging with SPECT tracers. J Nucl Cardiol. 2013;20(1):128–43.
2. Travin M. Cardiac radionuclide imaging to assess patients with heart failure. Semin Nucl Med. 2014;44(4):294–313.
3. Peix A, Mesquita CT, Paez D, Pereira CC, Felix R, Gutierrez C, Jaimovich R, Ianni BM, Soares Jr J, Olaya P, Rodriguez MV, Flotats A, Giubbini R, Travin M, Garcia EV. Nuclear medicine in the management of patients with heart failure: guidance from an expert panel of the International Atomic Energy Agency (IAEA). Nucl Med Commun. 2014;35(8):818–23.
4. Patel AD, Iskandrian AE. MIBG imaging. J Nucl Cardiol. 2002;9(1):75–94.
5. Yamashina S, Yamazaki J. Neuronal imaging using SPECT. Eur J Nucl Med Mol Imaging. 2007;34:939–50.
6. Flotats A, Carrio I, Agostini D, Le Guludec D, Marcassa C, Schaffers M, Somsen GA, Unlu M, Verberne HJ. Proposal for standardization of (123)I-metaiodobenzylguanidine (MIBG) cardiac sympathetic imaging by the EANM Cardiovascular Committee and the European Council of Nuclear Cardiology. Eur J Nucl Med Mol Imaging. 2010;37:1802–12.
7. Merlet P, Benvenuti C, Moyse D, Pouillart F, Dubois-Rande JL, Duval AM, Loisance D, Castaigne A, Syrota A. Prognostic value of MIBG imaging in idiopathic dilated cardiomyopathy. J Nucl Med. 1999;40:917–23.
8. Yamada T, Shimonagata T, Fukunami M, et al. Comparison of the prognostic value of cardiac iodine-123 mIBG imaging and heart rate variability in patients with chronic heart failure: a prospective study. J Am Coll Cardiol. 2003;41:231–8.
9. Verberne HJ, Brewster LM, Somsen GA, Eck-Smit BL. Prognostic value of myocardial 123I-metaiodobenzylguanidine (MIBG) parameters in patients with heart failure: a systematic review. Eur Heart J. 2008;29:1147–59.
10. Nakata T, Nakajima K, Yamashina S, Yamada T, Momose M, Kasama S, Matsui T, Matsuo S, Travin MI, Jacobson AF. A pooled analysis of multicenter cohort studies of I-123-mIBG cardiac sympathetic innervation imaging for assessment of long-term prognosis in chronic heart failure. JACC Cardiovasc Imaging. 2013;6:772–84.
11. Verschure DO, Veltman CE, Manrique A, Somsen GA, Koutelou M, Katsikis A, Agostini D, Gerson MC, van Eck-Smit BLF, Scholte AJHA, Jacobson AF, Verberne HJ. For what endpoint does myocardial ^{123}I-MIBG scintigraphy have the greatest prognostic value in patients with heart failure? Results of a pooled individual patient data meta-analysis. Eur Heart J Cardiovasc Imaging. 2014;15(9):996–1003.
12. Estorch M, Camprecios M, Flotats A, Mari C, Berna L, Catafau AM, Ballester M, Narula J, Carrio I. Sympathetic reinnervation of cardiac allografts evaluated by 123I-MIBG imaging. J Nucl Med. 1999;40:911–6.
13. Agostini D, Belin A, Amar MH, Darlas Y, Hamon M, Grollier G, Potier JC, Bouvard G. Improvement of cardiac neuronal function after carvedilol treatment in dilated cardiomyopathy: a 123I-MIBG scintigraphic study. J Nucl Med. 2000;41:845–51.
14. Kasama S, Toyama T, Kumakura H, Takayama Y, Ichikawa S, Suzuki T, Kurabayashi M. Effect of spironolactone on cardiac sympathetic nerve activity and left ventricular remodeling in patients with dilated cardiomyopathy. J Am Coll Cardiol. 2003;41:574–81.
15. Kasama S, Toyama T, Kumakura H, Takayama Y, Ichikawa S, Suzuki T, Kurabayashi M. Addition of valsartan to an angiotensin-converting enzyme inhibitor improves cardiac sympathetic nerve activity and left ventricular function in patients with congestive heart failure. J Nucl Med. 2003;44:884–90.
16. Kasama S, Toyama T, Kumakura H, Takayama Y, Ichikawa S, Suzuki T, Kurabayashi M. Effects of perindopril on cardiac sympathetic nerve activity in patients with congestive heart failure: comparison with enalapril. Eur J Nucl Med Mol Imaging. 2005;32:964–71.
17. Kasama S, Toyama T, Kumakura H, Takayama Y, Ichikawa S, Suzuki T, Kurabayashi M. Effects of candesartan on cardiac sympathetic nerve activity in patients with congestive heart failure and preserved left ventricular ejection fraction. J Am Coll Cardiol. 2005;45:661–7.
18. Cha YM, Oh J, Miyazaki C, Hayes DL, Rea RF, Shen WK, Asirvatham SJ, Kemp BJ, Hodge DO, Chen PS, Chareonthaitawee P. Cardiac resynchronization therapy upregulates cardiac autonomic control. J Cardiovasc Electrophysiol. 2008;19:1045–52.
19. Drakos SG, Athanasoulis T, Malliaras KG, Terrovitis JV, Diakos N, Koudoumas D, Ntalianis AS, Theodoropoulos SP, Yacoub MH, Nanas JN. Myocardial sympathetic innervation and long-term left ventricular mechanical unloading. JACC Cardiovasc Imaging. 2010;3:64–70.
20. Mcghie AI, Corbett JR, Akers MS, Kulkarni P, Sills MN, Kremers M, Buja LM, Durant-Reville M, Parkey RW, Willerson JT. Regional cardiac adrenergic function using I-123 meta-iodobenzylguanidine tomographic imaging after acute myocardial infarction. Am J Cardiol. 1991;67:236–42.
21. Yukinaka M, Nomura M, Ito S, Nakaya Y. Mismatch between myocardial accumulation of 123I-MIBG and 99mTc-MIBI and late ventricular potentials in patients after myocardial infarction: association with the development of ventricular arrhythmias. Am Heart J. 1998;136:859–67.
22. Simoes MV, Barthel P, Matsunari I, Nekolla SG, Schomig A, Schwaiger M, Schmidt G, Bengel FM. Presence of sympathetically denervated but viable myocardium and its electrophysiologic correlates after early revascularised, acute myocardial infarction. Eur Heart J. 2004;25:551–7.
23. Henneman MM, Bengel FM, Bax JJ. Will innervation imaging predict ventricular arrhythmias in ischaemic cardiomyopathy? Eur J Nucl Med Mol Imaging. 2006;33:862–5.
24. Bax JJ, Kraft O, Buxton AE, Fjeld JG, Parizek P, Agostini D, et al. 123 I-mIBG scintigraphy to predict inducibility of ventricular arrhythmias on cardiac electrophysiology testing: a prospective multicenter pilot study. Circ Cardiovasc Imaging. 2008;1:131–40.
25. Shapiro B, Wieland D, Brown LE, Nakajo M, Sisson JC, Beierwaltes WH. 131-meta-iodobenzylguanidine (MIBG) adrenal medullary scintigraphy. Interventional nuclear medicine. New York: Grune and Stratton, Inc; 1984. pp. 451–81.
26. Smets LA, Bout B, Wisse J. Cytotoxic and antitumor effects of the norepinephrine analogue Meta-Iodo-Benzylguanidine (MIBG). Cancer Chemother Pharmacol. 1988;21(1):9–13.
27. Ekelund S, Nygren P, Larsson R. Guanidino-Containing Drugs in Cancer Chemotherapy: Biochemical and Clinical Pharmacology. Biochem Pharmacol. 2001;61(10):1183–93.
28. Dae MW, De Marco T, Botvinick EH, O'Connell JW, Hattner RS, Huberty JP, Yuen-Green MS. Scintigraphic Assessment of MIBG uptake in globally denervated human and canine hearts--Implications for clinical studies. J Nucl Med. 1992;33(8):1444–50.
29. DeGrado TR, Zalutsky MR, Vaidyanathan G. Uptake Mechanisms of Meta-[^{123}I]Iodobenzylguanidine in Isolated Rat Heart. Nucl Med Biol. 1995;22(1):1–12.
30. Mangner TJ, Tobes MC, Wieland DW, Sisson JC, Shapiro B. Metabolism of Iodine-131 Metaiodobenzylguanidine in Patients With Metastatic Phaeochromocytoma. J Nucl Med. 1986;27(1):37–44.
31. Tobes MC, Fig LM, Carey J, Geatti O, Sisson JC, Shapiro B. Alterations of iodine-131 MIBG biodistribution in an anephric patient: Comparison to normal and impaired renal function. J Nucl Med. 1989;30(9):1476–82.

32. Kline RC, Swanson DP, Wieland DM, Thrall JH, Gross MD, Pitt B, Beierwaltes WH. Myocardial imaging in man with I-123 meta-iodobenzylguanidine. J Nucl Med. 1981;22:129–32.

33. Narula J, Sarkar K. A conceptual paradox of MIBG uptake in heart failure: retention with incontinence! J Nucl Cardiol. 2003;10(6):700–4.

34. Leimbach Jr WN, Wallin BG, Victor RG, Aylward PE, Sundlof G, Mark AL. Direct evidence from intraneural recordings for increased central sympathetic outflow in patients with heart failure. Circulation. 1986;73(5):913–9.

35. Bohm M, La Rosee K, Schwinger RH, Erdmann E. Evidence for reduction of norepinephrine uptake sites in the failing human heart. J Am Coll Cardiol. 1995;25(1):146–53.

36. Sisson JC, Wieland DM. Radiolabelled Meta-Iodobenzylguanidine: Pharmacology and clinical studies. Am J Physiol Imaging. 1986;1(2):96–103.

37. Inoue Y, Suzuki A, Shirouzu I, Machida T, Yoshizawa Y, Akita F, Ohnishi S, Yoshikawa K, Ohtomo K. Effect of collimator choice on quantitative assessment of cardiac iodine 123 MIBG uptake. J Nucl Cardiol. 2003;10:623–32.

38. Jacobson AF, Senior R, Cerqueira MD, Wong ND, Thomas GS, Lopez VA, et al. Myocardial Iodine-123 Meta-Iodobenzylguanidine Imaging and Cardiac Events in Heart Failure Results of the Prospective ADMIRE-HF (AdreView Myocardial Imaging for Risk Evaluation in Heart Failure) Study. J Am Coll Cardiol. 2010;55:2212–21.

39. Marshall A, Cheetham A, George RS, Mason M, Kelion AD. Cardiac iodine-123 metaiodobenzylguanidine imaging predicts ventricular arrhythmia in heart failure patients receiving an implantable cardioverter-defibrillator for primary prevention. Heart. 2012;98(18):1359–65.

40. Bengel FM, Schwaiger M. Assessment of cardiac sympathetic neuronal function using PET imaging. J Nucl Cardiol. 2004;11:603–16.

41. Estorch M, Carrio I, Mena E, Flotats A, Camacho V, Fuertes J, Kulisewsky J, Narula J. Challenging the neuronal MIBG uptake by pharmacological intervention: effect of a single dose of oral amitriptyline on regional cardiac MIBG uptake. Eur J Nucl Med Mol Imaging. 2004;31:1575–80.

42. Tamaki S, Yamada T, Okuyama Y, Morita T, Sanada S, Tsukamoto Y, Masuda M, Okuda K, Iwasaki Y, Yasui T, Hori M, Fukunami M. Cardiac iodine-123 metaiodobenzylguanidine imaging predicts sudden cardiac death independently of left ventricular ejection fraction in patients with chronic heart failure and left ventricular systolic dysfunction: results from a comparative study with signal-averaged electrocardiogram, heart rate variability, and QT dispersion. J Am Coll Cardiol. 2009;53:426–35.

43. Agostini D, Verberne HJ, Burchert W, Knuuti J, Povinec P, Sambuceti G, Unlu M, Estorch M, Banerjee G, Jacobson AF. I-123-mIBG myocardial imaging for assessment of risk for a major cardiac event in heart failure patients: insights from a retrospective European multicenter study. Eur J Nucl Med Mol Imaging. 2008;35:535–46.

44. Senior R, Agostini D, Travin M, Caldwell JH, Gerson MC, Jacobson AF. Imaging of myocardial sympathetic innervation for prediction of arrhythmic events in heart failure patients: Insights from the ADMIRE-HF trial (abstr). Presented at the American Heart Association 2009 Annual Meeting, Orlando.

45. Verberne HJ, Henzlova MJ, Jain D, Van Eck-Smit BLF, Carrió I, Jacobson AF, Travin M. 123I-mIBG and 99mTc-tetrofosmin SPECT for prediction of arrhythmic risk in ischemic heart failure patients (abstr). Presented at the Society of Nuclear Medicine 2014 Annual Meeting, St. Louis.

46. Boogers MJ, Borleffs CJ, Henneman MM, van Bommel RJ, van Ramshorst J, Boersma E, Dibbets-Schneider P, Stokkel MP, van der Wall EE, Schalij MJ, Bax JJ. Cardiac sympathetic denervation assessed with 123-iodine metaiodobenzylguanidine imaging predicts ventricular arrhythmias in implantable cardioverter-defibrillator patients. J Am Coll Cardiol. 2010;55:2769–77.

47. Shah AM, Bourgoun M, Narula J, Jacobson AF, Solomon SD. Influence of ejection fraction on the prognostic value of sympathetic innervation imaging with iodine-123 *meta*-iodobenzylguanidine (^{123}I-*m*IBG) in heart failure. JACC Cardiovasc Imaging. 2012;5:1139–46.

48. Levy WC, Mozaffarian D, Linker DT, Sutradhar SC, Anker SD, Cropp AB, et al. The Seattle Heart Failure Model: prediction of survival in heart failure. Circulation. 2006;113:1424–33.

49. Ketchum ES, Jacobson AF, Caldwell JH, Senior R, Cerqueira MD, Thomas GS, Agostini D, Narula J, Levy WC. Selective improvement in Seattle heart failure model risk stratification using Iodine-123 meta-iodobenzylguanidine imaging. J Nucl Cardiol. 2012;19:1007–16.

50. Jain KK, Hauptman PJ, Spertus JA, Kennedy KF, Bateman TM, Jacobson AF, Stolker JM. Incremental utility of iodine-123 Meta-Iodobenzylguanidine imaging beyond established heart failure risk models. J Card Fail. 2014;20:577–83.

51. Toyama T, Hoshizaki H, Yoshimura Y, Kasama S, Isobe N, Adachi H, Oshima S, Taniguchi K. Combined therapy with carvedilol and amiodarone is more effective in improving cardiac symptoms, function, and sympathetic nerve activity in patients with dilated cardiomyopathy: comparison with carvedilol therapy alone. J Nucl Cardiol. 2008;15:57–64.

52. Suwa M, Otake Y, Moriguchi A, Ito T, Hirota Y, Kawamura K, Adachi I, Narabayashi I. Iodine-123 metaiodobenzylguanidine myocardial scintigraphy for prediction of response to beta-blocker therapy in patients with dilated cardiomyopathy published erratum appears in Am Heart J 1997 Dec;134(6):1141¿. Am Heart J. 1997;133:353–8.

53. Yamazaki J, Muto H, Kabano T, Yamashina S, Nanjo S, Inoue A. Evaluation of beta-blocker therapy in patients with dilated cardiomyopathy--Clinical meaning of iodine 123-metaiodobenzylguanidine myocardial single-photon emission computed tomography. Am Heart J. 2001;141:645–52.

54. Kasama S, Toyama T, Hatori T, Sumino H, Kumakura H, Takayama Y, Ichikawa S, Suzuki T, Kurabayashi M. Evaluation of cardiac sympathetic nerve activity and left ventricular remodelling in patients with dilated cardiomyopathy on the treatment containing carvedilol. Eur Heart J. 2007;28:989–95.

5 PET Imaging and Quantitation of Cardiac Innervation

Stanley F. Fernandez, John M. Canty Jr, and James A. Fallavollita

Cardiac Autonomic Innervation

Disorders in cardiac autonomic function have been implicated in several cardiac diseases. Use of positron emission tomography (PET)-based radiotracers to quantify changes in cardiac autonomic innervation has provided insights into the effect and impact of these alterations on disease pathophysiology and long-term implications. Understanding the use of different radiotracers to evaluate autonomic innervation requires an understanding of the biochemical components of the cardiac autonomic system (Fig. 5.1).

V. Dilsizian, J. Narula (eds.), *Atlas of Cardiac Innervation*, DOI 10.1007/978-3-319-45800-7_5

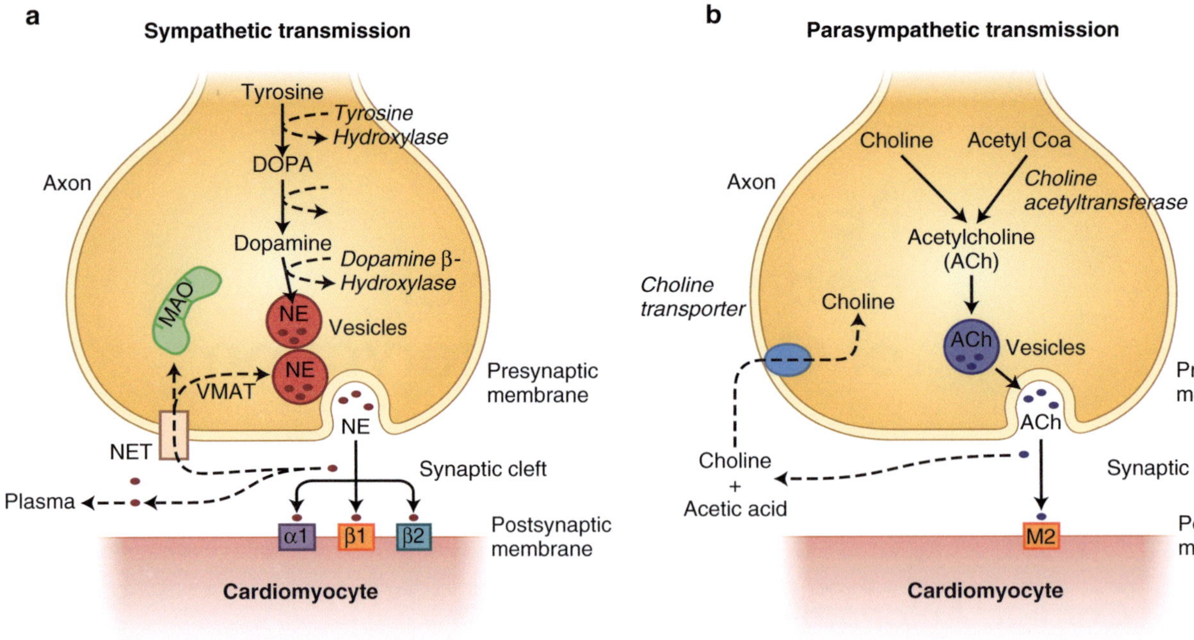

Figure 5-1. Schematic diagram of cardiac sympathetic and parasympathetic innervation. The cardiac network of neural innervation is composed primarily of two divisions, sympathetic (**a**) and parasympathetic (**b**). The sympathetic nervous system generally promotes positive inotropic and chronotropic responses through its major neurotransmitter, norepinephrine (NE), exerting its major cellular effects through binding to adrenergic receptors (predominantly β-receptors, β_1/β_2-receptors expressed in ~7:3 ratio). The parasympathetic nervous system generally suppresses cardiac inotropic and chronotropic responses through the release of its primary neurotransmitter, acetylcholine (ACh), binding to muscarinic receptors (M). (**a**) Within the presynaptic sympathetic nerve terminal, NE is synthesized through a series of enzymatic steps starting from the conversion of tyrosine to eventual formation of NE. Following presynaptic sympathetic nerve activation, docking of vesicles to the axonal membrane releases stored NE into the synaptic cleft. NE is actively recaptured from the synaptic cleft by NE transporter (NET) by the so-called uptake-1 mechanism. This saturable and ATP-dependent mechanism allows NE recycling and repackaging into vesicles. (**b**) Parasympathetic nerves are less abundant overall than sympathetic nerves, and primarily affect the atria rather than the ventricles. Stimulated parasympathetic postganglionic neurons release ACh, which binds and activates primarily M2 muscarinic receptors expressed in cardiomyocytes. ACh is enzymatically degraded by acetylcholinesterase. *DOPA* dihydroxyphenylalanine, *MAO* monoamine oxidase, *VMAT* vesicular monoamine transporter.

PET Radiotracers for Evaluation of Cardiac Autonomic Innervation

PET radiotracers used for imaging cardiac innervation may be classified based on their principal targets; that is, sympathetic versus parasympathetic nerve terminals and presynaptic versus postsynaptic components. The different radiotracers are summarized in Table 5.1.

Table 5-1. PET radiotracers for imaging cardiac innervation.

Nerve	Radiotracer	Description
Sympathetic		
Presynaptic	^{11}C-hydroxyephedrine (HED)	Most widely used PET-based radiotracer for cardiac sympathetic innervation
		NE analogue, accumulates through NET and transported to storage vesicles by VMAT2
		Not metabolized by MAO or COMT, excellent-quality images for quantitation
		Short half-life (20 min) isotope, requires on-site cyclotron
	^{11}C-epinephrine	Radiolabeled neurotransmitter that behaves similarly to NE
		Uptake, storage, and degradation mimic those of NE
		Cleared slowly because of its vesicular storage
	^{11}C-phenylephrine	Radiolabeled synthetic catecholamine with limited human studies
		Lower affinity for NET than HED
		Demonstrates vesicular leakage and enzymatic degradation by MAO, contributing to significant myocardial washout
	^{18}F-fluorodopamine	Longer half-life (2 h) isotope, permitting regional tracer synthesis
		Physiologic tracer forming labeled NE
		Difficult to manufacture and requires complex modeling
	^{18}F-LMI 1195	Accumulates through NET uptake
		Well-defined cardiac uptake, low washout, and low background activity
Postsynaptic	^{11}C-CGP 12177	Nonselective, hydrophilic β-receptor antagonist
		High specificity with low background activity
		Similar affinity for β_1- and β_2-receptors and lower affinity for β_3-receptor
		Difficult production of ^{11}C-phosgene, which is a required intermediate
Parasympathetic		
Presynaptic	Vesamicol derivatives	Selective inhibitors of vesicular acetylcholine transporter
		Low tracer retention, high nonspecific binding, and rapid washout
Postsynaptic	^{11}C-MQNB	M_2-receptor antagonist
		High receptor specificity in human studies

^{11}*C* carbon-11, *COMT* catechol-O-methyltransferase, ^{18}*F* fluorine-18, *MAO* monoamine oxidase, *MQNB* methiodide quinuclidinyl benzilate, *NE* norepinephrine, *NET* NE transporter, *VMAT2* vesicular monoamine transporter 2

Principles of PET Image Acquisition, Quantitation, and Interpretation

Cardiac PET imaging typically requires acquisition of a series of sequential dynamic images designed to provide information regarding tracer uptake, redistribution, decay, and dispersion. The sequence of images is designed to incorporate a minimum number of time frames that would allow analysis of tracer kinetics while ensuring adequate temporal resolution. Carbon-11 (^{11}C)-hydroxyephedrine (HED)-based imaging of sympathetic innervation is the most widely studied and therefore is used in the following section as a reference for discussion. Each of the following principles is applicable to other cardiac sympathetic markers, as well. Figure 5.2 describes the framework with which PET tracer kinetics may be used to probe physiologic systems.

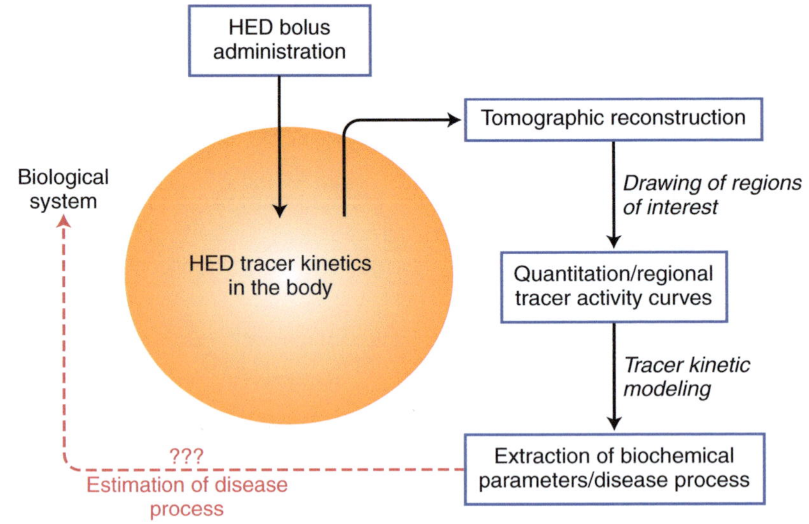

Figure 5-2. Framework for using sympathetic PET radiotracers for analyzing a biologic system. The initial step requires identification of an appropriate PET radiotracer to address a clinical question. The use of ^{11}C-hydroxyephedrine (*HED*) is well described and is the most frequently used radiotracer for probing sympathetic innervation. Following bolus intravenous administration of HED, its kinetics within the body reflects the summation of several physiologic processes within a specific biologic system (i.e., tracer distribution, retention, and washout). Its positron emission properties allow three-dimensional tomographic reconstruction and quantitation of dynamic time–activity curves. Based on the generated tracer activity, kinetic modeling may be applied to allow indirect estimation of different biochemical properties, such as tracer diffusion from blood to the interstitial layer or the rate of active uptake mechanism, among others. These estimated parameters derived from kinetic modeling may help define pathologic processes occurring within the biologic system.

Quantitation of Myocardial HED Uptake

Myocardial HED Radiotracer Time–Activity Curve

Image analysis may be approached several ways, from semiquantitative to the more sophisticated biochemical kinetic modeling. From the serial HED PET images, absolute myocardial tracer uptake may be obtained and analyzed. Following intravenous administration, HED rapidly accumulates in the myocardium and is cleared from the blood pool. Because of HED's rapid uptake and blood pool washout, emission data reflecting relative myocardial uptake of HED may be acquired within 40–60 min from the time of intravenous bolus administration. A dynamic sequence of image frames is obtained during the acquisition period (Fig. 5.3). Frequently, a shorter time interval between frames is ideal during the early time frame to capture the fast tracer uptake adequately. For the latter time frame, a longer time interval between images is typical to obtain sufficient photons as the tracer redistributes and decays. Raw data are obtained as a series of transaxial planes that may then be reconstructed into standard conventional tomographic views; that is, short axis, horizontal long, and vertical long axis views. Myocardial regions of interest may be identified and activity sampled over the entire indicated time frames, generating time–activity curves. Myocardial tracer activity is quantified as counts/pixel, which may be converted to megabecquerels per tissue volume from the machine calibration factor. To improve imaging accuracy, several corrections may be applied, including tissue attenuation correction using transmission scans of PET-emitting isotope source, partial volume correction to minimize systematic underestimation of small objects due to low camera spatial resolution [1, 2], and spillover corrections to account for heterogeneous uptake in adjacent structures.

HED Retention Index

Because the extent of HED tracer uptake depends on tracer availability, estimation of absolute HED uptake requires an arterial blood input function. The arterial input function typically is obtained from a blood pool region that has a high tracer concentration with minimal contributions from other adjacent organs. The left ventricular blood pool typically is used for this purpose. Alternatively, arterial input time–activity may be obtained from serial arterial sampling during image acquisition to determine plasma/blood HED activity. HED retention index is a frequently used quantitative parameter that can be computed easily and takes into account tracer availability (Fig. 5.4). It is estimated from the late myocardial tracer activity (i.e., final images acquired) normalized to the integrated blood pool time–activity or arterial input time–activity. This normalization corrects the HED retention for the total tracer delivered to the myocardium.

Standard Uptake Value

Standard uptake value is a simplified estimation, similar in principle to the retention index. Instead of the total integrated blood pool activity, myocardial tissue HED uptake is normalized to the total injected tracer dose (Fig. 5.5).

Polar Map Representation of Tracer Uptake

A polar map frequently is used to generate an overall volumetric representation of HED uptake distribution. This "bull's-eye" two-dimensional map is constructed from sequential circumferential or short axis rings extending from the base of the left ventricle to the apex. This allows representation of the left ventricle in its entirety. For a typical analysis, each short axis ring may be divided into several regions of interest (ROIs). For example, if eight short axis slices are each divided into 36 ROIs or angular sectors, then a total of 288 sectors would be available for analysis. The total number of sectors may be varied and depend on the specifics of reconstruction, analysis software, and intended purposes. Mean PET tracer counts in each sector may be normalized to the sector(s) with the maximum PET count(s). From these data, a polar map representation can be constructed from the stack of short axis rings with the apex in the center and basal region in the periphery of the circle. Sectors then may be grouped into the 17 standardized myocardial segments as recommended by the American Heart Association (Fig. 5.6). The extent of tracer uptake abnormalities may be expressed relative to the normal region. The region of the myocardium with the most intense or highest uptake typically represents the normal region, whereas the regions with relatively reduced uptake are considered abnormal. A semiquantitative scoring system also may be incorporated by using, for example, a score of 0–4, with 0 reflecting normal tracer uptake and 4 representing severe reduction. The scores from each segment may be added to represent the total abnormality.

Kinetic Modeling of Tracer Uptake and Disposition

Investigations into alterations in cardiac sympathetic function may be aided by accurate quantitation of biochemical parameters that may contribute to a diseased state. Estimation of biochemical properties such as neurotransmitter recycling, vesicular transport, and storage may help define some of the complex steps involved and characterize specific areas of dysregulation. The ultimate goal of kinetic modeling is to convert biologic systems into mathematical models for quantitative estimation. To achieve this, some of the necessary components include serial dynamic PET images of adequate quality to generate time-sensitive radiotracer uptake and distribution, in-depth knowledge of radiotracer-specific biologic processes, and mathematical kinetic models and computational methods to best fit the predicted and observed data. The fundamental concept is compartmental modeling, which is based on the overarching assumption that changes in tracer uptake, occurring over time, represent biologic shifts within different "compartments." Models may be constructed of varying complexity, from two to multiple compartment models. Increasing the number of compartments provides a more accurate physiologic characterization but consequentially increases the number of estimated parameters as well as statistical variability. The simplest is the two-compartment model, which assumes the arterial pool as the first compartment and the tissue as the second. Most neuronal tracers, however, are best described by a model with at least three compartments (Fig. 5.7). This area of investigation continues to evolve, but it has the potential to provide information on cellular processes that are not easily measured.

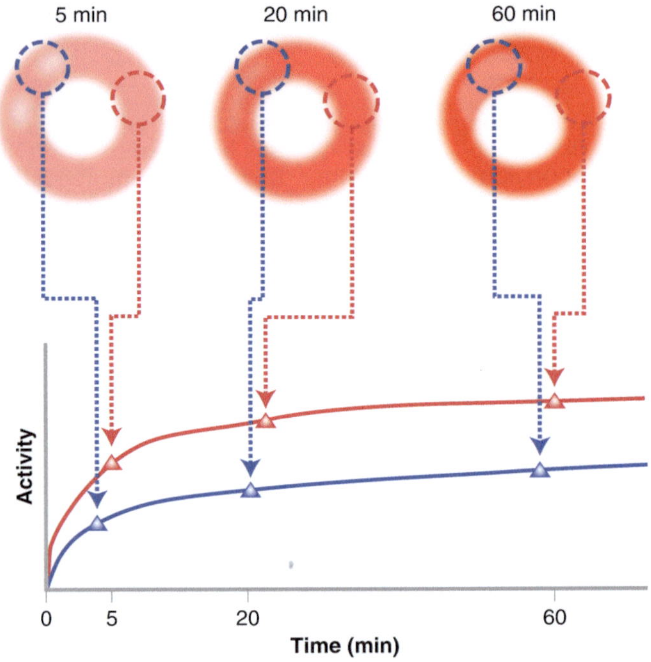

Figure 5-3. Schematic illustration for generating tracer time–activity curves. Specific regions of interest (ROIs) or "sectors" may be identified and marked, typically in the reconstructed standard short axis tomographic views. Based on the emission data acquired across a period of time, PET counts from the specified ROI may be quantified and plotted with respect to time. In this illustration, three time points are depicted (5, 20, and 60 min) from two different ROIs, the first from an area with relatively preserved tracer uptake (*red circle*) and the other ROI with reduced uptake (*blue circle*). Sequential acquisition of PET emission data from the two ROIs will then generate two distinct tracer time–activity curves reflecting the tracer uptake over time.

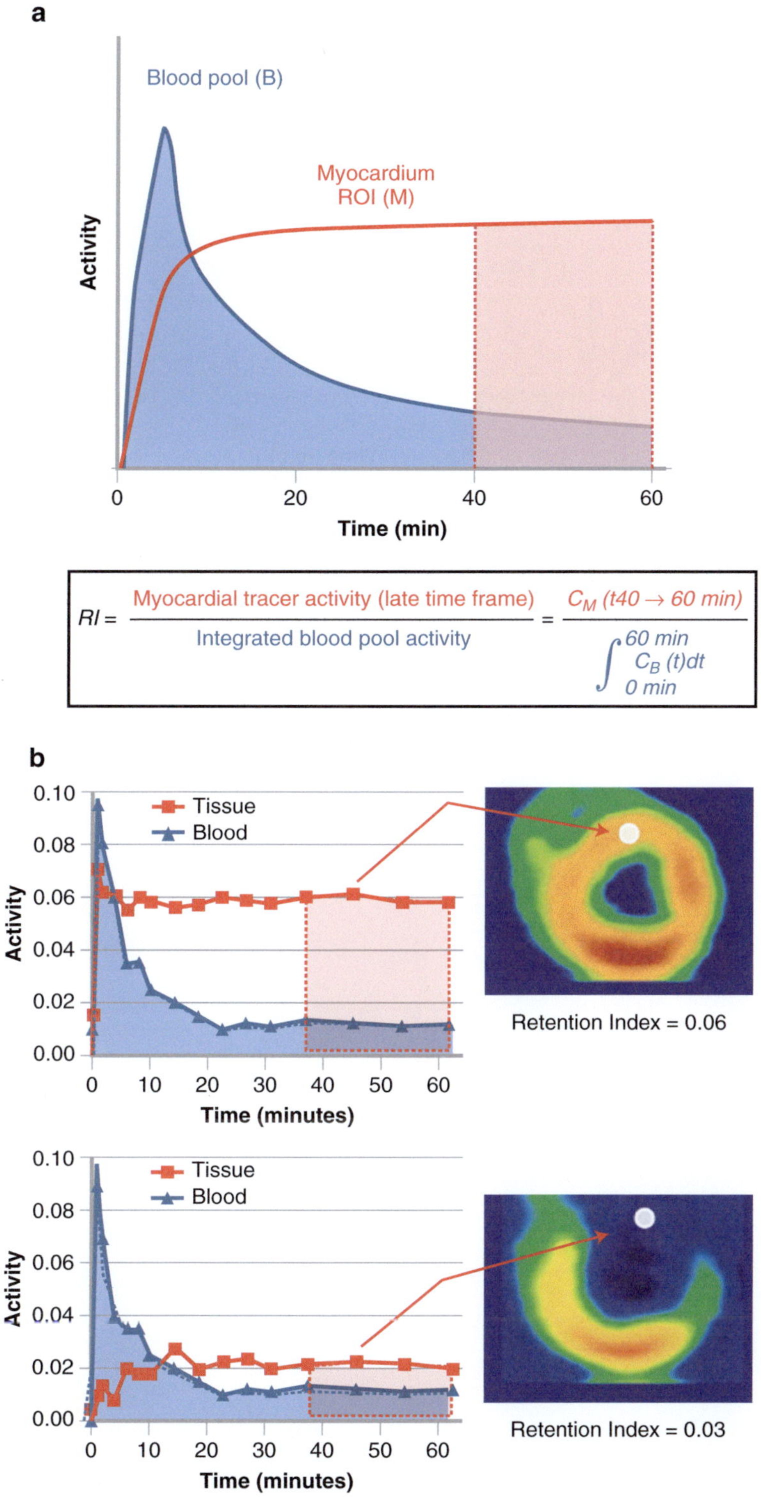

Figure 5-4. Myocardial HED retention index. (**a**), Retention index of a region of interest (*ROI*) is calculated from the tracer time–activity curve (*red line*) and normalized to the integrated blood pool time–activity curve (*blue line*). The later time frame emission data representing the net tracer uptake are used for calculation (*red vertical bar*), with the typical unit of measure milliliters of blood per minute per milliliter of tissue. (**b**) Examples of short axis tomograms of normal HED uptake (*upper image*) and significantly reduced HED uptake in an experimental model of myocardial infarction (*lower image*). The *white circle* represents the ROI, and the corresponding time–activity curve is indicated by the red line. The blood pool time–activity curve is indicated by the superimposed blue line. The retention index in infarcted myocardium was significantly reduced compared with that in normal myocardium (**b** adapted from Luisi et al. [3]).

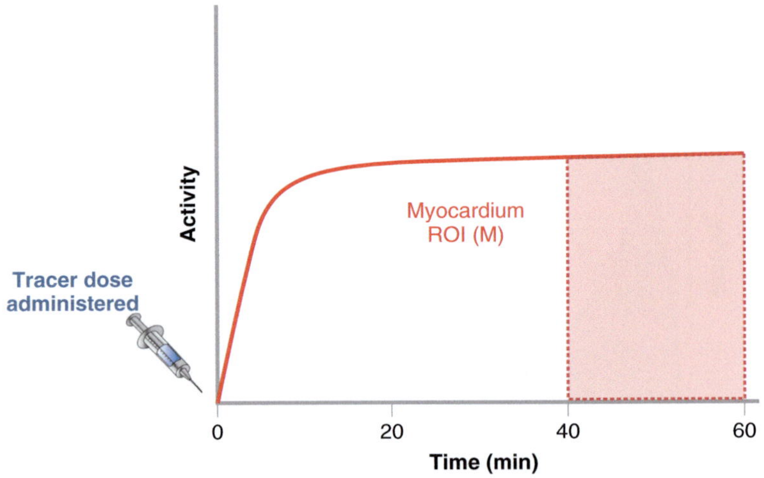

$$SUV = \frac{\text{Myocardial tracer activity (late time frame)}}{\text{Injected tracer dose / Patient weight}} = \frac{C_M(t)}{\text{Dose / Patient weight}}$$

Figure 5-5. Standard uptake value (*SUV*). SUV is similar in principle to the retention index quantitation. Analysis is simplified by using the injected tracer dose during the bolus administration to normalize the HED tracer uptake. This injected dose replaces the integrated blood pool time–activity (area under the curve) to represent correction for total tracer availability.

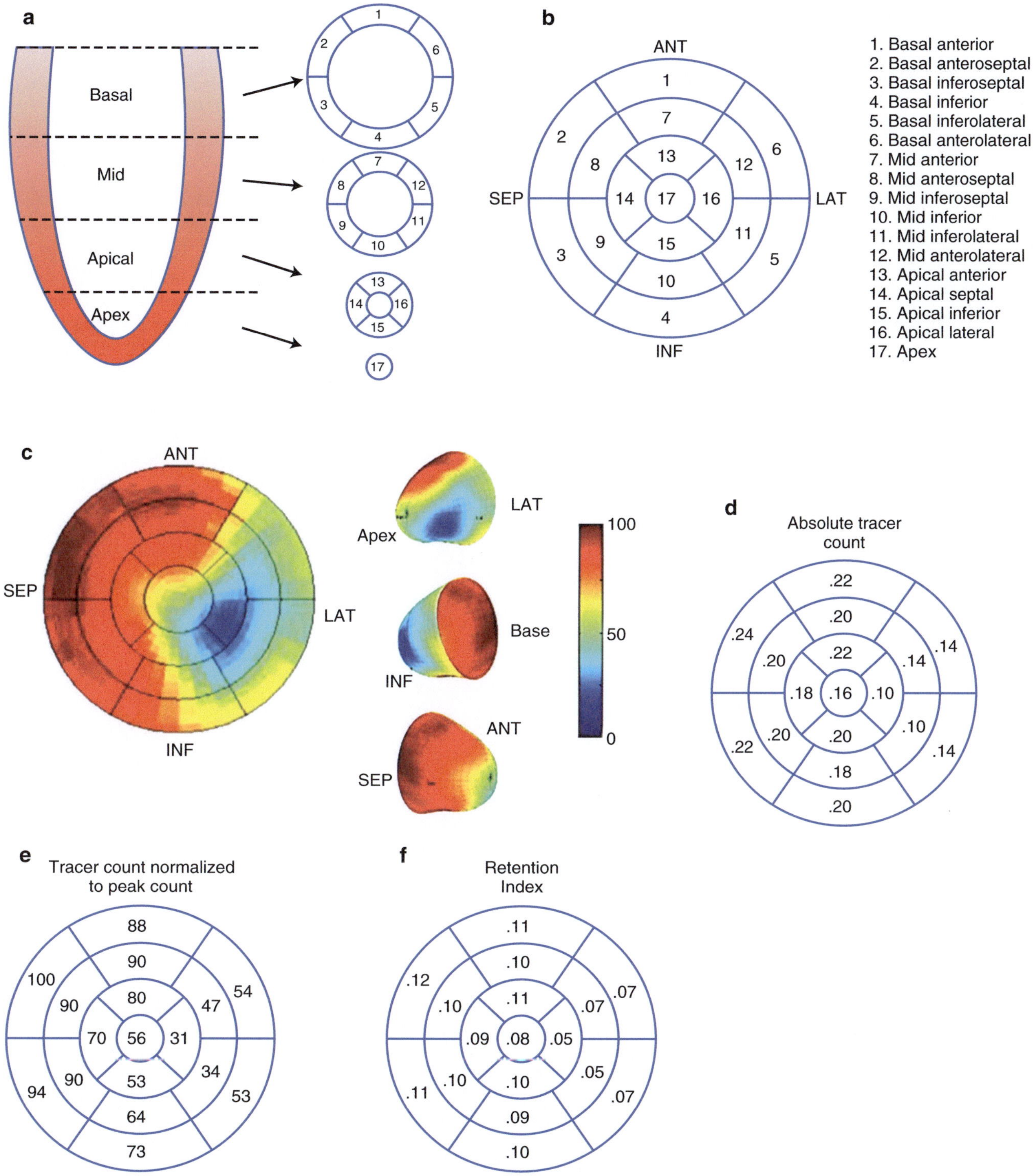

Figure 5-6. Polar map representation. Following quantitation of HED uptake using multiple ROIs from the series of short axis views to span the entire left ventricular myocardium, a polar map can be constructed. (**a**) Data from stacks of short axis views from the apex to the base are represented on a surface map with the apex at the center. The polar map is subdivided into a standardized 17-segment model. Each segment may contain a single ROI or be constructed from multiple ROIs. (**b**) A polar map representation of a patient with ischemic cardiomyopathy demonstrating reduced HED uptake in the lateral wall, consistent with partial regional sympathetic denervation (Adapted from Fallavollita et al. [4]). (**c**) Values are normalized to peak uptake, with the color palette representing uptake from 0 to 100% of peak. (**d–f**), Alternatively, tracer uptake from the different ROIs included in each segment may be averaged to generate a simplified numerical 17-segment dataset. Data may be reported based on averaged absolute tracer uptake (**d**, megabecquerels), normalized tracer uptake (**e**, average % of peak), or retention (**f**). *ANT* anterior, *INF* inferior, *LAT* lateral, *SEP* septal.

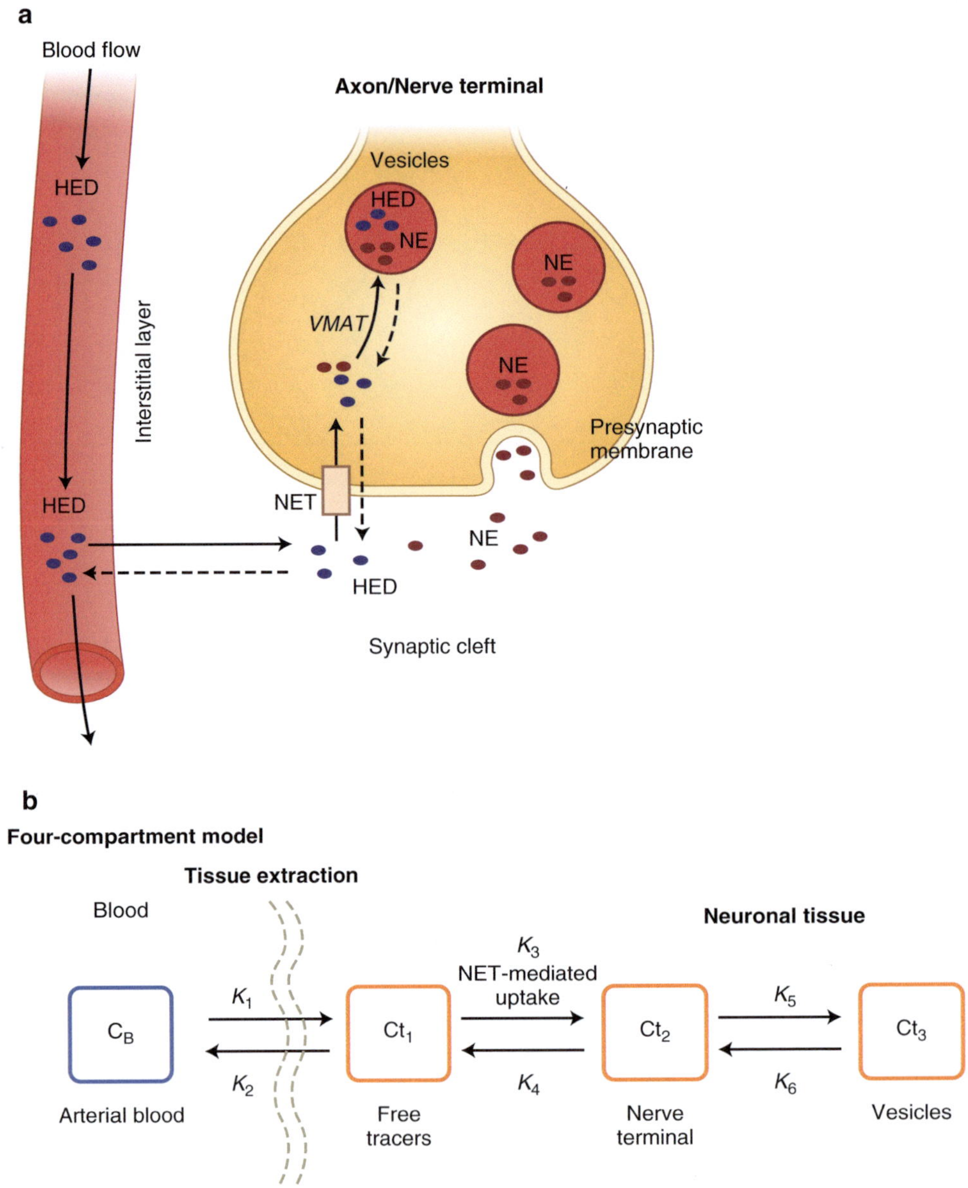

Figure 5-7. HED kinetic modeling. (**a**) Schematic illustration depicting HED uptake and distribution. HED delivered into the blood pool diffuses into the interstitial layer. HED in the interstitium and synaptic cleft has a fate similar to that of norepinephrine (*NE*) and may be actively transferred into the nerve terminal by the norepinephrine transporter (*NET*). HED subsequently is stored/sequestered in vesicles through the action of VMAT (vesicular monoamine transporter). (**b**) A four-compartment HED kinetic model [5] that includes the blood pool (C_B), interstitium (Ct_1), nerve terminal (Ct_2), and vesicular storage compartments (Ct_3). Based on this model, there are six estimated parameters (K_1… K_6). Rate parameters can be estimated from tracer activity curves after appropriate nonlinear curve fitting.

Graphic Method of β-Adrenergic Receptor Density Estimation

Estimation of receptor density using PET-based imaging involves complex analysis and nonlinear model fitting. Delforge et al. [6] published a graphic method of quantifying β-receptor density using a two-injection protocol of ^{11}C-CGP 12177 in experimental animals, with the initial injection using a high specific activity tracer dose followed by a second low specific activity tracer injection (admixed with unlabeled CGP; Fig. 5.8). The primary advantage of this approach is that it obviates the need for an arterial input function, which is affected by protein binding and metabolism of CGP. A similar approach was used by Ohte et al. [7] in clinical patients with prior myocardial infarction, demonstrating significant variability in β-adrenergic receptor density between remote and infarcted myocardium, as well as evidence for ongoing cardiac remodeling post infarction.

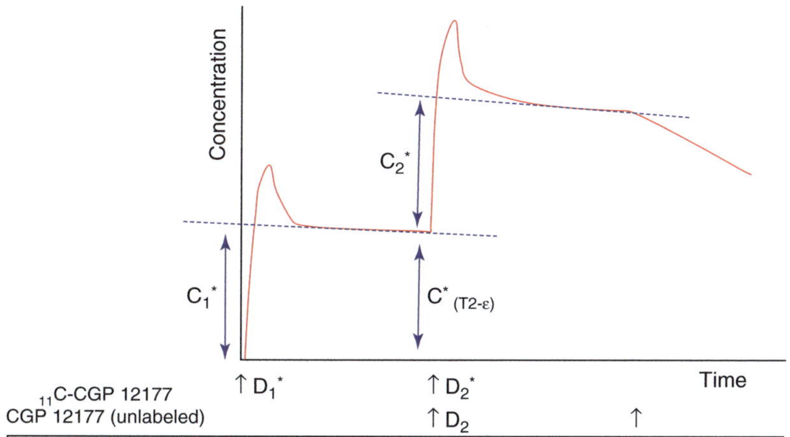

$$\left(B'_{max} - C^*_{(T2-\varepsilon)}\right)\left[1 - e^{\alpha\left(\frac{D_2 + D_2^*}{D_1^*}\right)\log\left(\frac{B'_{max} - C_1^*}{B'_{max}}\right)}\right] - C_2^*\,\frac{D_2 + D_2^*}{D_2^*} = 0$$

Figure 5-8. Graphic method of PET-based estimation of β-adrenergic receptors. Using a two-injection protocol, receptor density (B'_{max}) can be calculated from the equation, where D_1^* and D_2^* refer to first and second doses of radiolabeled CGP and D_2 is unlabeled CGP. C_1^*, C_2^*, and $C^*_{(T2-\varepsilon)}$ are obtained graphically from PET data generated from their respective plateau phase as indicated. A correction factor α is used to eliminate the need for arterial blood sampling (Adapted from Delforge et al. [6, 8]. This research was originally published in JNM. Delforge et al. [8]. Figure 2. © by the Society of Nuclear Medicine and Molecular Imaging, Inc.).

Acknowledgments We thank Robert deKemp, PhD, at the University of Ottawa for the use of FlowQuant® software, which has been used in our own PET research as well as some of the illustrations in this chapter. We also thank Anne Coe for her help with the preparation of the manuscript and figures.

References

1. Henze E, Huang SC, Ratib O, Hoffman E, Phelps ME, Schelbert HR. Measurements of regional tissue and blood-pool radiotracer concentrations from serial tomographic images of the heart. J Nucl Med. 1983;24(11):987–96.
2. Hoffman EJ, Huang SC, Phelps ME. Quantitation in positron emission computed tomography: 1. Effect of object size. J Comput Assist Tomogr. 1979;3(3):299–308.
3. Luisi Jr AJ, Suzuki G, deKemp R, Haka MS, Toorongian SA, Canty Jr JM, Fallavollita JA. Regional ^{11}C-hydroxyephedrine retention in hibernating myocardium: chronic inhomogeneity of sympathetic innervation in the absence of infarction. J Nucl Med. 2005;46(8):1368–74.
4. Fallavollita JA, Heavey BM, Luisi Jr AJ, Michalek SM, Baldwa S, Mashtare Jr TL, Hutson AD, de Kemp RA, Haka MS, Sajjad M, Cimato TR, Curtis AB, Cain ME, Canty Jr JM. Regional myocardial sympathetic denervation predicts the risk of sudden cardiac arrest in ischemic cardiomyopathy. J Am Coll Cardiol. 2014;63:141–9. doi:10.1016/j.jacc.2013.07.096.
5. Caldwell JH, Kroll K, Li Z, Seymour K, Link JM, Krohn KA. Quantitation of presynaptic cardiac sympathetic function with carbon-11-meta-hydroxyephedrine. J Nucl Med. 1998;39(8):1327–34.
6. Delforge J, Syrota A, Lançon JP, Nakajima K, Loc'h C, Janier M, Vallois JM, Cayla J, Crouzel C. Cardiac beta-adrenergic receptor density measured in vivo using PET, CGP 12177, and a new graphical method. J Nucl Med. 1991;32(4):739–48.
7. Ohte N, Narita H, Iida A, Fukuta H, Iizuka N, Hayano J, Kuge Y, Tamaki N, Kimura G. Cardiac beta-adrenergic receptor density and myocardial systolic function in the remote noninfarcted region after prior myocardial infarction with left ventricular remodelling. Eur J Nucl Med Mol Imaging. 2012;39(8):1246–53. doi:10.1007/s00259-012-2138-4.
8. Delforge J, Mesangeau D, Dolle F, Merlet P, Loc'h C, Bottlaender M, Trebossen R, Syrota A. In vivo quantification and parametric images of the cardiac beta-adrenergic receptor density. J Nucl Med. 2002;43(2):215–26.

6 Neuronal Imaging and Reverse Remodeling

Wataru Fujita, Kouji Kajinami, and Ichiro Matsunari

Introduction

Left ventricular (LV) remodeling, which refers to changes in chamber size, shape, and function of the heart, is known to be a marker of poor prognosis in patients with heart failure (HF). Reverse remodeling, on the other hand, is characterized as a reduction in LV end-diastolic and end-systolic volumes and an increase in LV ejection fraction (LVEF), which may occur in response to anti-HF therapies [1]. Reverse remodeling was first described in 1995 in a study by Kass et al. [2], in which the latissimus dorsi muscle was wrapped around the heart and chronically paced synchronously with ventricular systole in patients with dilated cardiomyopathy. Levin et al. [3] demonstrated reversal of chamber enlargement and normalization of cardiac structure due to unloading after LV assist device (LVAD) therapy. Reverse remodeling is clinically important because it generally is associated with a favorable prognosis and thus may serve as a surrogate end point [4]. It is known that reverse remodeling involves many alterations at the molecular, cellular, and myocardial tissue levels [5].

With regard to the β-adrenergic system, reverse remodeling is associated with normalization of excessive activation of β-adrenergic signaling and restoration of functional neuronal density and β-adrenergic receptors. Signals from the β-adrenergic system in the heart may be visualized and quantified in vivo by using cardiac neuroimaging techniques, such as iodine-123–metaiodobenzylguanidine (MIBG) imaging or carbon-11 (^{11}C)-hydroxyephedrine positron emission tomography (PET). Because reverse remodeling is closely related to changes in β-adrenergic signaling, neuronal imaging is expected to provide a clue for therapy monitoring, and even prediction of therapy response. Studies in patients undergoing LVAD have demonstrated that sympathetic neuronal function as measured by serial MIBG imaging improved "sympathetic reverse remodeling" in parallel to geometric, hemodynamic, functional, and biochemical improvement [6]. Among patients undergoing cardiac resynchronization therapy (CRT), sympathetic neuronal function likely will improve in responders but not in nonresponders [7]. Furthermore, patients with a preserved heart-to-mediastinum uptake (H/M) ratio, measured by MIBG imaging at baseline, likely will improve after CRT [7]. The power of MIBG imaging for predicting CRT response is enhanced further if it is combined with an index of mechanical dyssynchrony measured by speckle tracking echocardiography [8]. Such an imaging-based strategy also may apply to HF patients undergoing medical treatment that may induce reverse remodeling, such as β-blocker therapy. Several studies generally demonstrated an increase in H/M ratio, a decrease in MIBG washout rate (WR), and a decrease in single-photon emission computed tomography (SPECT) defect score after treatment [9–11], indicating that improved sympathetic activity—and hence, sympathetic reverse remodeling—occurs in response to medication. Similar to the results reported in the aforementioned CRT studies, a preserved H/M ratio and/or low MIBG WR at baseline predict subsequent functional recovery and reverse remodeling after medical treatment. It also is noteworthy that sympathetic remodeling, or sympathetic reverse remodeling, measured by serial MIBG

V. Dilsizian, J. Narula (eds.), *Atlas of Cardiac Innervation*, DOI 10.1007/978-3-319-45800-7_6

imaging may have prognostic value [12]. Finally, to date, only limited data are available regarding the use of neuronal PET in assessing reverse remodeling. However, a clinical study clearly demonstrated that myocardial β-adrenergic receptor density measured by ^{11}C-CGP12177 PET is closely related to carvedilol-induced functional improvement [13], indicating that neuronal PET may provide insight into the reverse remodeling–related pathophysiology. Thus, sympathetic neuronal imaging is a promising option for monitoring and even predicting reverse remodeling, which is closely related to patient outcome.

What Is Reverse Remodeling, and Why Is It Important?

Inhibition of the β-adrenergic system or renin–angiotensin–aldosterone system (RAAS) is known to induce reduction in LV chamber size and hence reverse remodeling. Cell transplantation may be a promising option for treating patients with end-stage HF who are resistant to conventional therapies. Device-based interventions such as CRT and LVAD implantation also may induce reverse remodeling and lead to a better prognosis. However, it should be noted that not all patients will show significant improvement in response to these therapeutic options. We expect that imaging-based biomarkers, such as those obtained by MIBG imaging, will provide clues for better patient selection and therapy monitoring.

Table 6-1. Clinical interventions that may induce reverse remodeling in patients with HF.

β-Blockers
Angiotensin-converting enzyme inhibitors
Angiotensin receptor blockers
Aldosterone inhibitors
Cell transplantation
Coronary arterial revascularization
Mitral valve repair/replacement
CRT
LVAD

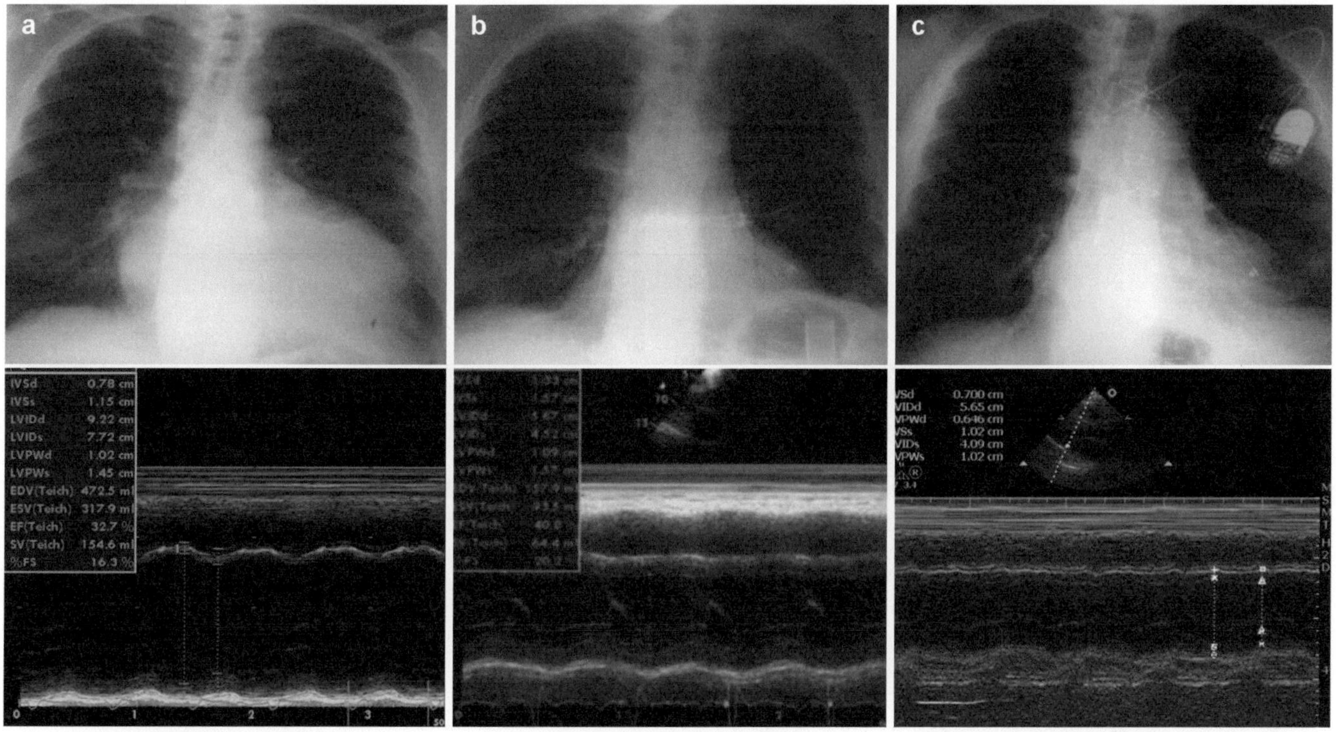

FIGURE 6-1. Representative example of reverse remodeling induced by LVAD therapy. Serial chest radiographs and echocardiograms (M mode, parasternal long-axis view) from a male patient with a multiyear history of idiopathic dilated cardiomyopathy and HF refractory to standard therapy, including inotropes (**a**–**c**). The patient underwent a combination of LVAD unloading and pharmacologic therapy and was weaned from the LVAD successfully 6 months after implantation. He continued on standard HF pharmacologic therapy and achieved a sustained functional recovery with no signs or symptoms of HF over a 7-year follow-up period. *EF* ejection fraction (*left ventricular*), *LVIDd* LV end-diastolic diameter (From Drakos et al. [14]; with permission).

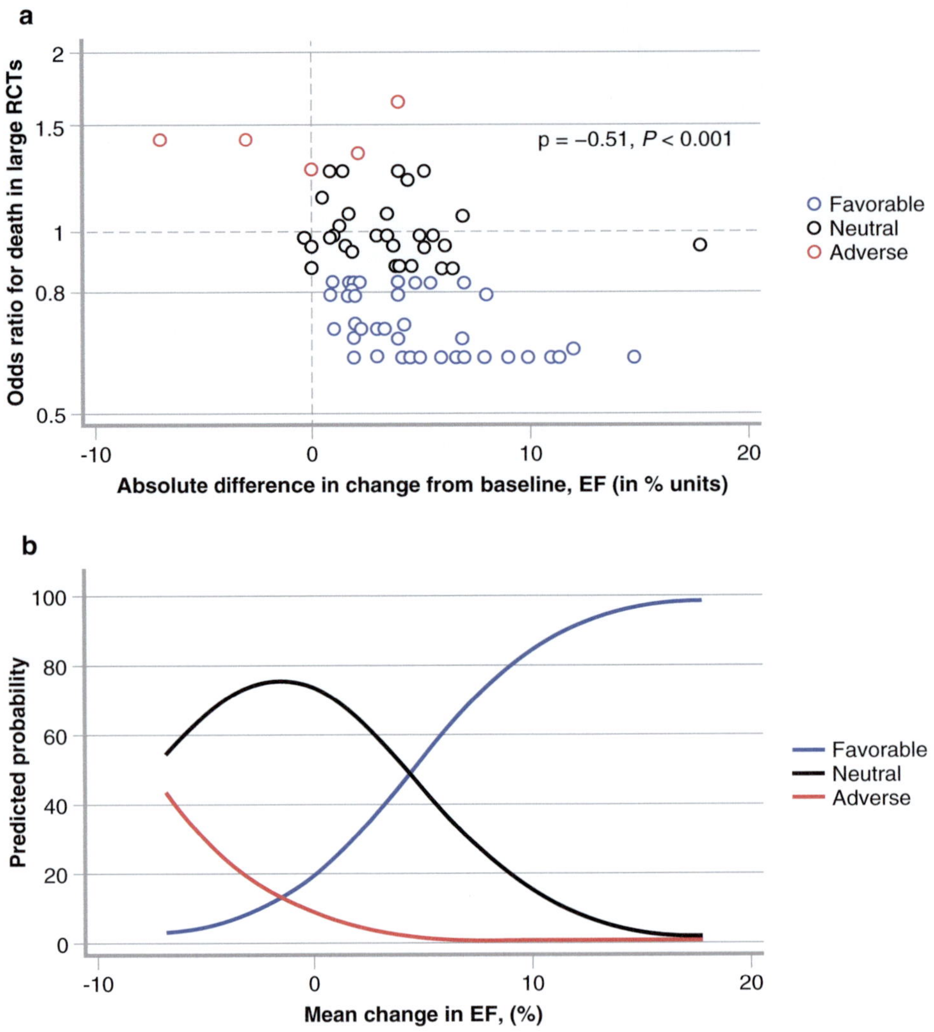

Figure 6-2. (**a**) Quantitative relationship between drug/device effects on ejection fraction (EF) and mortality: each data point represents a placebo-corrected change in EF from an individual remodeling trial plotted against the mortality odds ratio (OR) for the specific therapy. Color-coded mortality effect based on meta-analysis of published data. Interventions were classified as favorable (*blue circles*) if the upper limit of the 95% confidence interval (CI) of the OR for death from the mortality trials was less than 1, neutral (*black circles*) if the 95% CI crossed 1, and adverse (*red circles*) if the lower limit of the 95% CI was greater than 1. There was a significant correlation between short-term therapeutic effect on LVEF and longer-term therapeutic effect on mortality ($\rho = -0.51$, $P < 0.001$). Remodeling data were derived from analysis of 86 randomized controlled trials (RCTs) of 25 interventions involving 19,092 patients. (**b**) Predicted probability of a categorical mortality outcome based on drug/device effect on EF: the lines represent the likelihood of a categorical mortality outcome based on an intervention's trial-level effect on EF compared with placebo (unadjusted, weighted, ordered logistic regression). Color-coded mortality effect based on meta-analysis of published data. Definition of mortality effect for a given intervention is as described in **A**. The graph suggests that if the mean change in EF is 10% in the short-term studies, the probabilities that the long-term mortality studies will be significantly favorable (*blue line*), neutral (*black line*), or significantly unfavorable (*red line*) are approximately 85%, 15%, and 1%, respectively. As such, the degree of drug/device-induced reverse remodeling as reflected by EF change is a quantitative marker of favorable prognosis (Adapted from Kramer et al. [4]).

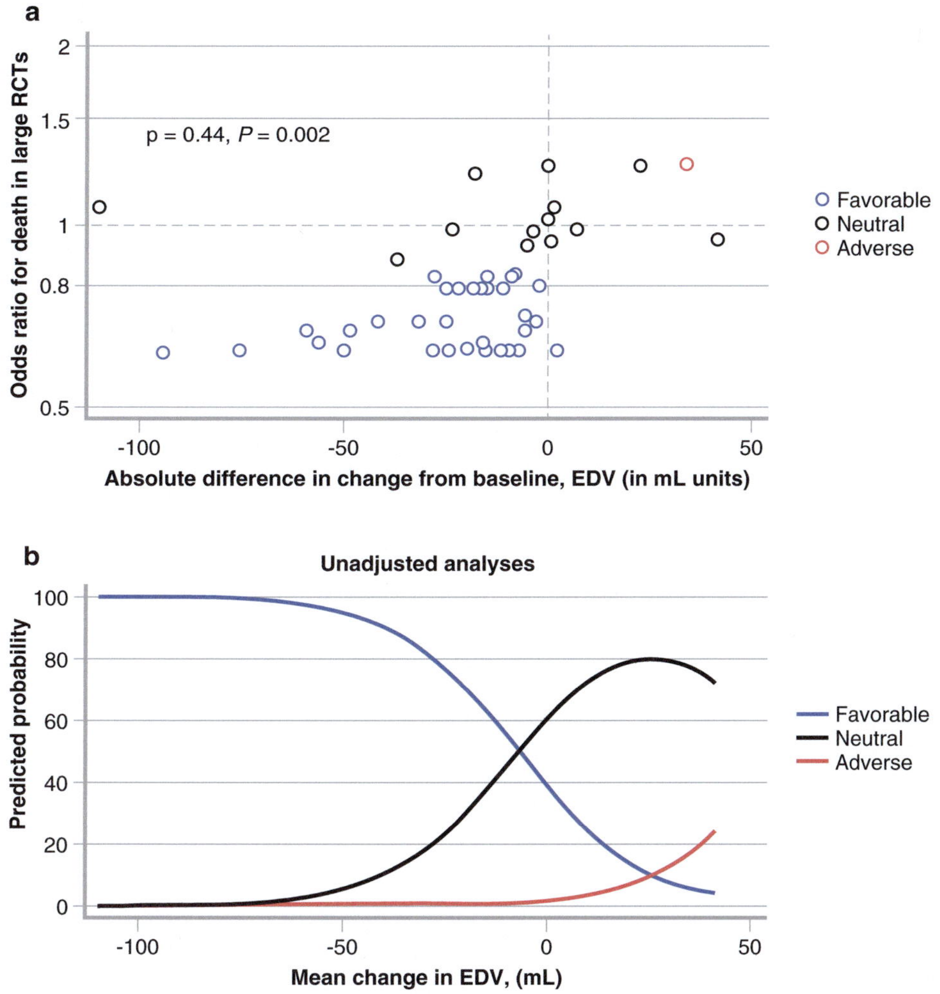

Figure 6-3. (**a**) Quantitative relationship between drug/device effects on end-diastolic volume (*EDV*) and mortality: each data point represents a placebo-corrected change in EDV from an individual remodeling trial plotted against the mortality OR for the specific therapy. Color-coded mortality effect based on meta-analysis of published data: favorable (*blue circles*), neutral (*black circles*), or adverse (*red circles*). Definition of mortality effect for a given intervention is as described in Fig. 6.2. There was a significant correlation between effect sizes in the mortality trials and mean therapy-induced changes in EDV ($\rho = 0.44$, $P = 0.002$). Remodeling data derived from analysis of 50 randomized controlled trials (RCTs) of 19 interventions, including 10,855 total patients. (**b**) Predicted probability of a categorical mortality outcome based on drug/device effect on EDV: the lines represent the likelihood of a categorical mortality outcome based on an intervention's trial-level effect on EDV compared with placebo (unadjusted, weighted, ordered logistic regression). Color-coded mortality effect based on meta-analysis of published data. Definition of mortality effect for a given intervention is as described in Fig. 6.2. The graph suggests that if the mean change in EDV is −10 mL in the short-term studies, the probability that the long-term mortality studies will be significantly favorable (*blue line*), neutral (*black line*), or significantly unfavorable (*red line*) is approximately 56%, 43%, and 1%, respectively. As such, the degree of drug/device-induced reverse remodeling as reflected by EDV change is a quantitative marker of favorable prognosis (Adapted from Kramer et al. [4]).

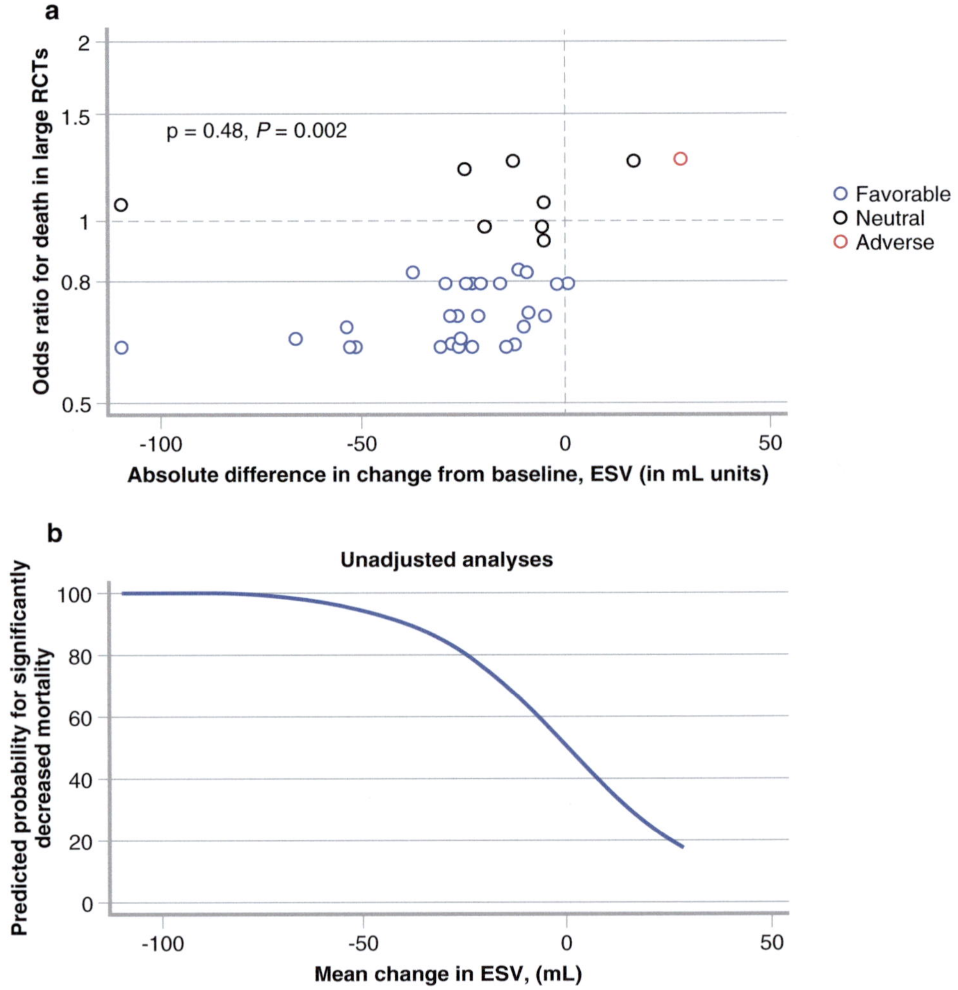

Figure 6-4. (**a**) Quantitative relationship between drug/device effects on end-systolic volume (*ESV*) and mortality: each data point represents a placebo-corrected change in ESV from an individual remodeling trial plotted against the mortality OR for the specific therapy. Color-coded mortality effect based on meta-analysis of published data: favorable (*blue circles*), neutral (*black circles*), or adverse (*red circles*). Definition of mortality effect for a given intervention is as described in Fig. 6.2. There was a significant correlation between effect sizes in the mortality trials and the effect sizes on ESV in the remodeling studies ($\rho = 0.48$, $P = 0.002$). Remodeling data are derived from analysis of 40 randomized controlled trials (*RCTs*) of 16 interventions, including 5,435 total patients. (**b**) Predicted probability of a favorable mortality outcome based on drug/device effect on ESV. The *blue line* represents the likelihood of a favorable mortality outcome based on an intervention's trial-level effect on ESV compared with placebo (unadjusted weighted logistic regression). There was insufficient remodeling data for ESV to model the probability for neutral or adverse outcomes individually. Color-coded mortality effect based on meta-analysis of published data. Definition of mortality effect for a given intervention is as described in Fig. 6.2. The graph suggests that if the mean change in ESV is +25 mL in the short-term studies, the probability that the long-term mortality studies will be significantly favorable is approximately 20%. This is equivalent to stating that the probability that the long-term mortality studies are neutral or significantly unfavorable is approximately 80% (100–20%). As such, the degree of drug/device-induced reverse remodeling as reflected by ESV change is a quantitative marker of favorable prognosis (Adapted from Kramer et al. [4]).

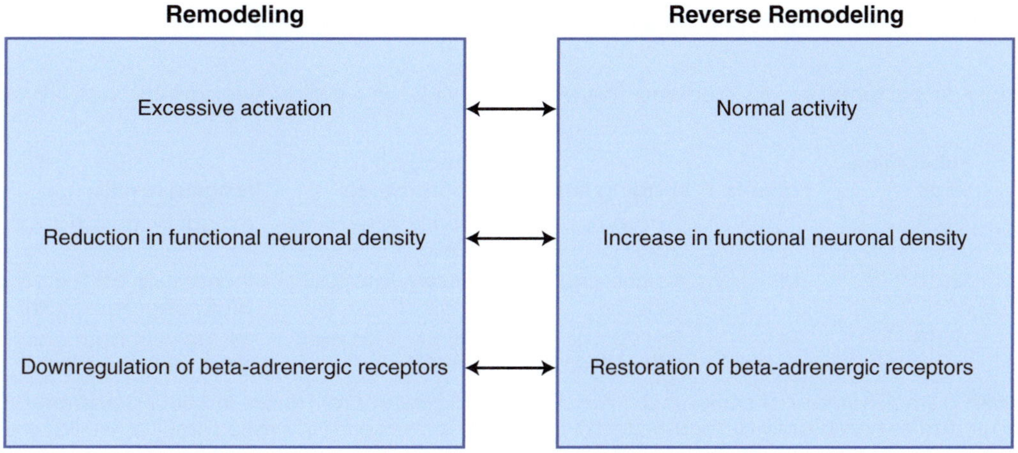

Figure 6-5. Schematic representation of the β-adrenergic system in the setting of remodeling and reverse remodeling. Remodeling is associated with excessive activation of sympathetic nerve activity [15], reduction in functional neuronal density [16, 17], and downregulation of β-adrenergic receptors [18–20]. It also is noteworthy that the degree of increase in sympathetic nerve activity is related to that of downregulation of β-adrenergic receptors [19]. Reverse remodeling, on the other hand, likely is associated with normalization of such adaptive or maladaptive changes.

Effects of LVADs on Sympathetic Neuronal Imaging

Table 6-2. Summary of published results assessing the effect of LVAD on cardiac sympathetic activity using serial MIB) imaging.

Authors	Publication year	Patients, n	Imaging time points	Imaging parameters	Imaging results
Miyagawa et al. [21]	2001	2 (10)[a]	2 months and >1 year	Early, late HMR; WR	No significant change
Drakos et al. [6]	2010	12	Before and at 3 months	Early, late HMR; WR	Increase in both early and late HMR, decrease in WR
George et al. [22]	2013	14	35±20 and 243±92 days	Early, late HMR; WR	Increase in both early and late HMR, decrease in WR

An early study with a small number of patients did not show significant improvement in MIBG parameters [21]. However, subsequent, larger studies consistently demonstrated a significant increase in H/M ratio (HMR) as well as a decrease in WR [6, 22], indicating improved sympathetic activity and hence, sympathetic reverse remodeling after LVAD support
[a]Two of 10 patients underwent serial MIBG imaging

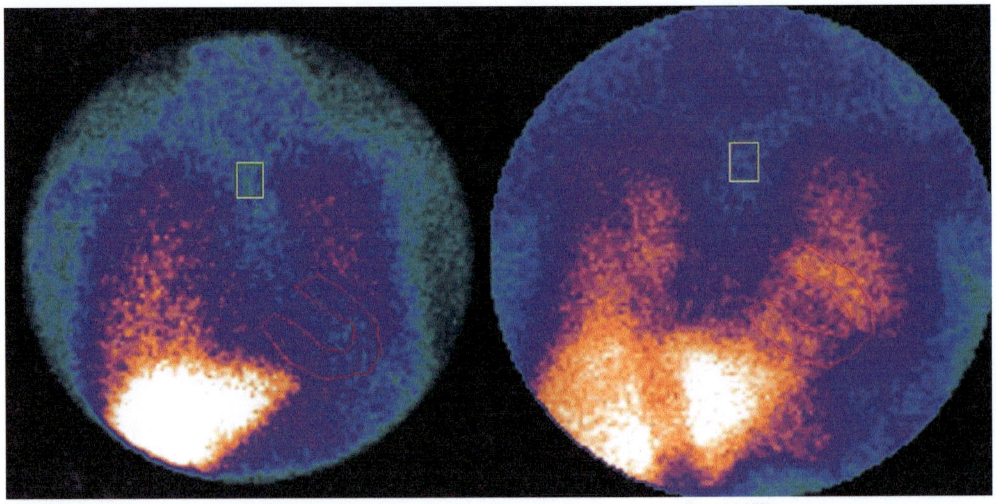

Figure 6-6. Effect of an LVAD on late MIBG imaging in a patient with dilated cardiomyopathy. There was an increase in cardiac MIBG uptake after 3 months of LVAD support, indicating sympathetic reverse remodeling (From Drakos et al. [6]; with permission).

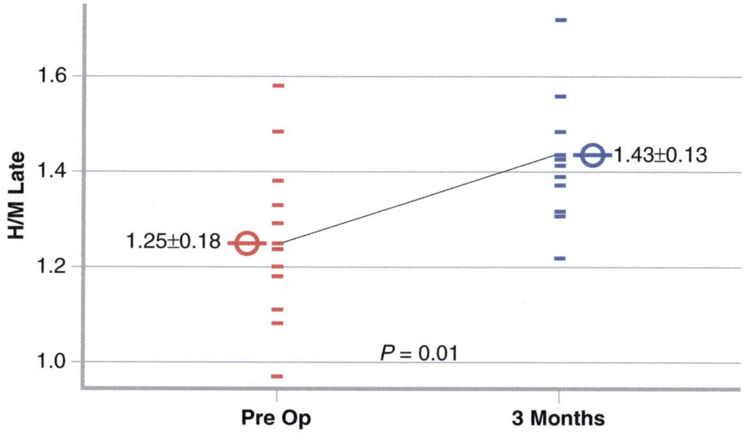

Figure 6-7. Effect of an LVAD on late heart-to-mediastinum MIBG uptake ratio (*H/M Late*). There was a significant increase in H/M Late after 3 months of LVAD support, which was associated with improved LV function and decreased LV size, indicating that sympathetic reverse remodeling is linked to geometric reverse remodeling (Adapted from Drakos et al. [6]).

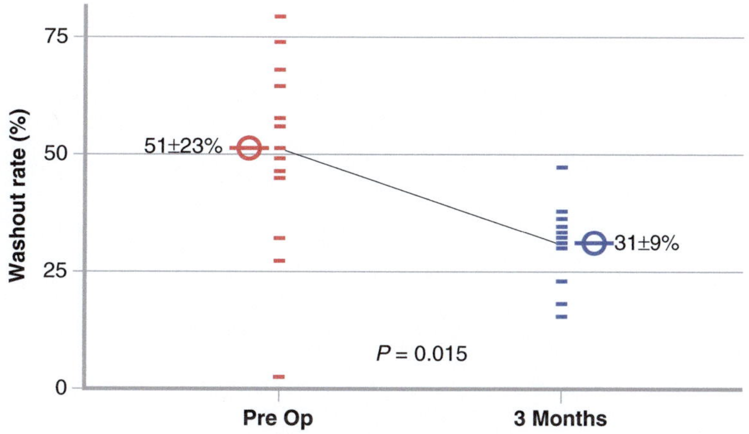

Figure 6-8. Effect of an LVAD on MIBG WR. The WR decreased significantly after 3 months of LVAD support, indicating improvement of excessive β-adrenergic activity (Adapted from Drakos et al. [6]).

Effects of CRT on Sympathetic Neuronal Imaging

Table 6-3. Summary of published results assessing the effect of CRT on cardiac sympathetic activity using serial MIBG imaging.

Authors	Publication year	Patients, n	Imaging time points	Imaging parameters	Imaging results
Erol-Yilmaz et al. [23]	2005	13	Before and at 6 months	Early, late HMR; WR	Increase in late HMR, and decrease in WR
Gould et al. [24]	2007	10	2 scans (CRT-on and CRT-off) with 2-week interval	Early, late HMR; WR	Increase in both early and late HMR
Nishioka et al. [7]	2007	30	Before and >3 months after	Early, late HMR; WR	Increase in both early and late HMR; decrease in WR only in responders
Burri et al. [25]	2008	16	Before and >6 months after	Early, late HMR; WR	Decrease in WR only in responders
Cha et al. [26]	2008	16	Before and at 6 months	Early, late HMR; WR	Increase in late HMR and decrease in WR
Cha et al. [27]	2011	45	Before and at 6 months	Early, late HMR; WR	Increase in late HMR; decrease in WR only in responders
Shinohara et al. [28]	2011	27	Before and at 6 months	Early, late HMR; WR	Increase in late HMR only in responders

The studies listed in this table generally demonstrated an increase in H/M ratio (HMR) and a decrease in WR in responders to CRT, indicating improved sympathetic activity and hence, CRT-induced sympathetic reverse remodeling

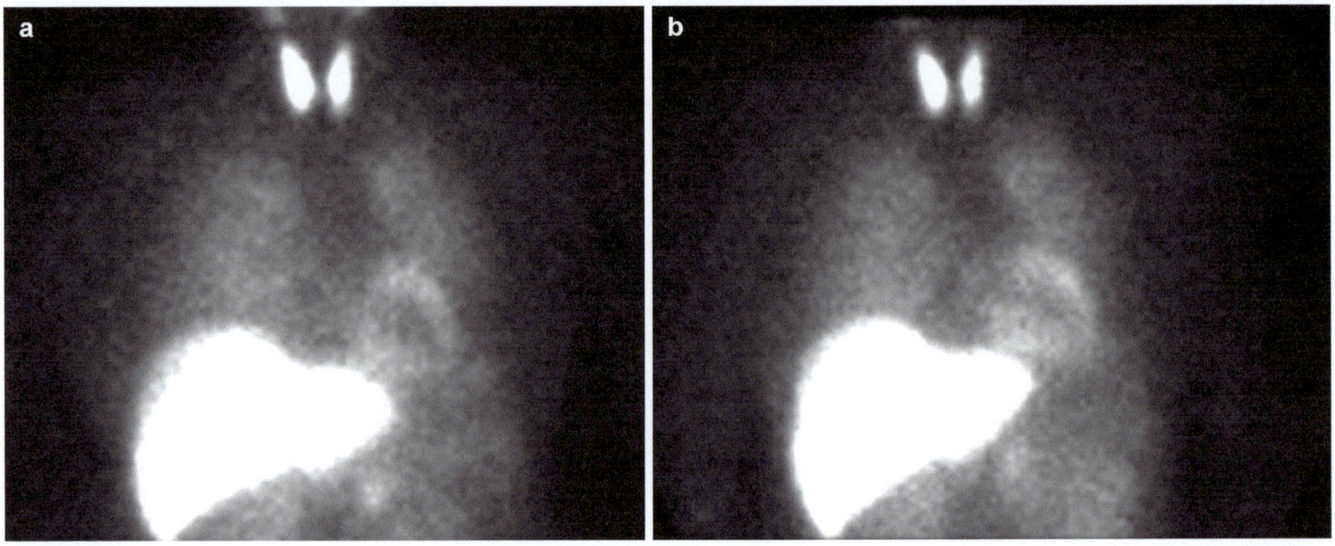

Figure 6-9. Effect of CRT on late MIBG imaging in a patient with HF. MIBG images before (**a**) and during CRT (**b**). Cardiac MIBG uptake increased after 2 weeks of CRT, indicating CRT-induced sympathetic reverse remodeling (From Gould et al. [24]; with permission).

Figure 6-10. Correlation between change in LVEF and change in MIBG washout (both in absolute terms) induced by CRT. There was a moderate but significant negative correlation between the two parameters, supporting the notion that sympathetic reverse remodeling is linked to geometric reverse remodeling (Adapted from Burri et al. [25]).

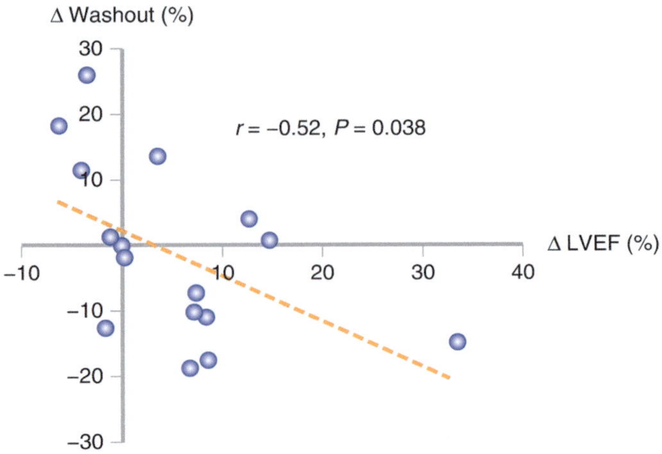

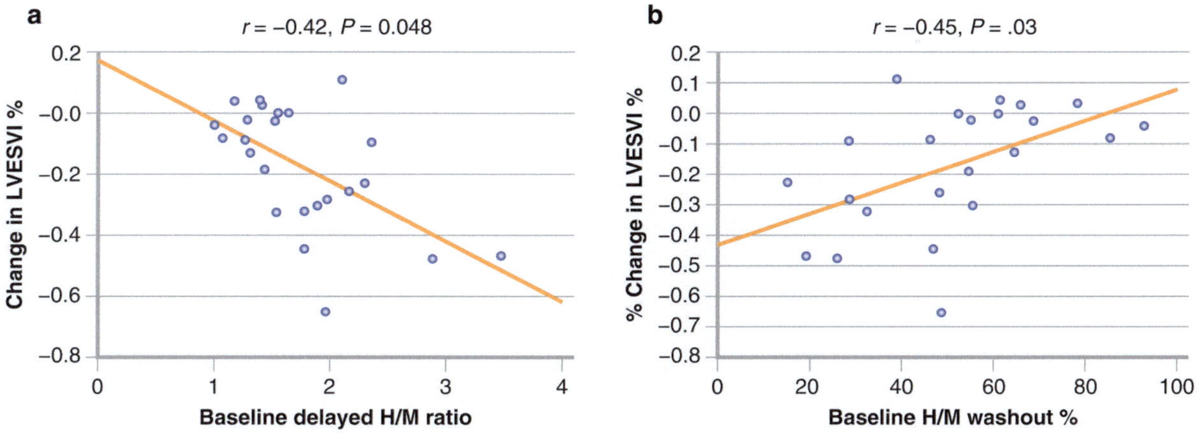

Figure 6-11. Correlation between change in LV systolic volume index (*LVESVI*) after CRT and baseline values of delayed H/M ratio (**a**) and WR (**b**). A high H/M ratio or low WR was related to reduction in LVESVI, and hence reverse remodeling, indicating that reverse remodeling after CRT is predictable by using baseline MIBG imaging (Adapted from Cha et al. [27]).

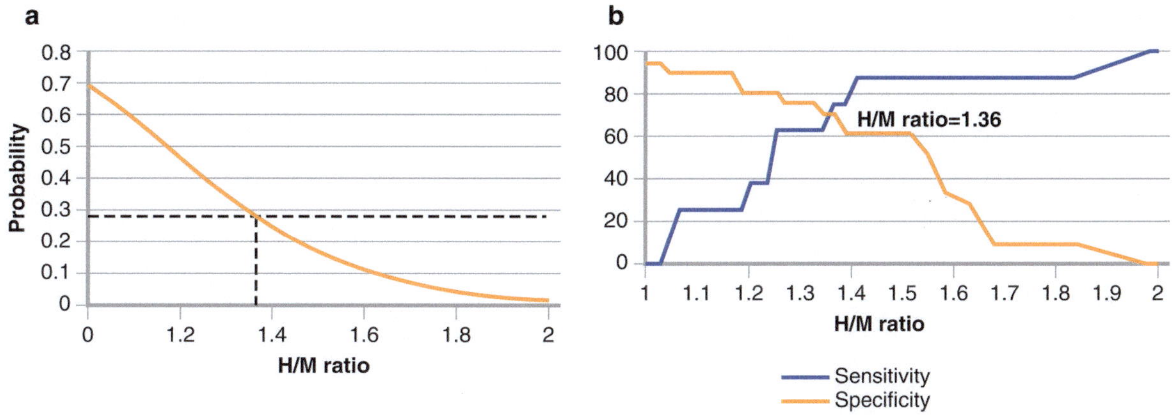

Figure 6-12. Receiver operating characteristic curves for the prediction of mortality or no response to CRT (**a**). The receiver operating characteristic curves showed a greater area under the curve for H/M ratio (before CRT). The optimal cutoff point of the H/M ratio was 1.36 (sensitivity, 75%; specificity, 71%) for the prediction of CRT response (**b**) (Adapted from Nishioka et al. [7]).

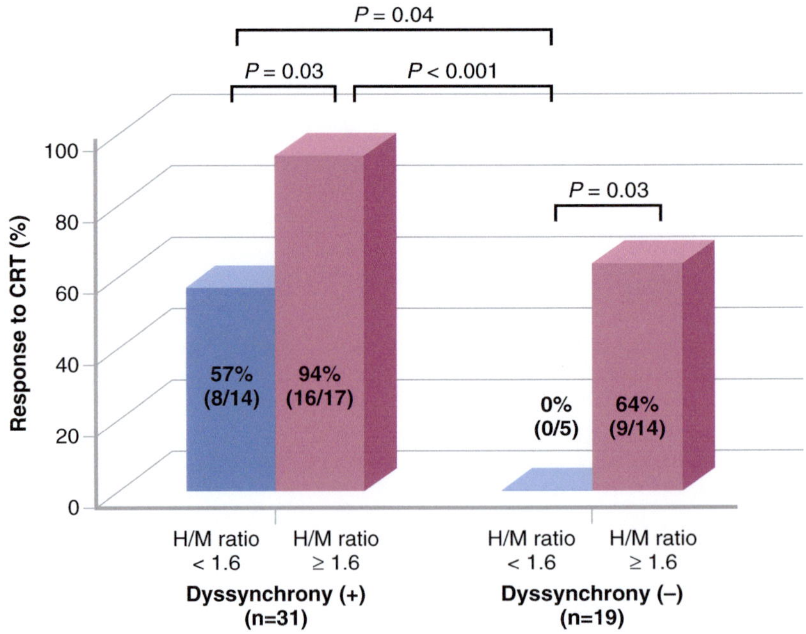

Figure 6-13. Bar graph showing the relationship between response rate to CRT and combined assessment of LV mechanical dyssynchrony, measured by speckle tracking echocardiography, and delayed H/M ratio measured by MIBG imaging. Patients with dyssynchrony and an H/M ratio ≥1.6 had a high degree of LV functional improvement, with a response rate of 94%. Patients without dyssynchrony and an H/M ratio <1.6, on the other hand, were more likely to show less LV functional improvement than the other patient subgroups. Thus, MIBG imaging combined with echocardiographic measurement of dyssynchrony can predict therapy response, and hence reverse remodeling, in patients undergoing CRT (Adapted from Tanaka et al. [8]).

Effects of Medical Therapy on Sympathetic Neuronal Imaging

Table 6-4. Summary of several published results assessing the effect of medications on cardiac sympathetic activity by using serial MIBG imaging.

Drug	Main imaging results
β-Blockers [9, 29]	Increase in late HMR, decrease in WR, and decrease in SPECT defect size
ACEIs/ARBs [30, 31]	Increase in late HMR, decrease in WR, and decrease in SPECT defect size
Aldosterone antagonists [32, 33]	Increase in late HMR, decrease in WR, and decrease in SPECT defect size
ATP-sensitive potassium channel openers [10, 34]	Increase in late HMR, decrease in WR, and decrease in SPECT defect size
Diuretics [35, 36]	Increase in late HMR, decrease in WR, and decrease in SPECT defect size
Calcium sensitizers [37]	Increase in HMR
Statins [38]	Increase in late HMR and decrease in WR
Amiodarone [11]	More decrease in WR and SPECT defect size than in the carvedilol-only group

Studies listed in this table, which for each medication are the two largest studies in which H/M MIBG uptake ratio (HMR) was calculated, generally demonstrated an increase in HMR and a decrease in WR in response to medical treatment, indicating improved sympathetic activity and hence, medication-induced sympathetic reverse remodeling. *ACEIs* angiotensin-converting enzyme inhibitors, *ARBs* angiotensin-receptor blockers, *ATP* adenosine triphosphate

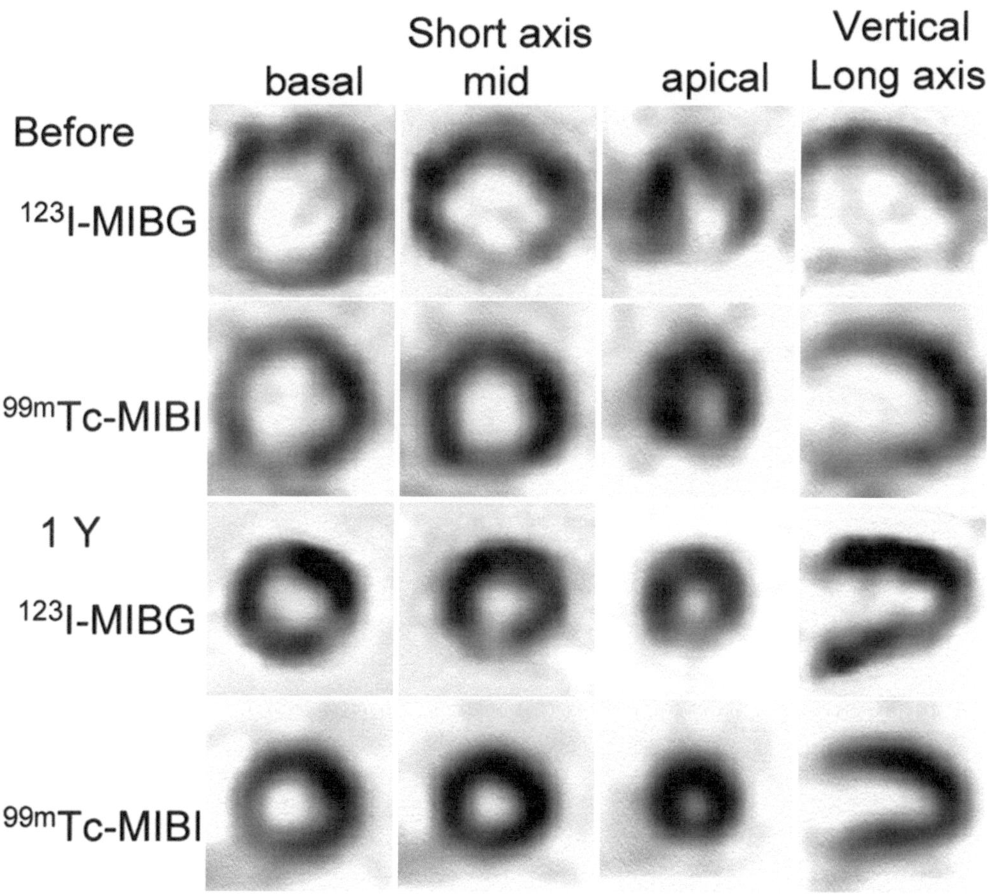

Figure 6-14. A representative case of MIBG and technetium-99 m methoxyisobutylisonitrile (^{99m}Tc-MIBI) SPECT images before and 1 year after carvedilol treatment. There is a decrease in LV chamber size, indicating carvedilol-induced reverse remodeling. Furthermore, the MIBG defect seen in the inferior wall decreased in both size and severity after treatment (Adapted from Toyama et al. [39]).

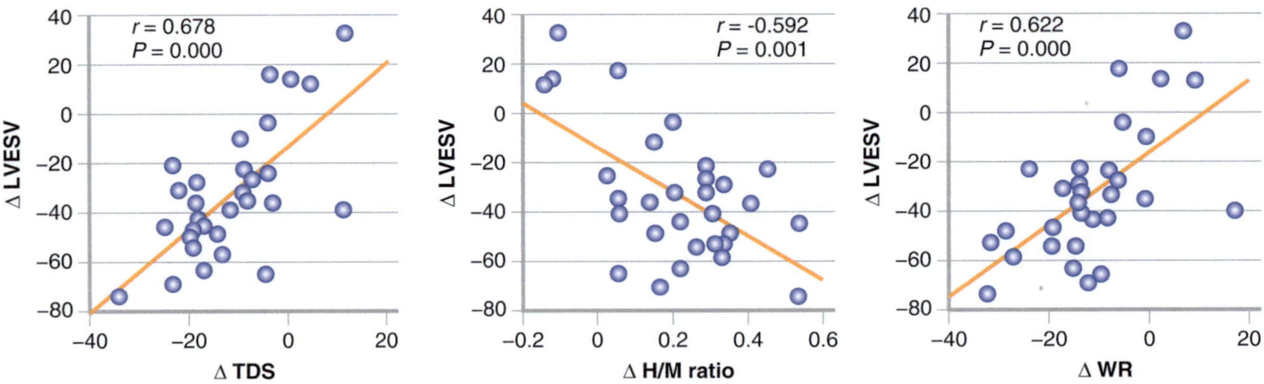

FIGURE 6-15. Correlations between the changes in MIBG scintigraphic findings and LV end-systolic volume (*LVESV*) after carvedilol treatment in 30 patients with dilated cardiomyopathy. There was a significant correlation between changes in MIBG scintigraphic parameters and those in LV parameters during treatment, indicating that the degree of sympathetic reverse remodeling measured by MIBG imaging reflects that of geometric reverse remodeling. *ΔLVESV* posttreatment LVESV minus pretreatment LVESV, *ΔTDS* posttreatment total defect score (*TDS*) minus pretreatment TDS, *ΔH/M ratio* posttreatment H/M ratio minus pretreatment H/M ratio, *ΔWR* posttreatment WR minus pretreatment WR (Adapted from Kasama et al. [29]).

Predicting Drug Response by Using Sympathetic Neuronal Imaging

Table 6-5. Summary of published results assessing MIBG imaging for predicting functional response to medical treatments.

Authors	Publication year	Drug	Main findings
Suwa et al. [40]	1997	β-Blocker	Late HMR >1.7 was a predictor of good functional response.
Fukuoka et al. [41]	1997	β-Blocker	Low regional WR on SPECT images at 1 month of treatment was a predictor of subsequent improvement in LV function at 3 months.
Kakuchi et al. [42]	1999	β-Blocker	Patients with successful β-blocker induction had a higher HMR and lower WR than those with induction failure.
Choi [43]	2001	β-Blocker	Low WR was a predictor of subsequent functional recovery.

The data indicate that preserved sympathetic innervation and/or normal or near normal sympathetic nerve activity, as reflected by a high H/M uptake ratio (HMR) and/or low WR, predict subsequent functional improvement and thus reverse remodeling before or during the early stages of β-blocker therapy

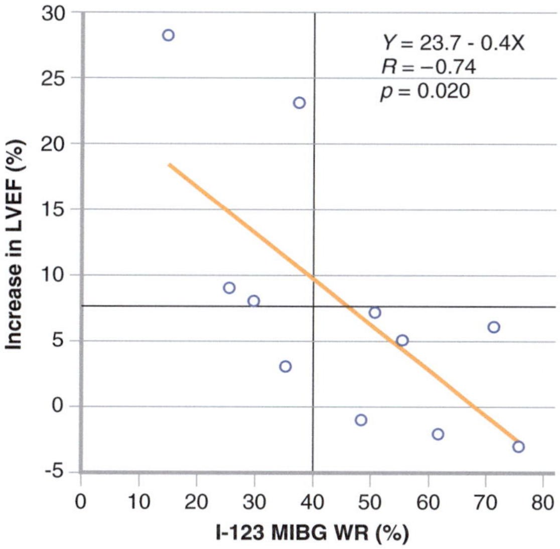

Figure 6-16. Scatterplot showing the relationship between myocardial MIBG WR and increases in LVEF between baseline and 1 year after carvedilol therapy. WR showed a significant inverse correlation with LVEF increase ($R = -0.74$), indicating that baseline MIBG imaging may predict β-blocker–induced functional recovery and reverse remodeling (Adapted from Choi et al. [43]).

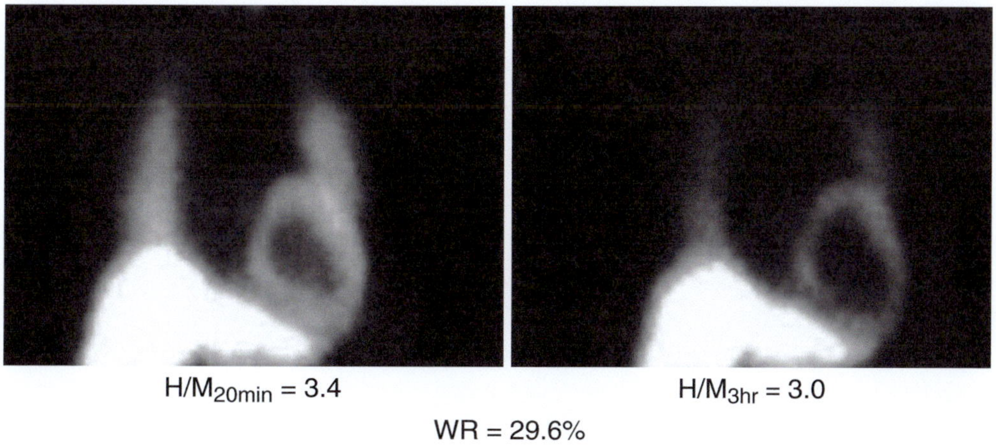

Figure 6-17. Early and late planar MIBG images of a patient with dilated cardiomyopathy. This patient showed a low WR and preserved H/M ratio, measured by MIBG imaging, and a subsequent increase in LVEF, from 21 to 29% 1 year after carvedilol therapy (Adapted from Choi et al. [43]).

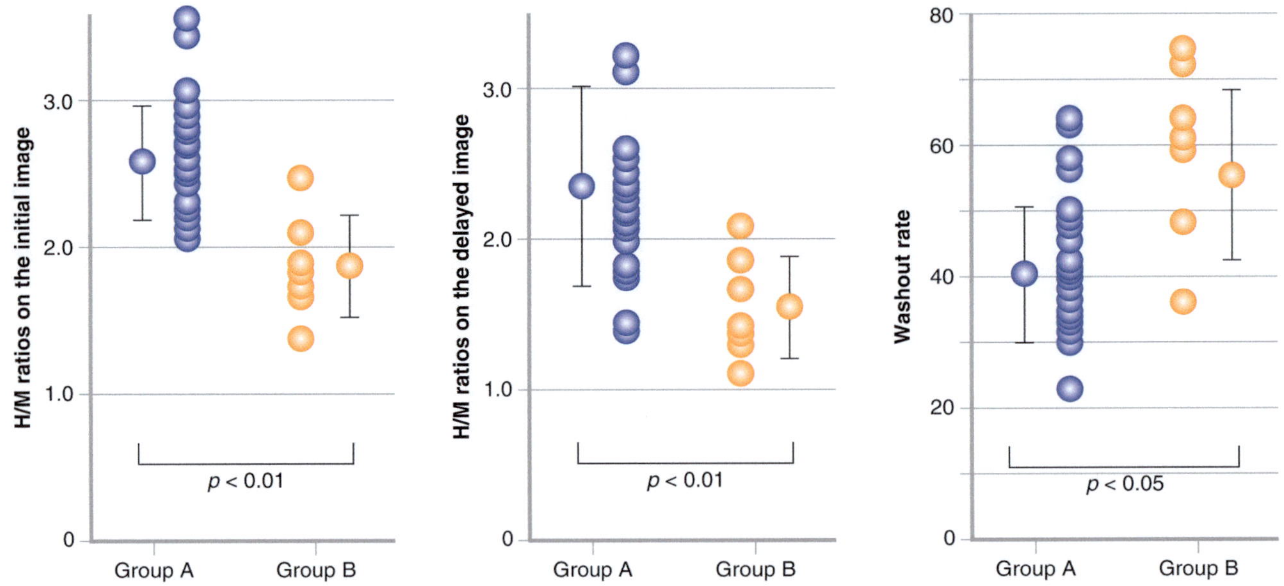

FIGURE 6-18. Baseline H/M ratios and WRs in patients with successful β-blocker induction (group A, *blue circles*) and in those with induction failure (group B, *orange circles*). Successful therapy induction was associated with higher H/M ratios and low WRs (Adapted from Kakuchi et al. [42]).

Prognostic Value of Sympathetic Reverse Remodeling

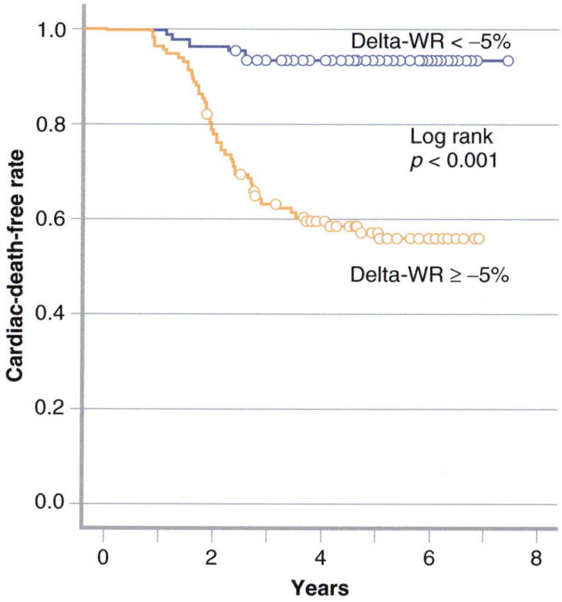

Figure 6-19. Kaplan–Meier survival curves of cardiac death–free rates in patients with chronic HF divided into two groups according to Delta-WR (difference in WR between baseline and 6 months), measured by serial MIBG imaging. Patients with a Delta-WR ≥25% had significantly greater cardiac death rates than their counterparts, indicating that worsening in MIBG WR is a marker of poor survival. Thus, sympathetic remodeling or sympathetic reverse remodeling measured by serial MIBG imaging may directly be related to prognosis and may serve as a clinical end point (Adapted from Kasama et al. [12]).

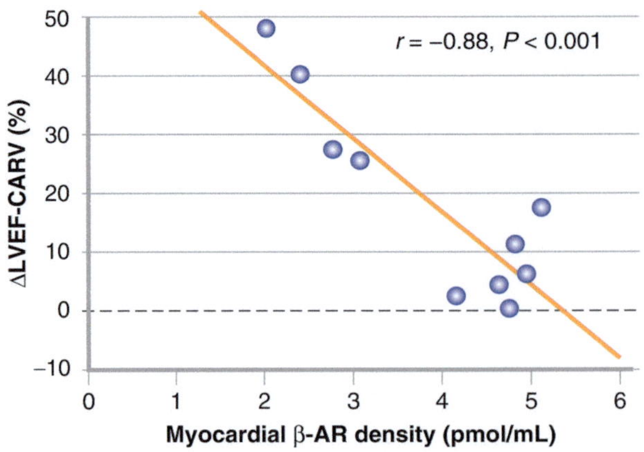

Figure 6-20. Relationship between carvedilol-induced changes in LVEF and baseline myocardial β-adrenergic receptor (β-AR) density measured by ^{11}C-CGP12177 positron emission tomography (PET) in patients with dilated cardiomyopathy. Myocardial β-AR density is closely related to improvement in LVEF and hence carvedilol-induced reverse remodeling, indicating that β-AR imaging with ^{11}C-CGP12177 PET may provide a clue for HF management (Adapted from Naya et al. [13]).

References

1. Mann DL, Barger PM, Burkhoff D. Myocardial recovery and the failing heart: myth, magic, or molecular target? J Am Coll Cardiol. 2012;60:2465–72.
2. Kass DA, Baughman KL, Pak PH, et al. Reverse remodeling from cardiomyoplasty in human heart failure. External constraint versus active assist. Circulation. 1995;91:2314–8.
3. Levin HR, Oz MC, Chen JM, et al. Reversal of chronic ventricular dilation in patients with end-stage cardiomyopathy by prolonged mechanical unloading. Circulation. 1995;91:2717–20.
4. Kramer DG, Trikalinos TA, Kent DM, et al. Quantitative evaluation of drug or device effects on ventricular remodeling as predictors of therapeutic effects on mortality in patients with heart failure and reduced ejection fraction: a meta-analytic approach. J Am Coll Cardiol. 2010;56:392–406.
5. Koitabashi N, Kass DA. Reverse remodeling in heart failure--mechanisms and therapeutic opportunities. Nat Rev Cardiol. 2012;9:147–57.
6. Drakos SG, Athanasoulis T, Malliaras KG, et al. Myocardial sympathetic innervation and long-term left ventricular mechanical unloading. JACC Cardiovasc Imaging. 2010;3:64–70.
7. Nishioka SA, MartinelliFilho M, Brandao SC, et al. Cardiac sympathetic activity pre and post resynchronization therapy evaluated by 123I-MIBG myocardial scintigraphy. J Nucl Cardiol. 2007;14:852–9.
8. Tanaka H, Tatsumi K, Fujiwara S, et al. Effect of left ventricular dyssynchrony on cardiac sympathetic activity in heart failure patients with wide QRS duration. Circ J. 2012;76:382–9.
9. Cohen-Solal A, Rouzet F, Berdeaux A, et al. Effects of carvedilol on myocardial sympathetic innervation in patients with chronic heart failure. J Nucl Med. 2005;46:1796–803.
10. Kasama S, Toyama T, Sumino H, et al. Long-term nicorandil therapy improves cardiac sympathetic nerve activity after reperfusion therapy in patients with first acute myocardial infarction. J Nucl Med. 2007;48:1676–82.
11. Toyama T, Hoshizaki H, Yoshimura Y, et al. Combined therapy with carvedilol and amiodarone is more effective in improving cardiac symptoms, function, and sympathetic nerve activity in patients with dilated cardiomyopathy: comparison with carvedilol therapy alone. J Nucl Cardiol. 2008;15:57–64.
12. Kasama S, Toyama T, Sumino H, et al. Prognostic value of serial cardiac 123I-MIBG imaging in patients with stabilized chronic heart failure and reduced left ventricular ejection fraction. J Nucl Med. 2008;49:907–14.
13. Naya M, Tsukamoto T, Morita K, et al. Myocardial beta-adrenergic receptor density assessed by 11C-CGP12177 PET predicts improvement of cardiac function after carvedilol treatment in patients with idiopathic dilated cardiomyopathy. J Nucl Med. 2009;50:220–5.
14. Drakos SG, Kfoury AG, Stehlik J, et al. Bridge to recovery: understanding the disconnect between clinical and biological outcomes. Circulation. 2012;126:230–41.
15. Imamura Y, Ando H, Mitsuoka W, et al. Iodine-123 metaiodobenzylguanidine images reflect intense myocardial adrenergic nervous activity in congestive heart failure independent of underlying cause. J Am Coll Cardiol. 1995;26:1594–9.
16. Bengel FM, Permanetter B, Ungerer M, et al. Relationship between altered sympathetic innervation, oxidative metabolism and contractile function in the cardiomyopathic human heart; a non-invasive study using positron emission tomography. Eur Heart J. 2001;22:1594–600.
17. Aoki H, Matsunari I, Nomura Y, et al. Myocardial sympathetic innervation, function, and oxidative metabolism in non-infarcted myocardium in patients with prior myocardial infarction. Ann Nucl Med. 2013;27:523–31.
18. Bristow MR, Ginsburg R, Minobe W, et al. Decreased catecholamine sensitivity and beta-adrenergic-receptor density in failing human hearts. N Engl J Med. 1982;307:205–11.
19. Tsukamoto T, Morita K, Naya M, et al. Decreased myocardial beta-adrenergic receptor density in relation to increased sympathetic tone in patients with nonischemic cardiomyopathy. J Nucl Med. 2007;48:1777–82.
20. Ohte N, Narita H, Iida A, et al. Cardiac beta-adrenergic receptor density and myocardial systolic function in the remote noninfarcted region after prior myocardial infarction with left ventricular remodelling. Eur J Nucl Med Mol Imaging. 2012;39:1246–53.
21. Miyagawa S, Sawa Y, Fukushima N, et al. Analysis of sympathetic nerve activity in end-stage cardiomyopathy patients receiving left ventricular support. J Heart Lung Transplant. 2001;20:1181–7.
22. George RS, Birks EJ, Cheetham A, et al. The effect of long-term left ventricular assist device support on myocardial sympathetic activity in patients with non-ischaemic dilated cardiomyopathy. Eur J Heart Fail. 2013;15:1035–43.
23. Erol-Yilmaz A, Verberne HJ, Schrama TA, et al. Cardiac resynchronization induces favorable neurohumoral changes. Pacing Clin Electrophysiol. 2005;28:304–10.
24. Gould PA, Kong G, Kalff V, et al. Improvement in cardiac adrenergic function post biventricular pacing for heart failure. Europace. 2007;9:751–6.
25. Burri H, Sunthorn H, Somsen A, et al. Improvement in cardiac sympathetic nerve activity in responders to resynchronization therapy. Europace. 2008;10:374–8.
26. Cha YM, Oh J, Miyazaki C, et al. Cardiac resynchronization therapy upregulates cardiac autonomic control. J Cardiovasc Electrophysiol. 2008;19:1045–52.
27. Cha YM, Chareonthaitawee P, Dong YX, et al. Cardiac sympathetic reserve and response to cardiac resynchronization therapy. Circ Heart Fail. 2011;4:339–44.
28. Shinohara T, Takahashi N, Saito S, et al. Effect of cardiac resynchronization therapy on cardiac sympathetic nervous dysfunction and serum C-reactive protein level. Pacing Clin Electrophysiol. 2011;34:1225–30.
29. Kasama S, Toyama T, Hatori T, et al. Evaluation of cardiac sympathetic nerve activity and left ventricular remodelling in patients with dilated cardiomyopathy on the treatment containing carvedilol. Eur Heart J. 2007;28:989–95.
30. Kasama S, Toyama T, Kumakura H, et al. Effects of candesartan on cardiac sympathetic nerve activity in patients with congestive heart failure and preserved left ventricular ejection fraction. J Am Coll Cardiol. 2005;45:661–7.
31. Kasama S, Toyama T, Hatori T, et al. Comparative effects of valsartan and enalapril on cardiac sympathetic nerve activity and plasma brain natriuretic peptide in patients with congestive heart failure. Heart. 2006;92:625–30.
32. Kasama S, Toyama T, Sumino H, et al. Additive effects of spironolactone and candesartan on cardiac sympathetic nerve activity and left ventricular remodeling in patients with congestive heart failure. J Nucl Med. 2007;48:1993–2000.
33. Kasama S, Toyama T, Sumino H, et al. Effects of mineralocorticoid receptor antagonist spironolactone on cardiac sympathetic nerve activity and prognosis in patients with chronic heart failure. Int J Cardiol. 2013;167:244–9.
34. Kasama S, Toyama T, Iwasaki T, et al. Effects of oral nicorandil therapy on sympathetic nerve activity and cardiac events in patients with chronic heart failure: subanalysis of our previous report using propensity score matching. Eur J Nucl Med Mol Imaging. 2014;41:144–54.

35. Kasama S, Toyama T, Hatori T, et al. Effects of torasemide on cardiac sympathetic nerve activity and left ventricular remodelling in patients with congestive heart failure. Heart. 2006;92:1434–40.
36. Hisatake S, Nanjo S, Fujimoto S, et al. Comparative analysis of the therapeutic effects of long-acting and short-acting loop diuretics in the treatment of chronic heart failure using (123) I-metaiodobenzylguanidinescintigraphy. Eur J Heart Fail. 2011;13:892–8.
37. Takeda N, Hayashi Y, Arino T, et al. Effect of pimobendan in patients with chronic heart failure. Exp Clin Cardiol. 2001;6:195–9.
38. Tsutamoto T, Sakai H, Ibe K, et al. Effect of atorvastatin vs. rosuvastatin on cardiac sympathetic nerve activity in non-diabetic patients with dilated cardiomyopathy. Circ J. 2011;75:2160–6.
39. Toyama T, Hoshizaki H, Seki R, et al. Efficacy of carvedilol treatment on cardiac function and cardiac sympathetic nerve activity in patients with dilated cardiomyopathy: comparison with metoprolol therapy. J Nucl Med. 2003;44:1604–11.
40. Suwa M, Otake Y, Moriguchi A, et al. Iodine-123 metaiodobenzylguanidine myocardial scintigraphy for prediction of response to beta-blocker therapy in patients with dilated cardiomyopathy. Am Heart J. 1997;133:353–8.
41. Fukuoka S, Hayashida K, Hirose Y, et al. Use of iodine-123 metaiodobenzylguanidine myocardial imaging to predict the effectiveness of beta-blocker therapy in patients with dilated cardiomyopathy. Eur J Nucl Med. 1997;24:523–9.
42. Kakuchi H, Sasaki T, Ishida Y, et al. Clinical usefulness of 123I meta-iodobenzylguanidine imaging in predicting the effectiveness of beta blockers for patients with idiopathic dilated cardiomyopathy before and soon after treatment. Heart. 1999;81:148–52.
43. Choi JY, Lee KH, Hong KP, et al. Iodine-123 MIBG imaging before treatment of heart failure with carvedilol to predict improvement of left ventricular function and exercise capacity. J Nucl Cardiol. 2001;8:4–9.

7 Neuronal Imaging, Ventricular Arrhythmias, and Device Therapy in Heart Failure

David M. Harris and Myron C. Gerson

Since the 1970s, cardiovascular mortality has decreased significantly as the result of identification and modification of cardiac risk factors, improvement in cardiovascular treatments, and advances in diagnostic imaging. One major advance was the introduction of the implantable cardiac defibrillator (ICD), which substantially increased survival in patients with cardiomyopathy. Unfortunately, however, accurate identification of patients who will develop sudden cardiac death (SCD) remains elusive. Many patients who meet criteria for ICD implantation never require device-administered therapy for ventricular tachyarrhythmias. Conversely, most patients who die suddenly do not meet current guideline criteria for ICD placement before their event. Therefore, a noninvasive test that can identify at-risk patients prospectively would be ideal. Data are mounting showing that radionuclide imaging with iodine-123 metaiodobenzylguanidine (^{123}I-MIBG) for single-photon emission computed tomography (SPECT) or carbon-11 hydroxyephedrine (^{11}C-HED) for positron emission tomography (PET) may provide important prognostic information regarding the development of SCD and might be used to risk stratify patients.

According to current estimates, the incidence of SCD in the United States ranges from 300,000 to 350,000 patients annually [1]. Ventricular tachycardia (VT) and ventricular fibrillation (VF) remain the leading etiology for arrhythmic mortality in patients with heart failure [2]. Initial pharmacologic therapy for SCD was based on the suppression of ventricular arrhythmias identified on Holter monitoring or provocative electrophysiology testing. Although some pharmacologic treatment strategies, such as amiodarone, have been shown to decrease arrhythmogenic deaths [3, 4], other treatments, including encainide, flecainide, moricizine, and sotalol, have been shown to increase mortality [5–7]. Additionally, pharmacologic therapy often is limited by drug toxicity or side effects and has a limited ability to decrease all-cause mortality in post–myocardial infarction patients. The development of ICDs profoundly improved survival for patients with SCD. In patients with ischemic cardiomyopathy in the second Multicenter Automatic Defibrillator Implantation Trial (MADIT II), ICD therapy decreased the relative risk of all-cause mortality by nearly 30% over 30 months in patients with a left ventricular ejection fraction (LVEF) <30% [8]. In the Sudden Cardiac Death in Heart Failure Trial (SCD-HeFT), ICD therapy was superior to optimal medical therapy with amiodarone [9]. Based in large part on these and other trials [10–12], current guidelines provide recommendations for an ICD for secondary prevention (after a life-threatening ventricular arrhythmia) or for primary prevention (optimally medically treated patients with New York Heart Association [NYHA] class II or III heart failure and an LVEF <35% or NYHA class I and an LVEF <30%) [13]. Although LVEF is an important predictor of SCD [8], it is imperfect, as only 35% of patients receive appropriate ventricular therapy within 3 years of implantation [14] and most SCDs occur in patients with an ejection fraction >35% [15].

V. Dilsizian, J. Narula (eds.), *Atlas of Cardiac Innervation*, DOI 10.1007/978-3-319-45800-7_7

Some guidelines recommend T-wave alternans, signal-averaged electrocardiography, baroreflex sensitivity (BRS), heart rate variability (HRV), and heart rate turbulence as potentially useful tools for diagnosing ventricular arrhythmias and risk stratifying patients [16]. Additionally, these guidelines recommend use of imaging modalities to investigate underlying structural abnormalities, cardiac function, or ischemia. Unfortunately, these techniques have not been as robust as previously hoped in predicting life-threatening arrhythmias.

Through the use of novel radiotracers, radionuclide imaging may further improve the risk stratification of patients at risk for SCD. This chapter outlines the background of existing imaging methods that have assessed ischemia and scar as markers for SCD. It then reviews the current literature supporting SPECT and PET sympathetic neural imaging for evaluating SCD and ICD placement.

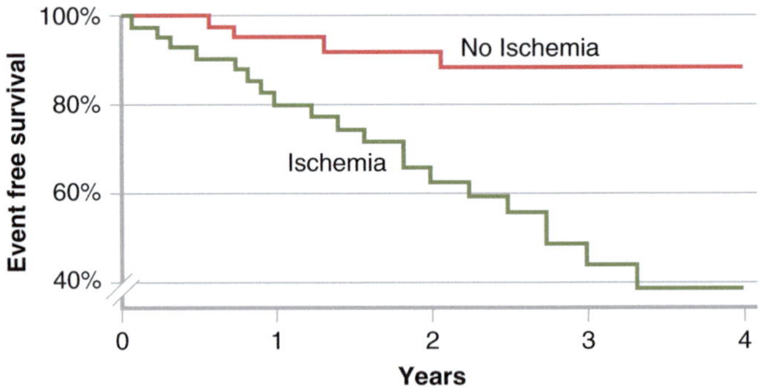

Figure 7-1. Myocardial ischemia is a well-established risk factor for the development of VT and SCD. In 90 patients who received an ICD, Elhendy et al. [17] showed by Kaplan–Meier analysis that myocardial ischemia detected by stress echocardiography was an independent predictor of SCD or appropriate ICD shock. Yet, myocardial ischemia is only one predictor of SCD. In a meta-analysis of patients with coronary artery disease and left ventricular dysfunction who underwent revascularization [18], those with nonviable myocardium had a significantly higher mortality than those with revascularized viable tissue, suggesting the importance of other factors, including myocardial scar (Adapted from Elhendy et al. [17].).

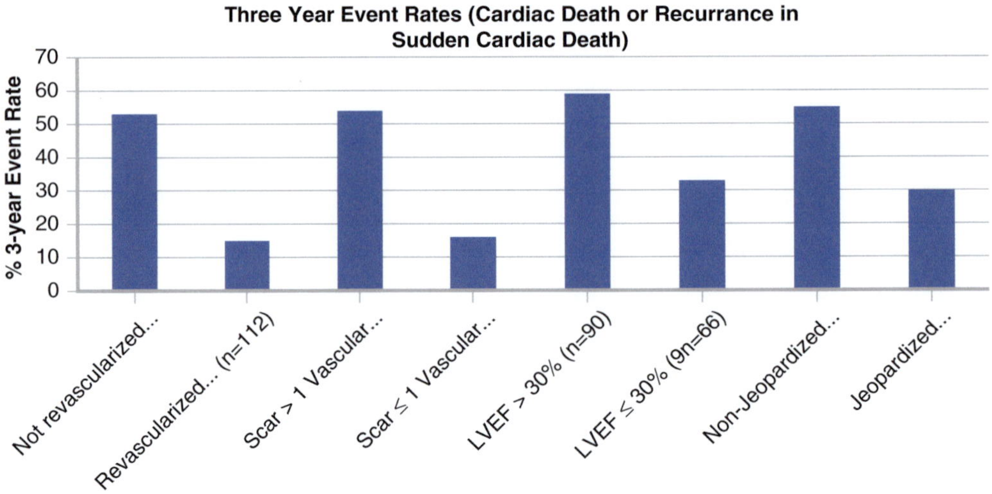

Figure 7-2. Myocardial remodeling after an infarction leads to the formation of scar tissue with islands of preserved myocytes. This remodeling allows development of conduction block and re-entrant circuits located within the scar, which act as a nidus for ventricular arrhythmias [19]. Cardiac magnetic resonance imaging (MRI), with its high spatial resolution, has helped detect previously unrecognized scar by using delayed gadolinium enhancement imaging and has been used for risk assessment in patients with or without ischemia [20, 21]. Scar size as determined by MRI is a predictor of VT during electrophysiologic induction testing [22], and the extent of tissue heterogeneity correlates with induction of ventricular arrhythmias [23] and spontaneous ventricular arrhythmias [24]. This figure shows the 3-year rate of cardiac death or recurrent SCD from a SPECT myocardial perfusion imaging study by van der Burg et al. [25]. It characterizes the association of scar burden, presence of jeopardized myocardium, and ejection fraction with cardiovascular events in 153 SCD survivors. On multivariable analysis, the only independent predictors of arrhythmic death were LVEF <30% and the presence of extensive scar tissue (Adapted from van der Burg et al. [25]).

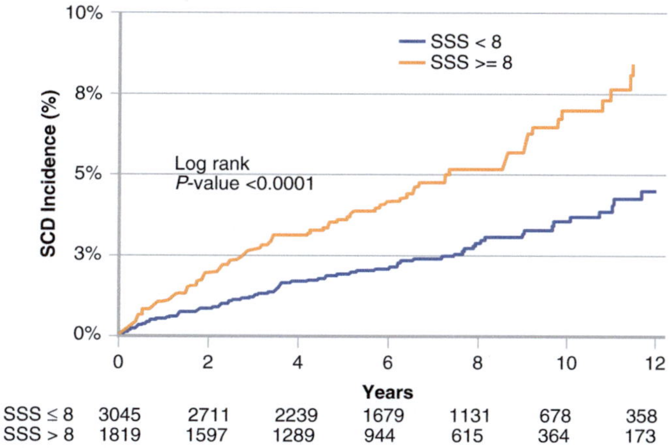

Figur 7-3. The combination of a large scar burden and the presence of ischemia has a synergistic effect and increases mortality and SCD [23] compared with either factor alone. In a cohort of more than 6000 patients with coronary artery disease who were evaluated with SPECT myocardial perfusion imaging, Piccini et al. [26] showed that infarct with ischemia, as represented by the summed stress score (SSS), was significantly associated with SCD. Compared with clinical variables, LVEF contributed 48.3% of the prognostic model content for estimating SCD. By comparison, the combination of ejection fraction and SSS contributed 51.6% of the prognostic model content for estimating SCD, with the addition of SSS providing a modest improvement in information content. This figure shows Kaplan–Meier curves using a SPECT SSS of 8 in predicting SCD. SSS-predicted SCD was independent of LVEF and clinical variables [27] (Adapted from Piccini et al. [27]).

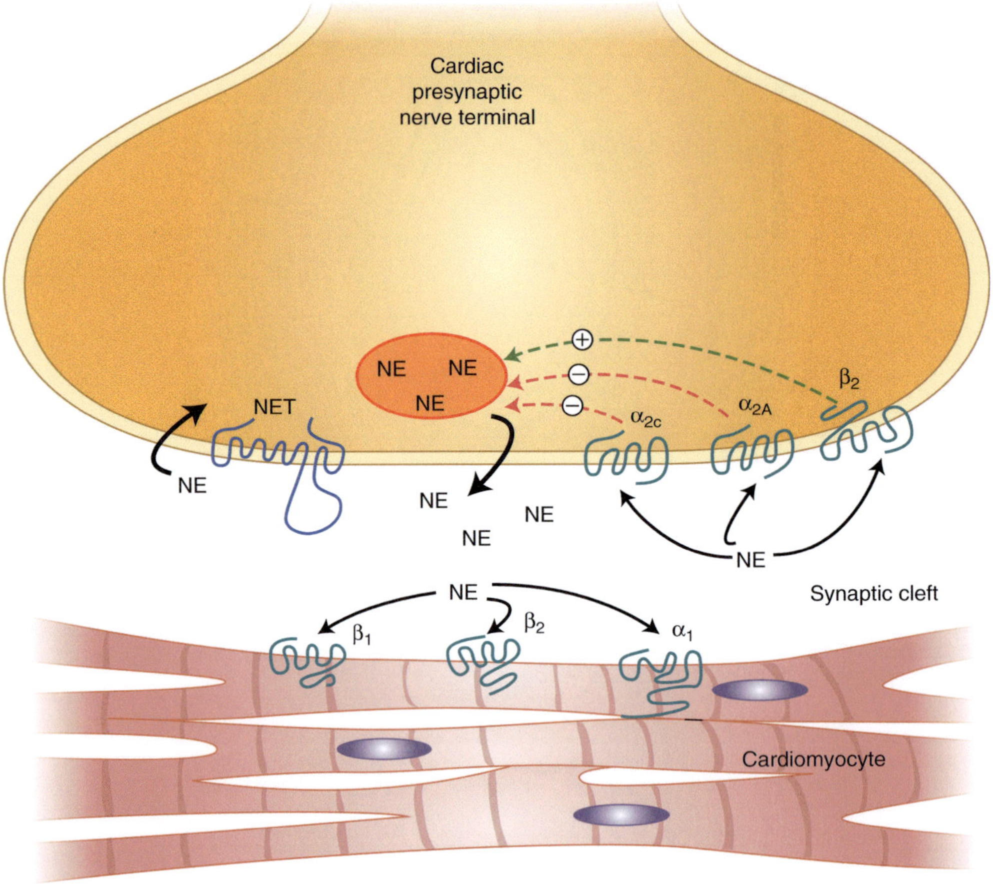

Figure 7-4. Although perfusion, scar, and ejection fraction have been beneficial in evaluating patients at risk for SCD, additional discrimination is required because most patients with an ICD never require defibrillation and many with a normal ejection fraction develop SCD. The introduction of ^{123}I-MIBG has facilitated investigation into myocardial sympathetic innervation and function. ^{123}I-MIBG allows direct analysis of cardiac sympathetic function, as it is structurally similar to norepinephrine (NE) and is transported into the cardiac sympathetic neurons by human NE transporter 1 (hNET1), contained on the presynaptic nerve terminus [28]. ^{123}I-MIBG requires an intact cardiac sympathetic nervous system for normal uptake, is stored in the presynaptic vesicles, and is released by stimulation from NE [29]. Experimental manipulation of cardiac sympathetic function alters MIBG uptake and distribution [30–33]. In both ischemic and dilated cardiomyopathy, increased sympathetic nerve activity results in a decrease in the number and function of myocardial β-adrenergic receptors [34, 35]. Chronically increased catecholamine levels trigger a cascade of events leading to altered β-adrenergic receptor regulation, impaired NE reuptake and calcium regulation, depletion of presynaptic NE stores, and cardiac fibrosis and remodeling. This figure illustrates the synaptic cleft, showing the uptake and regulation of NE. ^{123}I- MIBG follows the same uptake and regulation as those of NE, but is not metabolized by monoamine oxidase or catechol-O-methyltransferase.

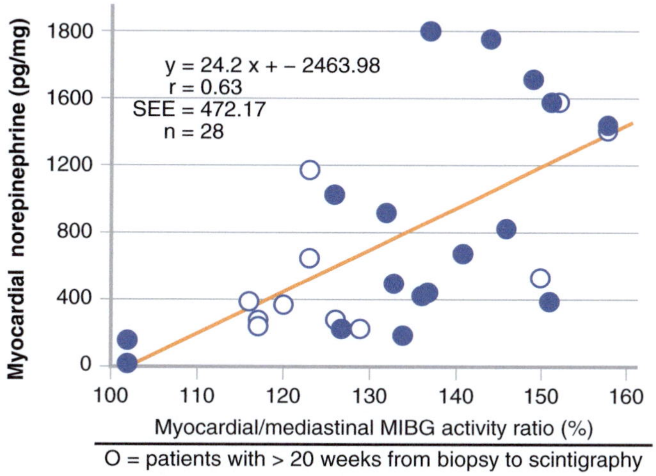

FIGURE 7-5. Planar image acquisition after ^{123}I-MIBG injection enables evaluation of sympathetic activation. Early and delayed measurement of the heart-to-mediastinum (H/M) ratio assesses the initial uptake and washout of the tracer. In 28 patients with NYHA I to IV dilated cardiomyopathy, the H/M ratio correlated with myocardial NE concentration on cardiac biopsies. *SEE* standard error of the estimate (Adapted from Schofer et al. [36]).

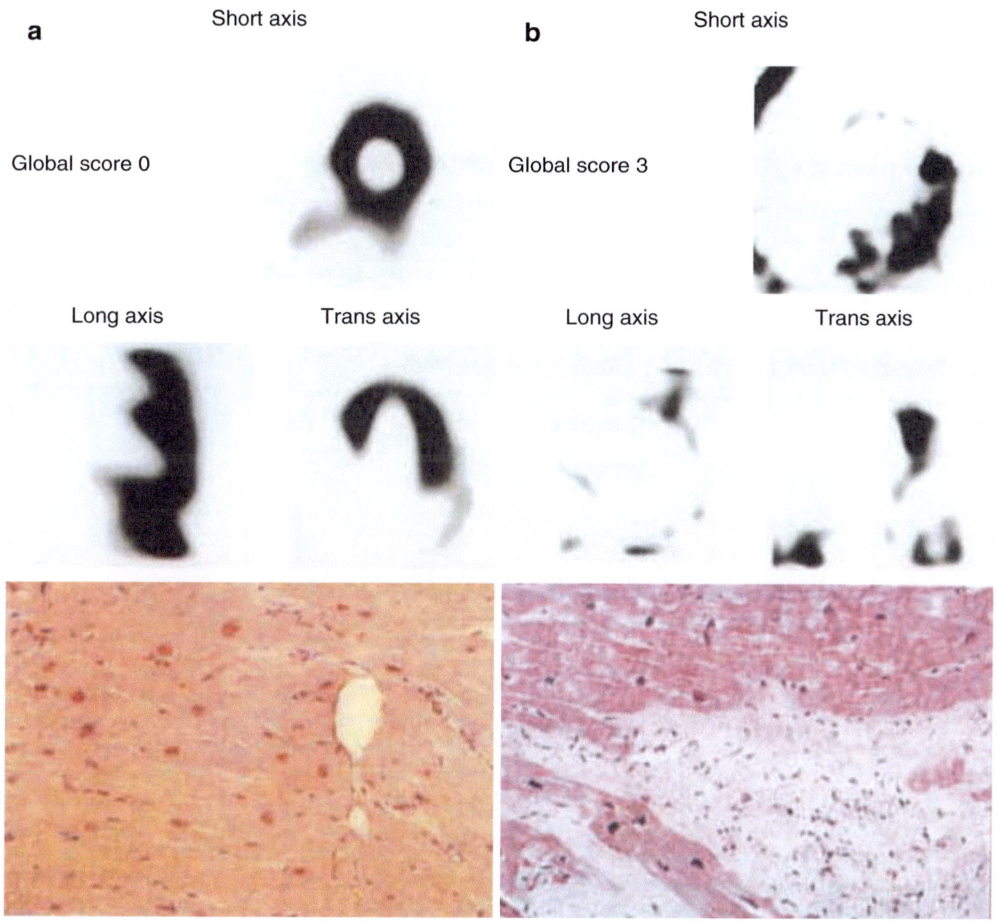

FIGURE 7-6. Fibrotic myocardial tissue has reduced neuronal NE content and decreased ^{123}I-MIBG uptake. Murata et al. [37] showed that ^{123}I-MIBG uptake in 24 patients with dilated cardiomyopathy, as measured by a 0 to 3 grading system for normal to no uptake, respectively, correlated with the level of histologic abnormalities, including myocyte hypertrophy, myocardial fibrotic change, myocyte degeneration, mononuclear cell infiltration, and myocyte disarray [37]. This figure shows two patients, one with normal uptake and a global score of 0 (**a**) and one with severely decreased uptake and a global score of 3 (**b**) (From Murata et al. [37]; with permission).

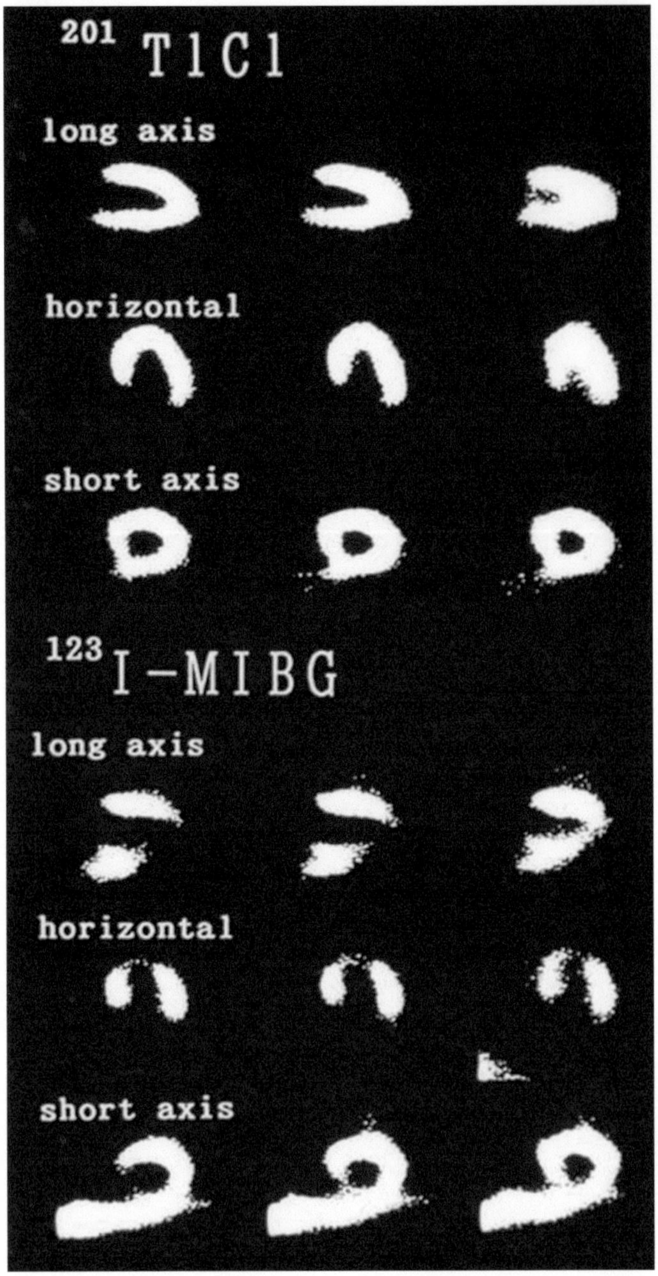

Figure 7-7. A substrate for ventricular arrhythmias in patients with coronary artery disease is the presence of myocardium that is denervated but remains viable after an acute coronary event. The extent of decreased myocardial ^{123}I-MIBG uptake has been shown to extend beyond the infarcted territory and to be present after an ischemic insult without persistent perfusion abnormalities [38]. This innervation–perfusion mismatch likely represents the at-risk myocardium and has been characterized as a marker for myocardial ischemic memory [39]. These areas of decreased ^{123}I-MIBG uptake represent denervated myocardium, which is at an increased risk for augmented early afterdepolarizations in response to catecholamines [40] and increased arrhythmogenicity [41]. As a marker of myocardial fibrosis, reduced ^{123}I-MIBG H/M ratio has been correlated with reduced LVEF [**36**]. With its relationship to myocardial fibrosis, LVEF, peri-infarction ischemia, and electrically abnormal myocardium, the extent and distribution of reduced ^{123}I-MIBG in the myocardium has consistently predicted SCD. The figure displays thallium myocardial perfusion images and ^{123}I-MIBG images obtained after resolution of a 6-h episode of ischemic chest pain. The perfusion images are normal, but the ^{123}I-MIBG images show a defect predominantly in the apical, anterior, and inferior walls. On left heart catheterization, there were 75% left anterior descending and right coronary artery lesions [39]. ^{201}*TlCl* thallium-201 chloride (From Tomoda et al. [39]; with permission).

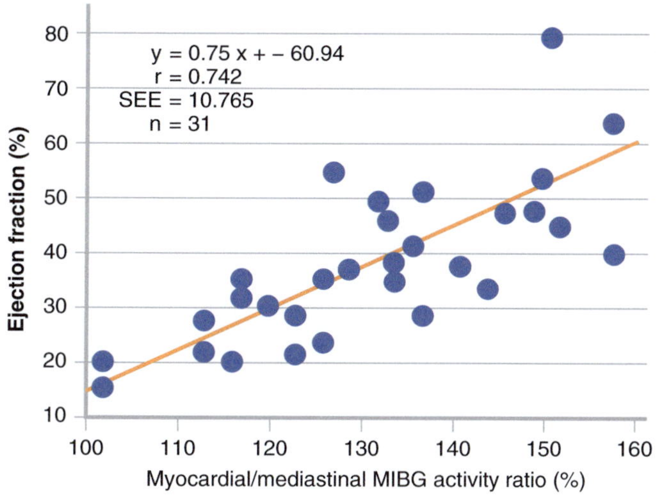

Figure 7-8. As a marker of myocardial fibrosis, ^{123}I-MIBG H/M ratio is directly correlated with reduced LVEF [**36**]. *SEE* standard error of the estimate (Adapted from Schofer et al. [**36**]).

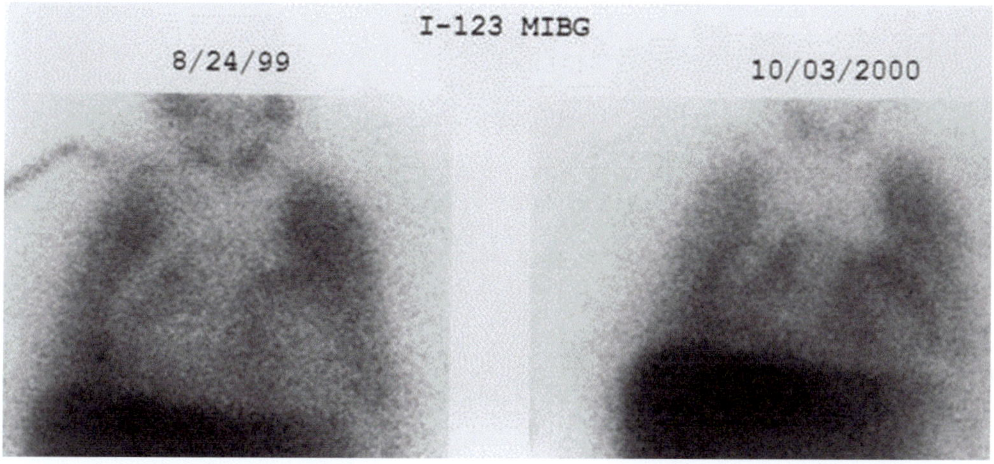

Figure 7-9. During recent decades, the mortality from heart failure has decreased because of earlier and better therapies, including pharmacologic treatments, revascularization, and resynchronization. Intuitively, as clinical status improves with treatment, MIBG uptake and washout also should improve. In 2002, Gerson et al. [**42**] studied 22 patients with idiopathic cardiomyopathy by using ^{123}I-MIBG scintigraphy before and after carvedilol treatment. Ten patients had severe myocardial sympathetic impairment with an H/M ratio <1.4. In this group, LVEF increased from 25.4 to 37.3% with a concomitant increase in H/M ratio from 1.26 to 1.39 [**42**]. Other investigators reported similar responses with β-blockers [**43, 44**]. Improvement in ^{123}I-MIBG H/M ratio also has been documented in response to antiarrhythmic therapy with amiodarone [**45–47**]. Whether the presence or absence of a favorable response of cardiac neuronal measurements to guideline-based heart failure therapies can stratify risk for sudden cardiac death needs further documentation. Shown here are planar ^{123}I MIBG images from a patient with heart failure before and after treatment with carvedilol. There is a visually apparent increase in myocardial ^{123}I-MIBG uptake 10 months after the initiation of treatment. *H* heart, *M* mediastinum (From Gerson et al. [**42**]).

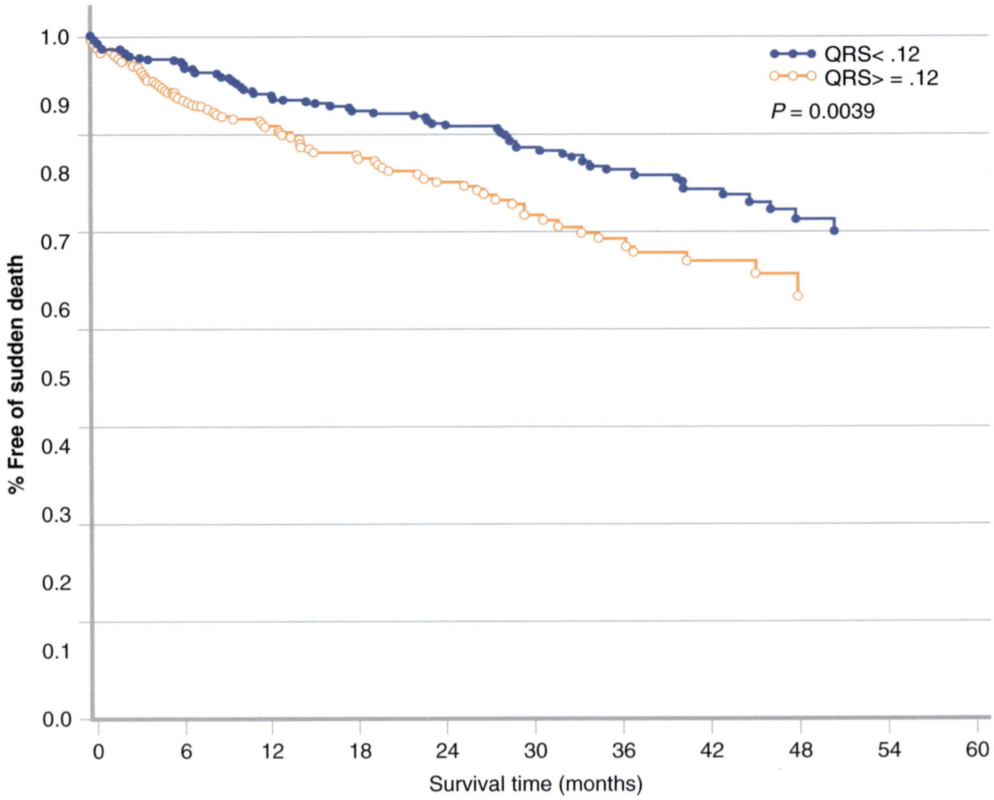

Figure 7-10. Patients with systolic heart failure, wide QRS complexes, and a left bundle branch block pattern are at an increased risk for SCD and overall mortality compared with patients with heart failure and a narrow QRS complex [**48**]. Cardiac resynchronization therapy (CRT) has been shown to lead to a reduction in SCD and a 36% relative risk reduction in overall mortality, compared with medical therapy alone [**49**] (Adapted from Iuliano et al. [**48**]).

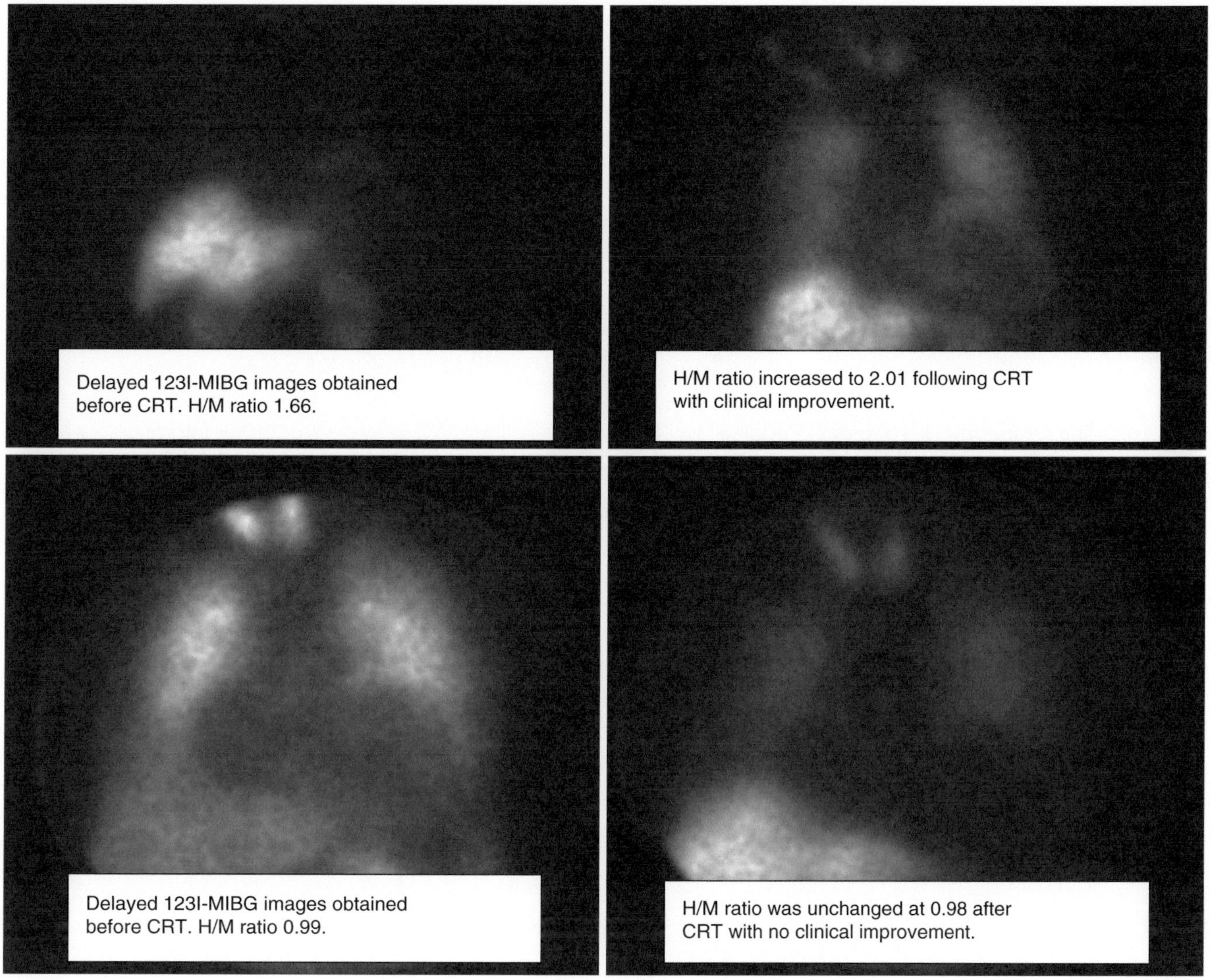

Figure 7-11. Delayed ^{123}I-MIBG images obtained before and after CRT. In the patient in the upper images, who had a favorable clinical response to resynchronization therapy, the H/M ratio before CRT was 1.66 (*left*) and increased to 2.01 after resynchronization (*right*). The lower images are from a patient with no clinical improvement after CRT, with an H/M ratio of 0.99 before (*left*) and 0.98 after therapy (*right*). Nishioka et al. [**50**] showed that the ^{123}I-MIBG H/M ratio and washout rate are associated with response to resynchronization therapy and that the H/M ratio may be useful in predicting which patients will respond to CRT (From Nishioka et al. [**50**]).

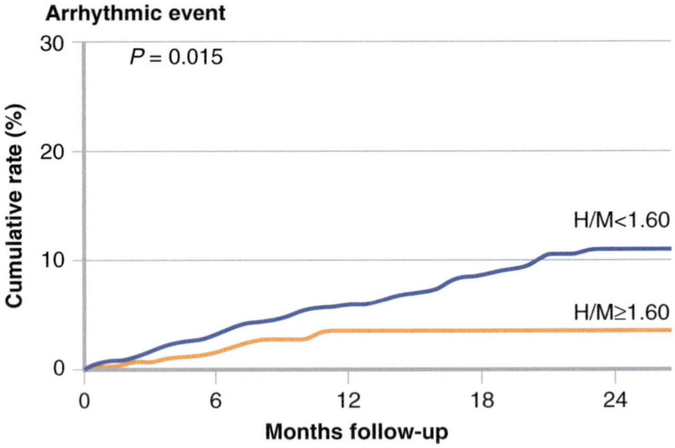

FIGURE 7-12. The AdreView Myocardial Imaging for Risk Evaluation in Heart Failure (ADMIRE-HF) study investigated the potential role of ^{123}I-MIBG H/M ratio in predicting life-threatening ventricular arrhythmias [**51**]. This large prospective trial used a ^{123}I-MIBG H/M ratio of less 1.6 for predicting cardiovascular events in patients with symptomatic heart failure. The study enrolled 961 patients (NYHA class II–III) with severe systolic heart failure (LVEF ≤35%). More than 90% of the patients were receiving β-blockers, angiotensin-converting enzyme inhibitors, or angiotensin receptor blockers. Those with a ventricular pacemaker, history of defibrillation, ICD, acute myocardial infarction, or serum creatinine >3.0 mg/dL were excluded. LVEF was measured primarily by echocardiography at the enrolling site. The patients were divided into two prespecified groups (H/M ratio >1.6 and H/M ratio <1.6). Eighty-six participants had major arrhythmic events: 63 nonfatal events, including sustained VT, aborted cardiac arrest, and ICD firing, and 23 SCDs. The Kaplan–Meier curves show a significant increase in the rate of major arrhythmic events for patients with an H/M ratio <1.6 (Adapted from Jacobson et al. [**51**]).

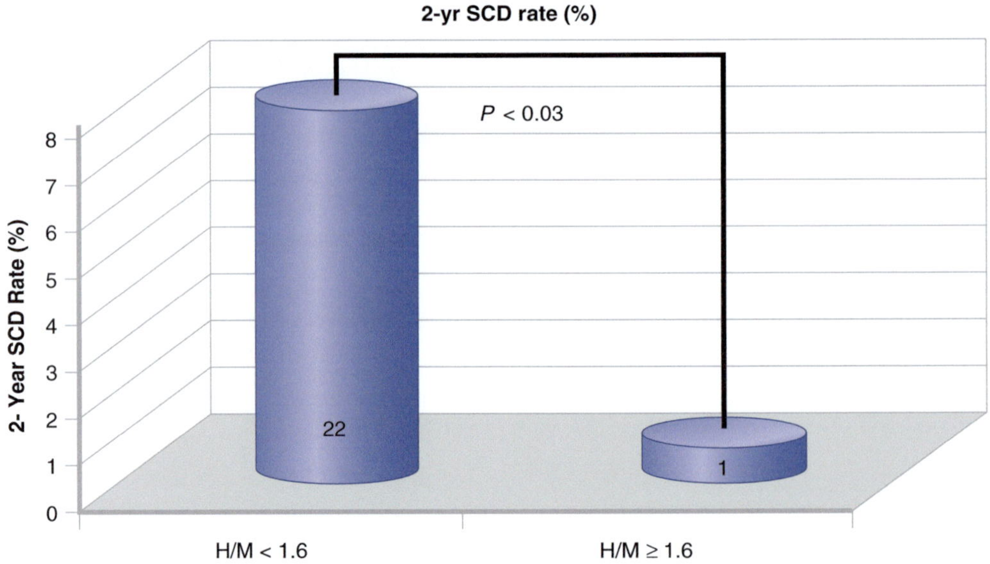

FIGURE 7-13. Sudden cardiac death rate during 2-year follow-up. SCD occurred in 22 subjects with an H/M ratio <1.6 and in only 1 subject with an H/M ratio ≥ 1.6 [**51**] (Adapted from the ADMIRE-HF study, courtesy of Arnold Jacobson MD, PhD).

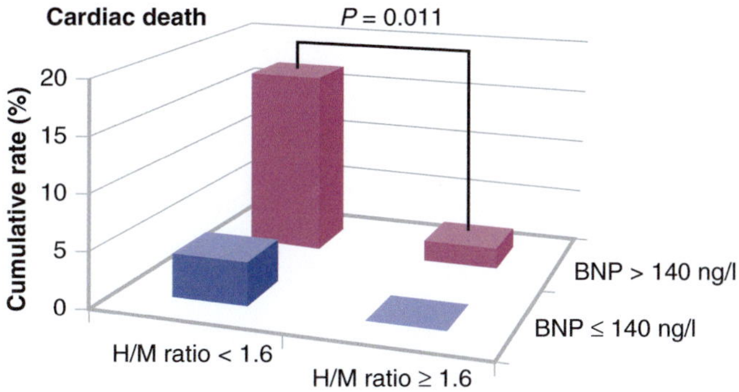

FIGURE 7-14. In ADMIRE-HF, the ^{123}I-MIBG H/M ratio provided additional risk stratification for cardiac death when compared with a brain natriuretic peptide (BNP) level >140 ng/L or LVEF <30% and was an independent predictor of cardiac death. The Kaplan–Meier survival curves in this figure depict the significantly increased rate of cardiac death for patients with BNP >140 ng/L and an H/M ratio <1.6. In those with BNP <140 ng/L the addition of H/M ratio did not predict an increased event rate [**51**] (Adapted from Jacobson et al. [**51**]).

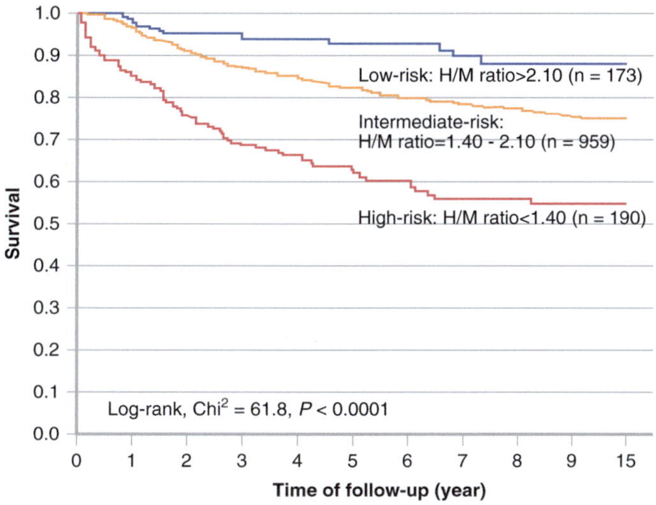

FIGURE 7-15. Sudden cardiac death and progressive heart failure are responsible for most deaths in patients with severe heart failure and left ventricular dysfunction. Nakata et al. [**52**] pooled data from six prospective cohort trials involving 1322 patients to investigate all-cause mortality in patients with heart failure. Mean follow-up was 5 years, and the mean LVEF was 37%. In this cohort, 326 patients had a lethal event, and the mortality rate was 5.6%, 11.3%, and 19.7% at 1-, 2-, and 5-year follow-up, respectively. Based on a multivariate Cox model, age, NYHA class, late H/M ratio, and LVEF were independent predictors of survival. An analysis separating the cohort into three groups—low risk, H/M >2.1; intermediate risk, H/M 1.4–2.1; and high risk, H/M <1.4—showed a significant decrease in survival with worsening MIBG late H/M ratio. Thresholds of 1.68 for H/M ratio and 43% for the washout rate were determined by receiver operator analysis to predict an increased risk for all-cause mortality ($P<0.0001$ for both) (Adapted from Nakata et al. [**52**]).

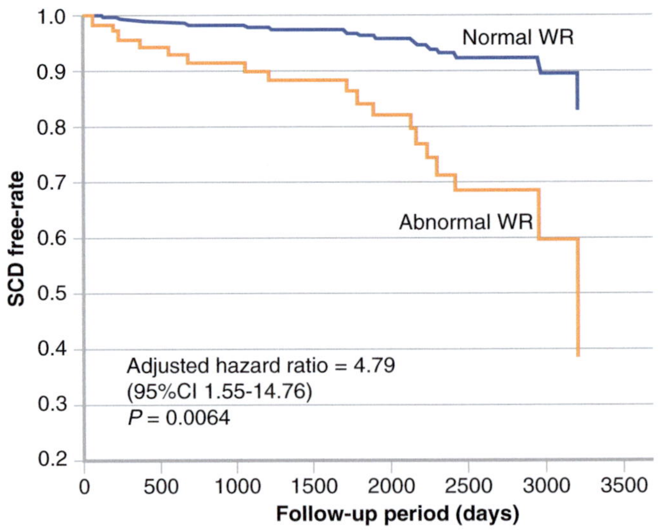

Figure 7-16. In addition to H/M ratio, the washout rate (WR) is an important predictor of SCD. Myocardial washout of ^{123}I-MIBG is defined by the following equation: early ^{123}I-MIBG counts per pixel minus late ^{123}I-MIBG counts per pixel divided by early ^{123}I-MIBG counts per pixel. Tamaki et al. [**53**] followed up 106 consecutive heart failure patients with an LVEF <40. SCD was defined as witnessed cardiac arrest and death within 1 h of the acute onset of symptoms. An abnormal MIBG washout rate, defined as <27 %, was a significant predictor of SCD after adjustment for age, gender, and LVEF. Signal-averaged ECG, HRV, and QT dispersion were not independent predictors of SCD in this study. Furthermore, ^{123}I-MIBG washout rate may be used to further risk stratify patients with stable cardiomyopathy who are on medical therapy [**54**]. The ^{123}I-MIBG washout rate in patients with chronic heart failure was shown to be an independent predictor of SCD and provided additional risk stratification when compared with the Seattle Heart Failure Model alone [**55**] (Adapted from Tamaki et al. [**53**]).

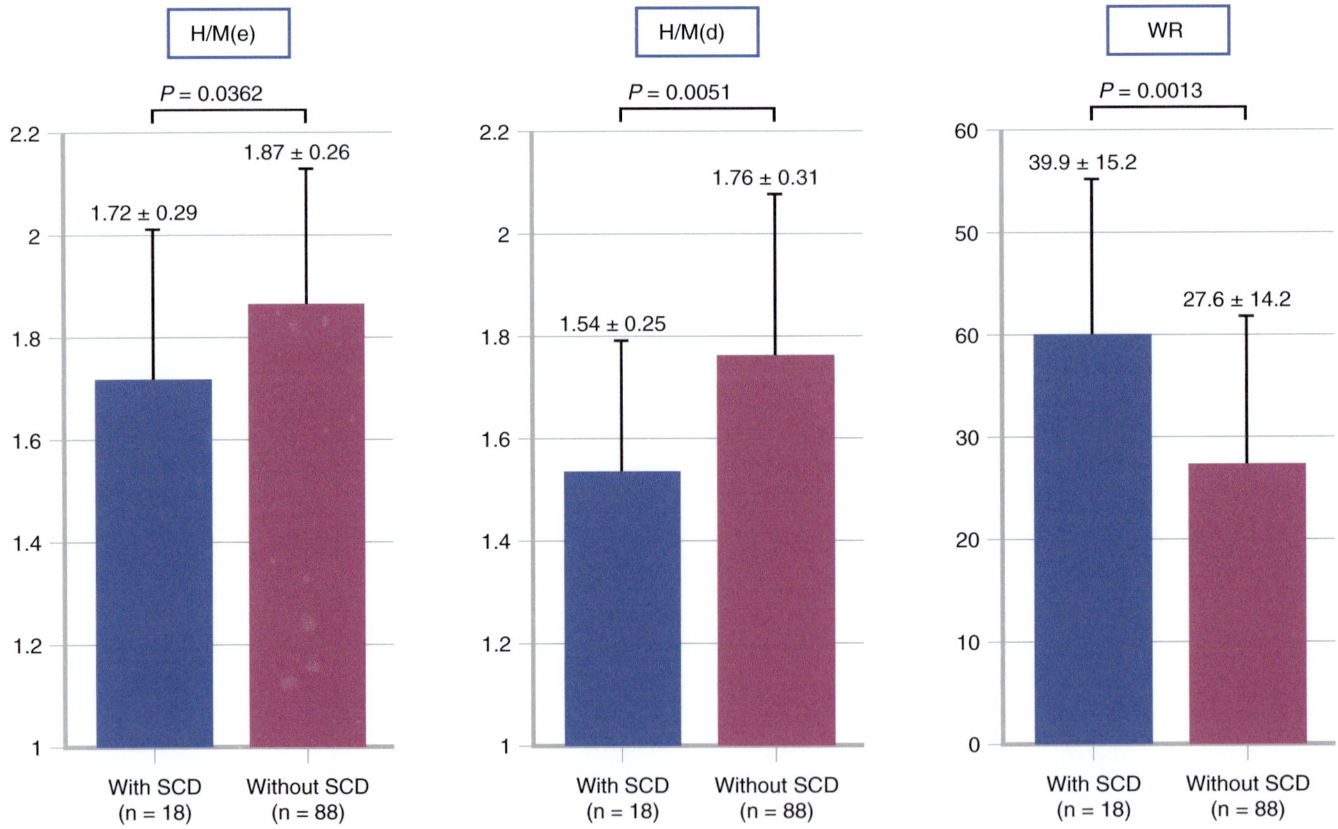

Figure 7-17. Mean H/M ratios and washout rates for patients with and without SCD [**53**]. The ^{123}I-MIBG washout rate was comparable to the delayed H/M ratio in comparing SCD at 5 years (Adapted from Tamaki et al. [**53**]).

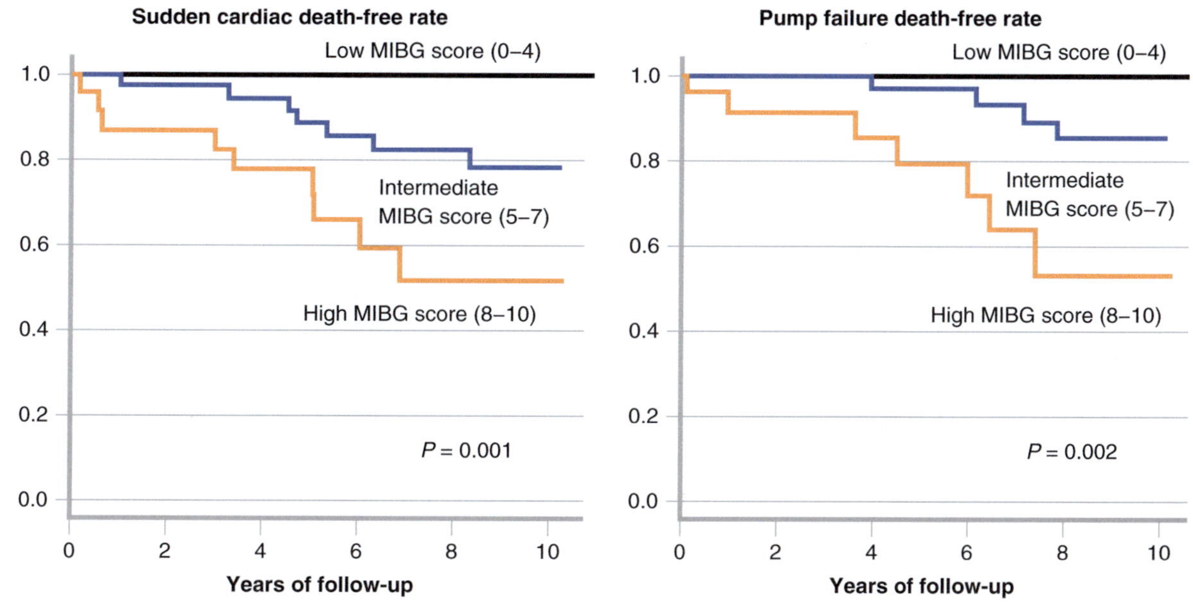

	Sudden cardiac death: No. at risk						Pump failure death: No. at risk					
Low	19	19	18	16	10	9	19	19	18	16	10	9
Intermediate	37	35	33	27	21	17	37	35	33	27	21	17
High	25	19	14	9	4	4	25	19	14	9	4	4
Positive predictive value(%)		100	100	100	100	100		100	100	100	100	100
Negative predictive value(%)		6	11	21	24	26		3	6	10	18	18

Figure 7-18. It has been suggested that both the ^{123}I-MIBG delayed H/M ratio and the washout rate provide additive value in predicting SCD. Kawai et al [**56**] classified patients into low-, medium-, and high-risk groups based on the sum of the deviation of both H/M ratios and washout rates from the mean values in a control population. They studied 81 patients with NYHA class I, II, or III heart failure and an LVEF <35%. No patients had an ICD or biventricular pacemaker at study entry. Exclusion criteria included renal dysfunction, insulin-dependent diabetes mellitus, and autonomic neuropathy. During a mean follow-up of 6.9±3.1 years, 16 SCDs occurred, but none of the 19 patients in the low-risk group died (P=0.001). The authors concluded that an MIBG score including H/M ratio and washout rate may identify heart failure patients at very low risk for SCD (Adapted from Kawai et al. [**56**]).

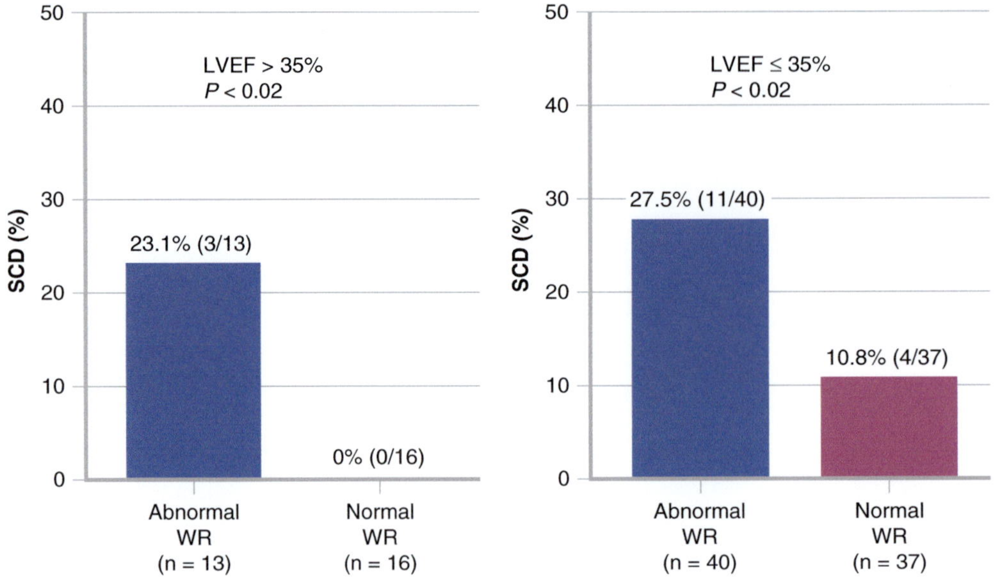

Figure 7-19. Patients with cardiomyopathy and an LVEF >35% require special attention because they do not meet the criteria for primary prevention ICD implantation but represent most patients who have SCD. ^{123}I-MIBG data are limited in this patient population. The figure shows patients with an LVEF >35% (*left*) and those with an LVEF ≤35% (*right*) grouped by a normal (<27%) or an abnormal (>27%) washout rate (WR). An abnormal washout rate was shown to be significantly associated with SCD by the log-rank test, regardless of LVEF (*P* values are shown above) (Adapted by Tamaki et al. [**53**]).

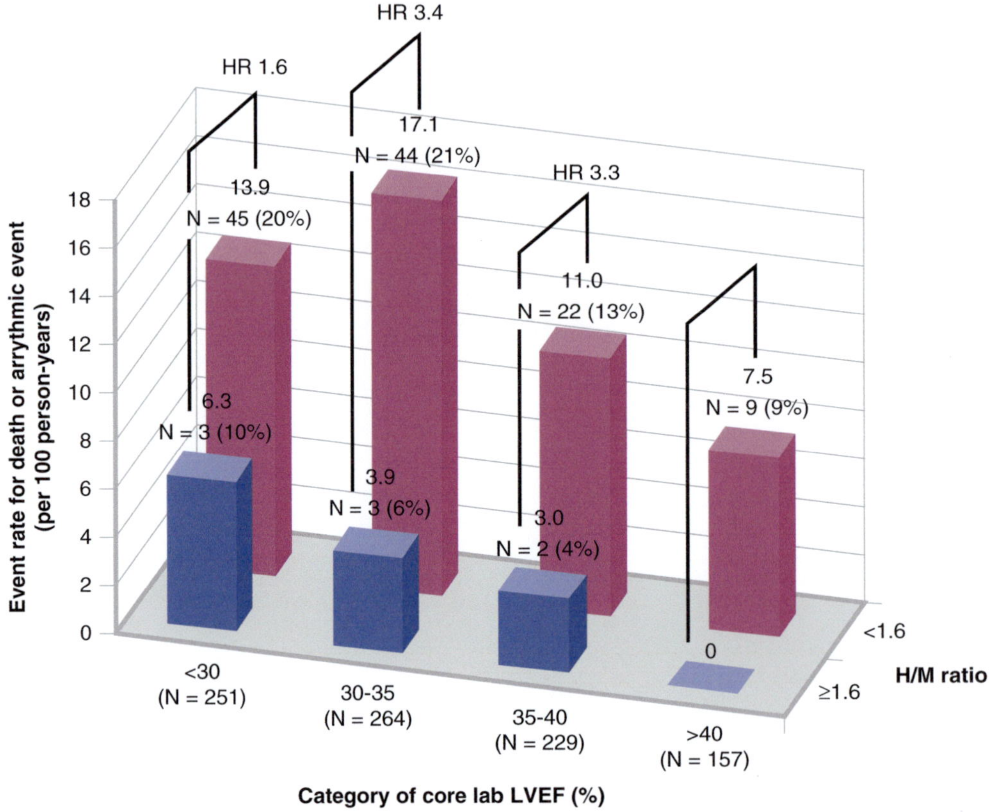

Figure 7-20. A subgroup analysis of the ADMIRE-HF trial showed a significant SCD association for patients with an H/M ratio <1.6, regardless of baseline LVEF [**57**]. Although LVEF ≤35% was an inclusion criterion for ADMIRE-HF, significant interobserver variability exists. On core laboratory review, 386 of 901 patients whose LVEFs were available for evaluation were found to have an LVEF >35% (overall mean, 34%±7%). The ADMIRE-HF patients were then grouped according to LVEF and H/M ratio <1.6 (high risk) or ≥1.6 (low risk). Regardless of ejection fraction, the risk of death or arrhythmic events was significantly increased (Adapted by Shah et al. [**57**]).

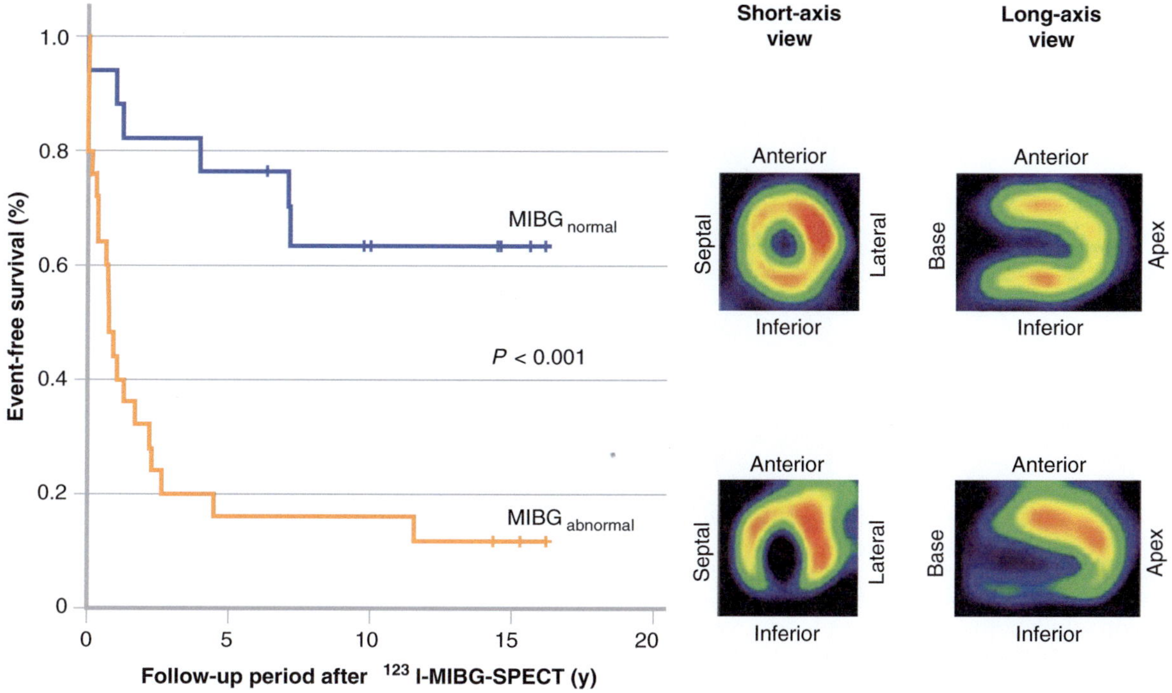

Event-free survivors at time	0 y	5y	10y	15 y of follow-up
MIBG $_{normal}$, n	17	13	9	5
MIBG $_{abnormal}$, n	25	4	4	2

Figure 7-21. Although ischemic and nonischemic cardiomyopathy are common causes of life-threatening ventricular arrhythmias, channelopathies such as arrhythmogenic right ventricular cardiomyopathy (ARVC), Brugada syndrome, and congenital long QT syndrome require specific attention. ARVC is a predominantly autosomal dominant inherited cardiomyopathy afflicting 1 in 5000 people [**58**]. Pathophysiologic characteristics, including myocardial fatty infiltration and fibrosis, result in nonhomogeneous refractory periods and provide a substrate for ventricular arrhythmias and SCD. This arrhythmogenic potential is exacerbated further by catecholamines, which increase the refractory dispersion. In some series, ARVC accounted for approximately 22% of SCDs in athletes [**59**]. Current guidelines recommend ICD implantation for secondary prevention in ARVC patients with VT or VF and for primary prevention in patients with extensive disease, left ventricular involvement, a family history of SCD, or undiagnosed syncope [**16**]. Screening is imperfect, and additional techniques are needed for risk stratification in this high-risk population. The figure shows representative ^{123}I-MIBG images [**60**] from a control subject (*upper right*) and a patient with ARVC (*lower right*) with decreased inferoseptal activity. The survival curves (*left*) show significantly decreased event-free survival for ARVC patients with an abnormal scan (Adapted from Paul et al. [**60**]).

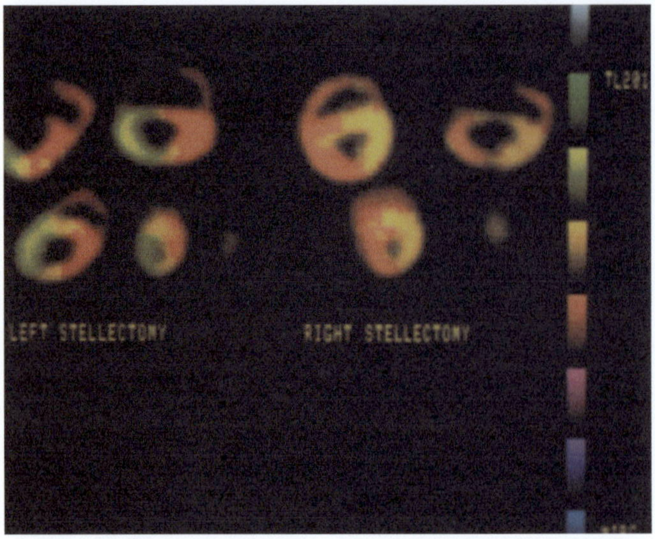

Figure 7-22. In patients with channelopathies, it has been postulated that heterogeneous cardiac sympathetic innervation contributes to life-threatening ventricular arrhythmias. In a canine model, Dae et al [**33**] showed that stellate nerve ablation can produce regional variation in sympathetic innervation that is independent of regional myocardial perfusion. The left stellate ganglion innervates the right ventricle and the left ventricular inferior and inferoseptal walls, whereas the right stellate ganglion innervates the anterior and lateral walls. The figure shows MIBG and thallium-201 dual-isotope SPECT images after stellectomy. Equal innervation and perfusion are displayed in red, decreased MIBG relative to perfusion in yellow to green, and increased innervation relative to perfusion in blue. The myocardial slices show denervation of the inferior and inferoseptal left ventricle after left stellectomy and anterior denervation of the left ventricle after right stellectomy (From Dae et al. [**33**]; with permission).

Table 7-1. Neuronal imaging reported findings in ion channel disorders linked to sudden cardiac death.

Clinical disorder	Onset	Global norepinephrine reuptake	β-Receptors	Regional reuptake
ARVC [60–62]	Stress	↓ by MIBG, trend only by PET	↓ by PET	↓ by MIBG inferoseptal walls, trend only by PET
Brugada syndrome [63, 64]	Rest	↑ by PET but not by MIBG	No change	↓ by MIBG inferoseptal walls, trend only by PET
Long QT syndrome [65–70]	Stress	↓ or no change	No data	↓ anteroseptal ± lateral in most but not all reports
RVO-VT [71–73]	Stress	↓	↓	↓ inferior or septal by MIBG, uniform by PET

In a cohort of 48 patients with ARVC, Wichter et al. [**61**] showed a pattern of regional sympathetic denervation in the basal inferoseptal segments in 83% and in the right ventricle in 100%. Significant coronary artery disease was excluded in all patients with stress and rest myocardial perfusion images and coronary angiography. The sympathetic image findings were in contrast to those of nine patients with idiopathic ventricular tachycardia, seven of whom had uniform ^{123}I-MIBG radiotracer distribution, as did all of the control participants. Further ^{123}I-MIBG evaluation in 42 ARVC patients, followed up for a mean of 11.9 years, showed that of 25 patients with abnormal MIBG uptake—defined as at least three adjacent segments with a >2-SD decrease in ^{123}I-MIBG counts—22 had life-threatening ventricular tachyarrhythmias, compared with 6 of 17 patients with normal ^{123}I-MIBG scans ($P<0.0005$) (Fig. 7.21) [**60**]. The decreased uptake was in the septum (32%), inferior wall (31%), and anterior walls (29%). Although *PKP2* mutations were identified in 17 patients, plakophilin-2 positivity did not correlate with the degree of ^{123}I-MIBG uptake

Eight of 17 patients with Brugada syndrome studied by Wichter et al. [**63**] had significantly decreased left ventricular inferior and septal MIBG uptake

People with idiopathic right ventricular outflow tract VT (RVO-VT) or idiopathic VF have significantly decreased ^{123}I-MIBG uptake, predominantly in the left ventricular inferior wall (Fig. 7.23) [**71**]

Patients with another channelopathy, long QT syndrome, have segmental decreases in ^{123}I-MIBG uptake. In 28 patients with a long QT interval and a history of syncope [**18**] or SCD [**10**], ^{123}I-MIBG uptake was decreased in the anterior septum, independent of long QT genetic subtype or heart rate–corrected QTc interval (Fig. 7.24) [**65**]. Other investigators, however, have reported different regional distributions of radiotracer

In these channelopathies that cause life-threatening ventricular arrhythmias, ^{123}I-MIBG imaging is reported to have a characteristic pattern of abnormal regional uptake. This regional inhomogeneity of ^{123}I-MIBG has predicted ventricular arrhythmias

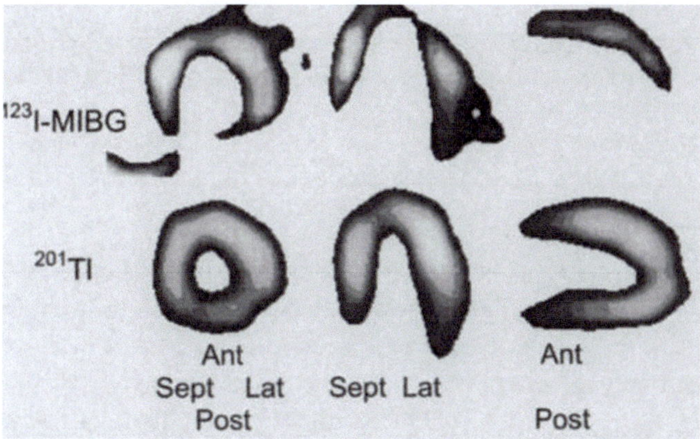

Figure 7-23. People with idiopathic right ventricular outflow tract tachycardia or idiopathic VF have significantly decreased regional MIBG uptake, predominantly in the left ventricular inferior wall [**71**]. Shown here are MIBG and thallium-201 (^{201}Tl) perfusion images (short axis, horizontal long axis, and vertical long axis) from a patient with idiopathic right ventricular outflow tract tachycardia. The perfusion images show normal resting uptake, whereas the MIBG images show decreased uptake in the left ventricular inferior wall (This research was originally published in JNM. Schäfers et al. [**71**]. Figure 1. © by the Society of Nuclear Medicine and Molecular Imaging, Inc.).

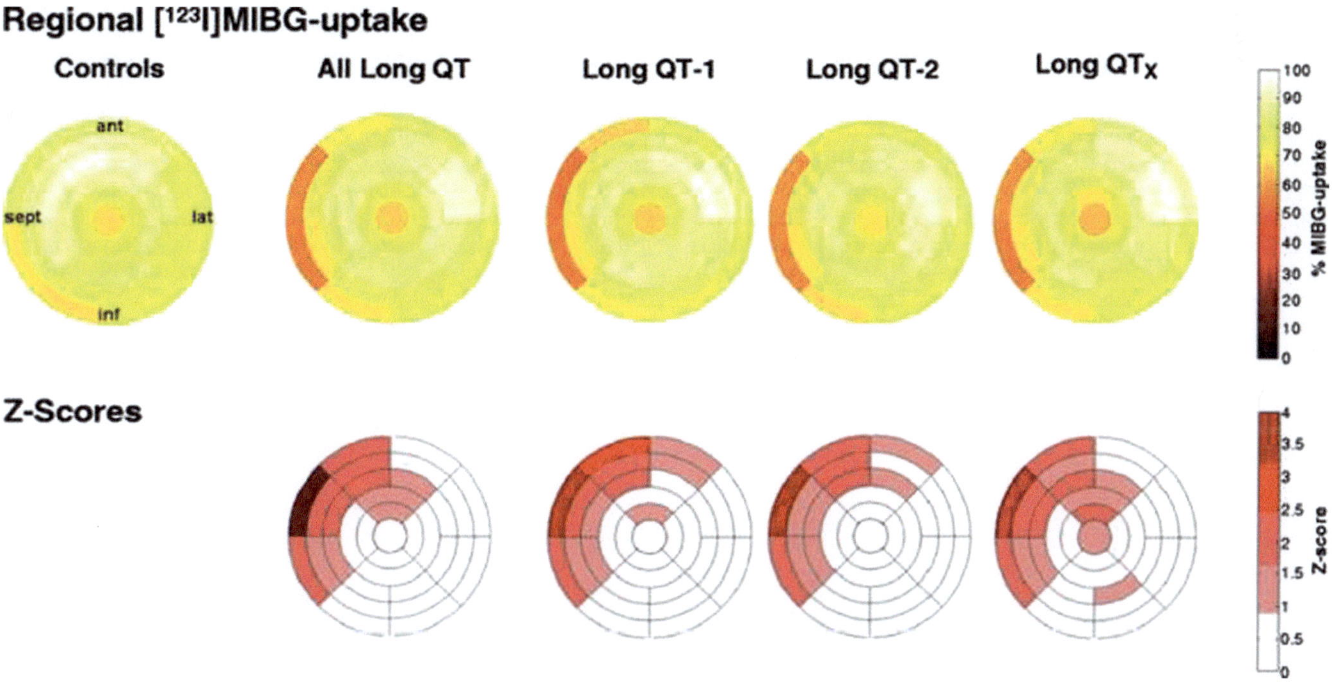

Figure 7-24. Yellow polar maps showing the relative uptake of MIBG per segment for controls, a composite of all long QT subtypes, and individual subtypes of long QT. The bottom polar maps represent the Z-score for the composite of all long QT subtypes and individual subtypes of long QT relative to the control. There is significantly decreased ^{123}I-MIBG uptake, predominantly in the anterior septum. This pattern was independent of long QT subtype [**65**] (From Kies et al. [**65**]).

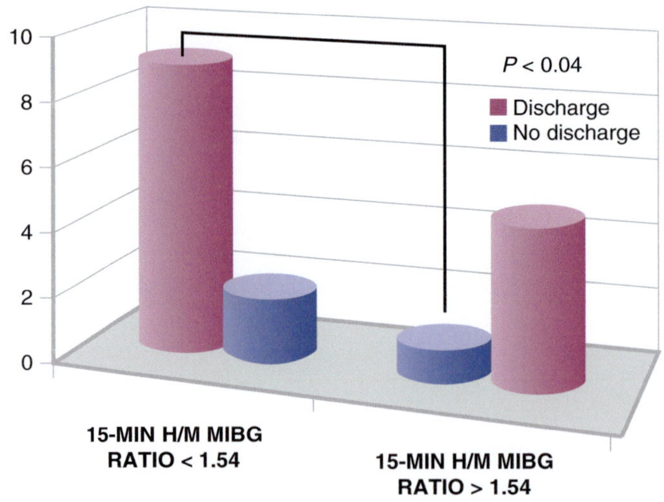

Figure 7-25. Dysfunction of myocardial sympathetic innervation is associated with ICD discharge. Arora et al. [**74**] performed an early ^{123}I-MIBG study in ICD patients, 10 with at least one appropriate defibrillation and 7 without defibrillation. Patients with a ^{123}I-MIBG H/M ratio <1.54 were significantly more likely to have an appropriate ICD discharge than those with a higher H/M ratio. When combined with HRV, all patients (four of four) with an MIBG uptake <1.54 and a 5-min low-frequency HRV <443 ms^2 had an appropriate ICD discharge whereas none of the patients (zero of three) with an H/M ratio >1.54 and a 5-min low-frequency HRV >443 ms^2 had an ICD discharge. The Arora study was followed by a prospective study by Nagahara et al. [**75**] in which 54 patients requiring ICD placement for diverse indications were characterized with baseline ^{123}I-MIBG H/M ratio, plasma concentration of brain natriuretic peptide (BNP), and LVEF. The patients were followed up for 15 months. The group was separated into patients with appropriate ICD discharge (n=21) and those without an appropriate discharge (n=33). On multivariate analysis, late H/M ratio was an independent predictor of ICD discharge. Combining BNP (>187 pg/mL) or LVEF (<50%) with the late H/M ratio (<1.95) was associated with a positive predictive value of 82% and 58%, respectively. Improvement in risk stratification also was investigated by Koutelou et al. [**76**], who used HRV, baroreflex sensitivity (BRS), and ^{123}I-MIBG imaging in 25 patients with ischemic or nonischemic NYHA class I to II heart failure who had recently had an ICD implanted for secondary prevention. The ^{123}I-MIBG washout rate, two HRV parameters (power in the low-frequency range and the square root of the mean of the squared differences between successive RR intervals over a 24-h period), and BRS were independently associated with ventricular tachyarrhythmias with a cycle length <330 ms. These variables reflect both the sympathetic and parasympathetic function and characterize different facets of autonomic regulation, allowing for improved risk stratification (Adapted from Arora et al. [**74**]).

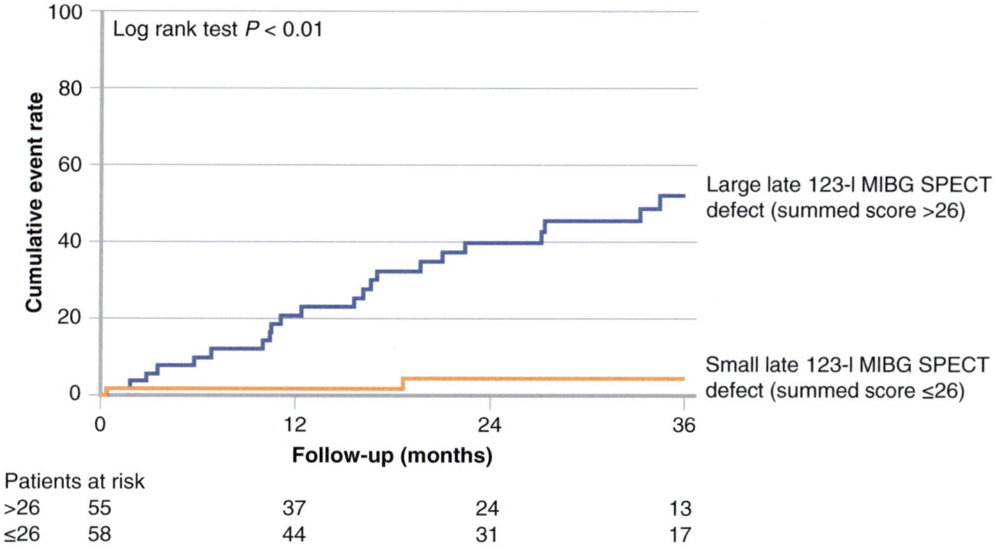

Figure 7-26. Boogers et al. [**77**] obtained ^{123}I-MIBG images and technetium-99 m tetrofosmin stress and resting myocardial perfusion scans in 116 heart failure patients before ICD implantation. Over approximately 2 years, 24 patients required appropriate ICD therapy, the primary end point, and 32 had cardiac death, the secondary end point. Appropriate therapy consisted of 44 episodes of antitachycardia pacing in 16 patients and 42 defibrillations in 15 patients. On univariate analysis, early ^{123}I-MIBG SPECT defect score ($P<0.01$), late ^{123}I-MIBG SPECT defect score ($P<0.01$), summed perfusion difference score ($P<0.12$), and MIBG/perfusion mismatch score ($P<0.01$) were associated with appropriate therapy. The extent of decreased uptake for ^{123}I-MIBG was greater than that of the rest SPECT perfusion defect. This mismatch is discussed further in Fig. 7.29 and likely represents the area with the greatest arrhythmogenic potential, although the extent of the denervation/perfusion mismatch was not a statistically significant predictor of ICD therapy on multivariate analysis in the Boogers study. Upon multivariate analysis, late ^{123}I-MIBG defect score was significantly associated with appropriate ICD therapy. This figure shows ICD therapy in patients with a late ^{123}I-MIBG defect score that was higher (>26; 28 patients [51 %]) or lower (≤26; 4 patients [7 %]). The risk for appropriate ICD therapy was eightfold greater in patients with a high ^{123}I-MIBG defect score (8.28 [95% CI, 2.91–23.6]; $P<0.01$) (Adapted from Boogers et al. [**77**]).

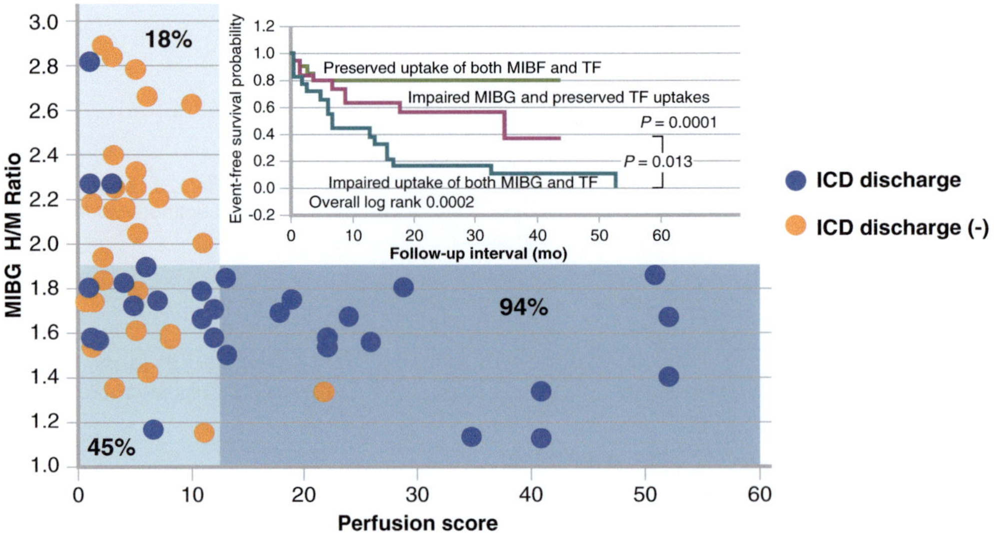

Figure 7-27. The combination of ^{123}I-MIBG neural imaging and myocardial perfusion imaging may enhance prediction of ICD therapy delivery. Nishisato et al. [**78**] studied 60 patients with cardiac defibrillators implanted for diverse indications. The combination of a resting summed perfusion defect score >12 and an H/M ratio <1.9 identified patients with ICD discharge (P<0.0001). This scatter plot delineates the percentage of patients with ICD discharge on follow-up by three patient subsets: high ^{123}I-MIBG H/M ratio and low resting perfusion summed score (18% with ICD discharge), low ^{123}I-MIBG H/M ratio and low resting perfusion summed score (45% with ICD discharge), and low ^{123}I-MIBG H/M ratio and high resting perfusion summed score (94% with ICD discharge). No patient had an ^{123}I-MIBG H/M ratio >1.9 and a resting perfusion score >12. The upper right portion of the image shows the Kaplan–Meier curves generated for these groups, with impaired uptake of both MIBG and tetrofosmin (TF) conferring the greatest risk of defibrillation. Subgroup analysis of patients with an LVEF >50% (31 patients) showed that 100% of those with a low MIBG H/M ratio and high tetrofosmin resting summed defect score (three of three patients) had an appropriate ICD discharge (P<0.0138). A subanalysis of patients with nonischemic cardiomyopathy in the ADMIRE-HF trial further supports the utility of combining a high summed rest hypoperfusion score (>8) and a low H/M ratio (<1.6) for prediction of ICD therapy [**79**] (Adapted from Nishisato et al. [**78**]).

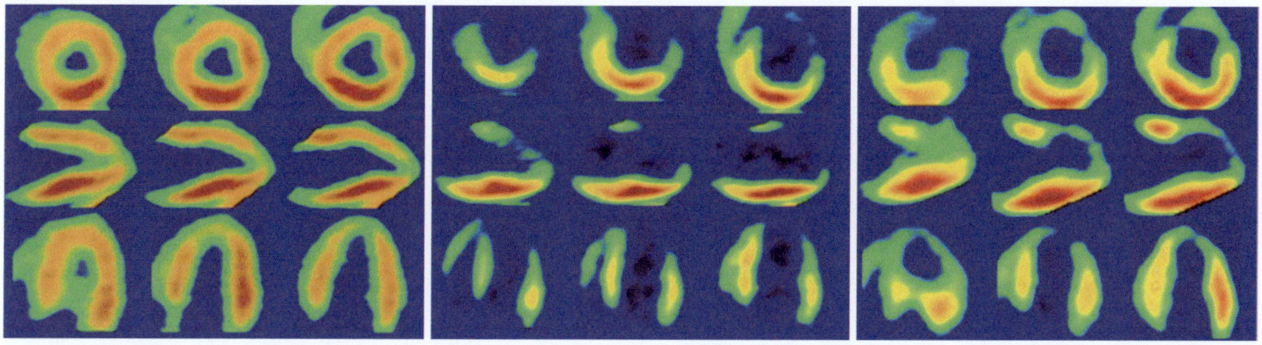

FIGURE 7-28. Cardiac PET has added important dimensions to cardiac sympathetic imaging, including better spatial resolution, improved regional tracer distribution analysis, wider sympathetic radiotracer selection, and detailed kinetic analysis. The most widely used PET cardiac sympathetic imaging tracer has been ^{11}C-HED. Disruption in myocardial sympathetic innervation is hypothesized to be a cause of SCD and has been shown to occur after an ischemic insult [**80**]. The sympathetic abnormalities often are larger than the underlying infarcted territory and may even be present without underlying irreversible myocardial injury [**81**, **82**]. Therefore, the area of denervation likely represents the underlying jeopardized ischemic territory. Evaluation of chronic ischemia (hibernating myocardium) in swine indicated that hibernating myocardium is a risk factor for development of SCD independent of coronary artery stenosis severity, acute myocardial necrosis, or scar [**83**]. Additionally, disruption in the sympathetic innervation in hibernating myocardium of swine with chronic left anterior descending (LAD) artery stenosis, as seen by ^{11}C-HED uptake on PET imaging, may contribute to SCD [**84**]. Shown here are reconstructed ^{11}C-HED images from pigs with normal (**a**), hibernating (**b**), and infarcted (**c**) myocardium. Standard views demonstrate homogeneous HED uptake in a healthy control animal. In contrast, a severe and extensive HED defect involving LAD distribution is seen in the pig with hibernating myocardium, consistent with sympathetic dysinnervation. In the animal with subendocardial infarction in the LAD distribution, the defect in HED uptake is similar to that in hibernating myocardium. HED activity is color coded from red, with the greatest activity, to blue–black, with the least. *HLA* horizontal long axis, *SA* short axis, *VLA* vertical long axis. (This research was originally published in JNM. Luisi et al. [**84**]. Figure 1. © by the Society of Nuclear Medicine and Molecular Imaging, Inc.).

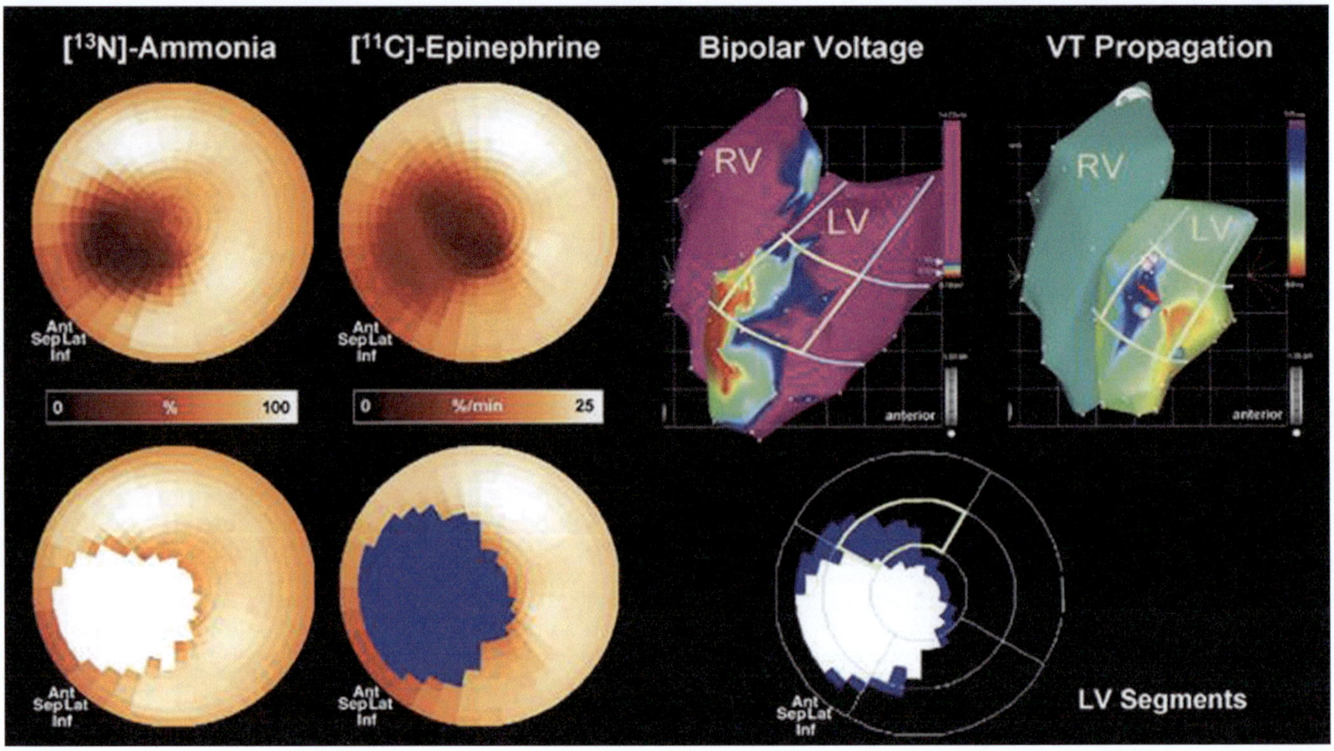

Figure 7-29. Mismatch between myocardial innervation and perfusion has been proposed as an important substrate for ventricular arrhythmias and SCD. Experimental evidence in a porcine model of coronary artery occlusion was provided by Sasano et al. [**85**] using PET. The upper polar maps show perfusion (nitrogen-13 [^{13}N]-ammonia) and innervation (^{11}C-epinephrine) defect size [**84**]. (*Lower left*), the extent of hypoperfusion >2 SD below the normal range is shown in white and the corresponding area of sympathetic denervation in blue. (*Lower right*), the extent of the denervation zone is larger than the area of hypoperfusion, highlighting the area of mismatch in the ischemic border zone. The mismatched area was larger in the group with inducible VT than in the group without inducible tachycardia. (*Upper right*), the mismatch area was shown to be the site for inducible VT in this model. These results suggest that denervation/perfusion mismatch may be useful in identifying patients at risk for ventricular arrhythmias. (From Sasano et al. [**85**]; with permission).

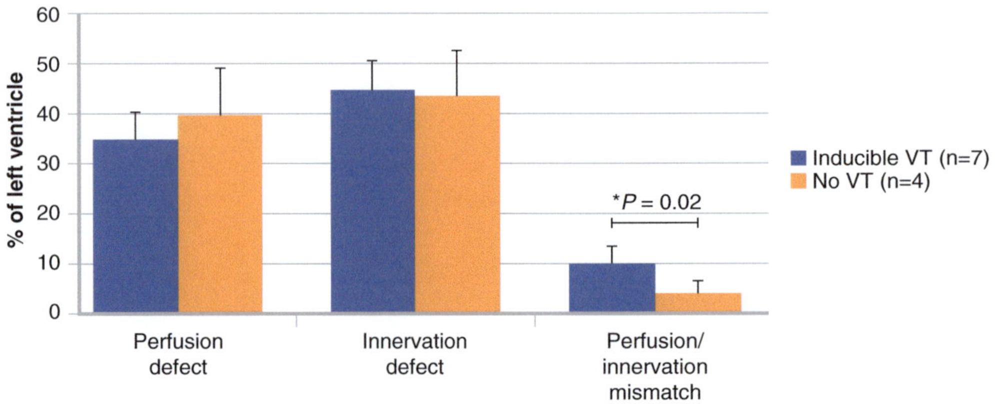

Figure 7-30. Perfusion defect, innervation defect, and perfusion/innervation mismatch in animals after a mid–left anterior descending artery occlusion with and without inducible VT. There was no significant difference in the perfusion or innervation defect in the inducible animals, but the perfusion/innervation mismatch was significantly larger in the inducible population [**85**] (Adapted from Sasano et al. [**85**]).

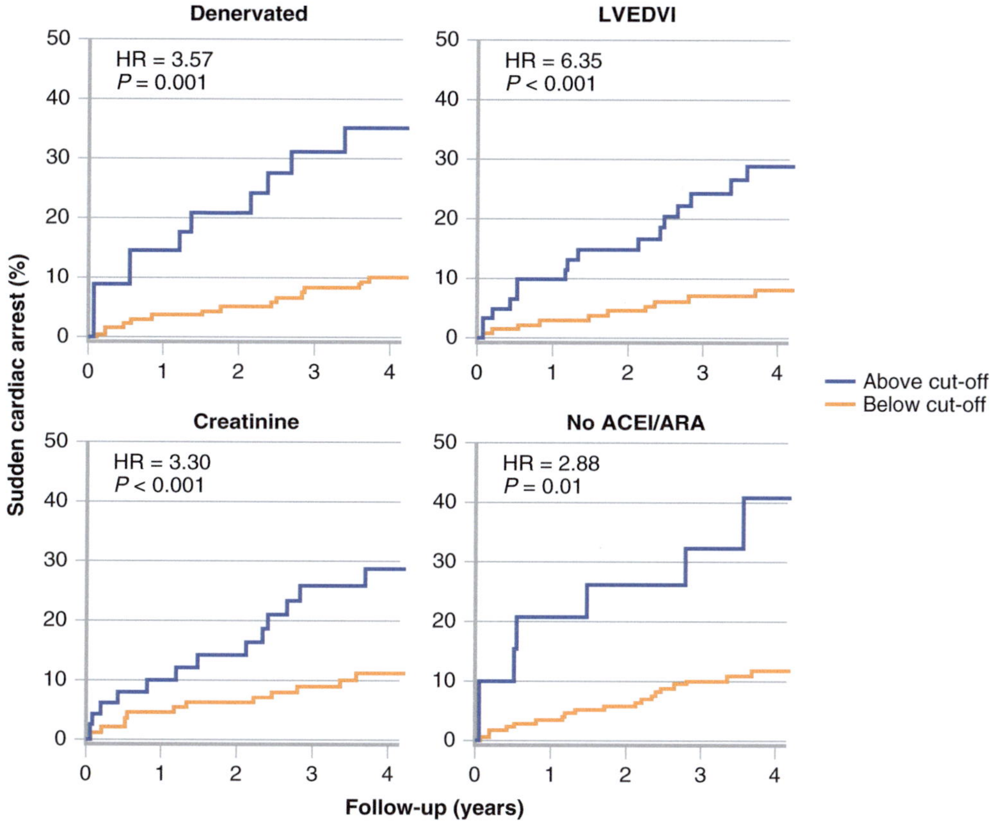

Figure 7-31. The Prediction of Arrhythmic Events with Positron Emission Tomography (PAREPET) study examined the association between myocardial sympathetic innervation and sudden cardiac arrest (SCA), defined as arrhythmic death or ICD discharge for VF or VT >240 bpm. PAREPET prospectively followed up 204 patients with ischemic cardiomyopathy and a primary prevention indication for ICD implantation [**86**]. Myocardial perfusion, viability, and sympathetic denervation were quantified with ^{13}N-ammonia, fluorine-18 2-deoxyglucose, and ^{11}C-HED PET, respectively. Over a median of 4.1 years, 33 SCAs occurred (22 arrhythmic deaths and 11 ICD discharges). Variables associated with SCA were volume of denervation and volume of viable denervated myocardium, whereas the volumes of hibernating myocardium and infarcted myocardium were not associated with SCA. The highest tertile of denervation conferred a 6.7% per year event rate compared with the moderate and low tertile groups of 2.2 and 1.2% per year, respectively. Multivariate analysis identified the volume of denervated myocardium, left ventricular end-diastolic volume index (LVEDVI), creatinine, and lack of angiotensin-converting enzyme inhibitor (ACEI) or angiotensin receptor antagonist (ARA) therapy as risk factors for the development of SCA (Adapted from Fallavollita et al. [**86**]).

Table 7-2. Summary and future directions.

Neurocardiac imaging studies using ^{123}I-MIBG for SPECT and ^{11}C-HED for PET provide prognostic data regarding cardiac death [51, 52], ventricular arrhythmia potential [76, 77], and appropriate ICD therapy.
Additional data are needed to clarify the underlying mechanisms for and regulation of myocardial autonomic dysfunction in relation to various cardiomyopathies and SCD.
PET imaging techniques for molecular receptor mapping may provide further insights into the relationships between receptor density and regulation and SCD.
Current guidelines regarding ICD placement are limited in their ability to differentiate patients at high from those at low risk for SCD. The addition of nuclear myocardial sympathetic imaging to guideline-accepted risk factors for the development of SCD (LVEF, T-wave alternans, signal-averaged ECG, BRS, HRV) has been shown to improve risk stratification for both SCD and appropriate ICD therapy.
Based on the growing strength of the data supporting the utility of ^{123}I-MIBG and ^{11}C-HED, these techniques merit consideration of a more prominent role in future guidelines for predicting ventricular arrhythmias and implanting cardiac defibrillators.

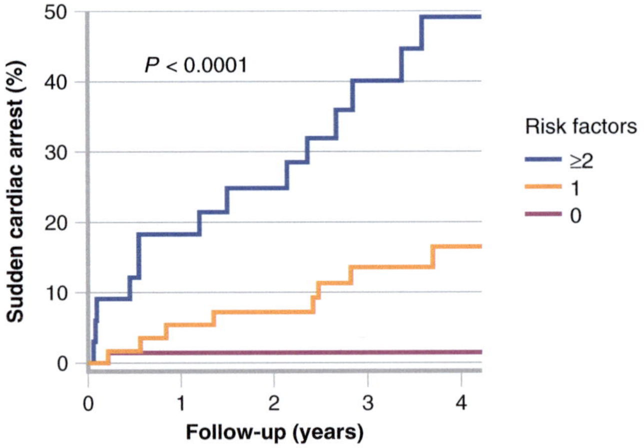

Figure 7-32. Kaplan–Meier curves characterizing the risk of SCA as delineated by the number of risk factors outlined in the preceding figure. Cut points for the risk factors were >37.6% of myocardial volume for denervation, >99 mL/m² for LVEDVI, >1.49 mg/dL for creatinine, and no angiotensin therapy. Patients with two or more of these risk factors had a 12% annual risk of SCA versus <1% in patients with none of these risk factors. This study demonstrates the utility of characterizing myocardial sympathetic denervation to predict SCA [**86**] (Adapted from Fallavollita et al. [**86**]).

References

1. Myerburg RJ, Kessler KM, Castellanos A. Sudden cardiac death: epidemiology, transient risk, and intervention assessment. Ann Intern Med. 1993;119:1187–97.
2. Greenberg H, Case RB, Moss AJ, Brown MW, Carroll ER, Andrews ML. Analysis of mortality events in the Multicenter Automatic Defibrillator Implantation Trial (MADIT-II). J Am Coll Cardiol. 2004;43:1459–65.
3. Julian DG, Camm AJ, Frangin G, Janse MJ, Munoz A, Schwartz PJ, et al. Randomised trial of effect of amiodarone on mortality in patients with left-ventricular dysfunction after recent myocardial infarction: EMIAT. European Myocardial Infarct Amiodarone Trial Investigators. Lancet. 1997;349:667–74.
4. Boutitie F, Boissel JP, Connolly SJ, Camm AJ, Cairns JA, Julian DG, et al. Amiodarone interaction with beta-blockers: analysis of the merged EMIAT (European Myocardial Infarct Amiodarone Trial) and CAMIAT (Canadian Amiodarone Myocardial Infarction Trial) databases The EMIAT and CAMIAT Investigators. Circulation. 1999;99:2268–75.
5. Echt DS, Liebson PR, Mitchell LB, Peters RW, Obias-Manno D, Barker AH, et al. Mortality and morbidity in patients receiving encainide, flecainide, or placebo. The Cardiac Arrhythmia Suppression Trial. N Engl J Med. 1991;324:781–8.
6. Effect of the antiarrhythmic agent moricizine on survival after myocardial infarction. The cardiac arrhythmia suppression trial II investigators. N Engl J Med. 1992;327:227–33.
7. Waldo AL, Camm AJ, deRuyter H, Friedman PL, MacNeil DJ, Pauls JF, et al. Effect of d-sotalol on mortality in patients with left ventricular dysfunction after recent and remote myocardial infarction. The SWORD Investigators. Survival with Oral d-Sotalol. Lancet. 1996;348:7–12.
8. Moss AJ, Zareba W, Hall WJ, Klein H, Wilber DJ, Cannom DS, et al. Prophylactic implantation of a defibrillator in patients with myocardial infarction and reduced ejection fraction. N Engl J Med. 2002;346:877–83.
9. Bardy GH, Lee KL, Mark DB, Poole JE, Packer DL, Boineau R, et al. Amiodarone or an implantable cardioverter-defibrillator for congestive heart failure. N Engl J Med. 2005;352:225–37.
10. A comparison of antiarrhythmic-drug therapy with implantable defibrillators in patients resuscitated from near-fatal ventricular arrhythmias. The Antiarrhythmics versus Implantable Defibrillators (AVID) Investigators. N Engl J Med. 1997;337:1576–83.
11. Kuck KH, Cappato R, Siebels J, Ruppel R. Randomized comparison of antiarrhythmic drug therapy with implantable defibrillators in patients resuscitated from cardiac arrest : the Cardiac Arrest Study Hamburg (CASH). Circulation. 2000;102:748–54.
12. Connolly SJ, Gent M, Roberts RS, Dorian P, Roy D, Sheldon RS, et al. Canadian implantable defibrillator study (CIDS): a randomized trial of the implantable cardioverter defibrillator against amiodarone. Circulation. 2000;101:1297–302.
13. Epstein AE, DiMarco JP, Ellenbogen KA, Estes 3rd NA, Freedman RA, Gettes LS, et al. ACC/AHA/HRS 2008 guidelines for device-based therapy of cardiac rhythm abnormalities: a report of the American college of cardiology/American heart association task force on practice guidelines (writing committee to revise the ACC/AHA/NASPE 2002 guideline update for implantation of cardiac pacemakers and antiarrhythmia devices): developed in collaboration with the American association for thoracic surgery and society of thoracic surgeons. Circulation. 2008;117:e350–408.
14. Moss AJ, Greenberg H, Case RB, Zareba W, Hall WJ, Brown MW, et al. Long-term clinical course of patients after termination of ventricular tachyarrhythmia by an implanted defibrillator. Circulation. 2004;110:3760–5.
15. Stecker EC, Vickers C, Waltz J, Socoteanu C, John BT, Mariani R, et al. Population-based analysis of sudden cardiac death with and without left ventricular systolic dysfunction: two-year findings from the Oregon sudden unexpected death study. J Am Coll Cardiol. 2006;47:1161–6.
16. Zipes DP, Camm AJ, Borggrefe M, Buxton AE, Chaitman B, Fromer M, et al. ACC/AHA/ESC 2006 guidelines for management of patients with ventricular arrhythmias and the prevention of sudden cardiac death: a report of the American college of cardiology/American heart association task force and the European society of cardiology committee for practice guidelines (writing committee to develop guidelines for management of patients with ventricular arrhythmias and the prevention of sudden cardiac death): developed in collaboration with the European heart rhythm association and the heart rhythm society. Circulation. 2006;114:e385–484.
17. Elhendy A, Chapman S, Porter TR, Windle J. Association of myocardial ischemia with mortality and implantable cardioverter-defibrillator therapy in patients with coronary artery disease at risk of arrhythmic death. J Am Coll Cardiol. 2005;46:1721–6.
18. Allman KC, Shaw LJ, Hachamovitch R, Udelson JE. Myocardial viability testing and impact of revascularization on prognosis in patients with coronary artery disease and left ventricular dysfunction: a meta-analysis. J Am Coll Cardiol. 2002;39:1151–8.
19. Lo R, Hsia HH. Ventricular arrhythmias in heart failure patients. Cardiol Clin. 2008;26:381–403.
20. Wu E, Judd RM, Vargas JD, Klocke FJ, Bonow RO, Kim RJ. Visualisation of presence, location, and transmural extent of healed Q-wave and non-Q-wave myocardial infarction. Lancet. 2001;357:21–8.
21. Gulati A, Jabbour A, Ismail TF, Guha K, Khwaja J, Raza S, et al. Association of fibrosis with mortality and sudden cardiac death in patients with nonischemic dilated cardiomyopathy. JAMA. 2013;309:896–908.
22. Bello D, Fieno DS, Kim RJ, Pereles FS, Passman R, Song G, et al. Infarct morphology identifies patients with substrate for sustained ventricular tachycardia. J Am Coll Cardiol. 2005;45:1104–8.
23. Schmidt A, Azevedo CF, Cheng A, Gupta SN, Bluemke DA, Foo TK, et al. Infarct tissue heterogeneity by magnetic resonance imaging identifies enhanced cardiac arrhythmia susceptibility in patients with left ventricular dysfunction. Circulation. 2007;115:2006–14.
24. Roes SD, Borleffs CJ, van der Geest RJ, Westenberg JJ, Marsan NA, Kaandorp TA, et al. Infarct tissue heterogeneity assessed with contrast-enhanced MRI predicts spontaneous ventricular arrhythmia in patients with ischemic cardiomyopathy and implantable cardioverter-defibrillator. Circ Cardiovasc Imaging. 2009;2:183–90.
25. van der Burg AE, Bax JJ, Boersma E, Pauwels EK, van der Wall EE, Schalij MJ. Impact of viability, ischemia, scar tissue, and revascularization on outcome after aborted sudden death. Circulation. 2003;108:1954–9.
26. Piccini JP, Horton JR, Shaw LK, Al-Khatib SM, Lee KL, Iskandrian AE, et al. Single-photon emission computed tomography myocardial perfusion defects are associated with an increased risk of all-cause death, cardiovascular death, and sudden cardiac death. Circ Cardiovasc Imaging. 2008;1:180–8.
27. Piccini JP, Starr AZ, Horton JR, Shaw LK, Lee KL, Al-Khatib SM, et al. Single-photon emission computed tomography myocardial perfusion imaging and the risk of sudden cardiac death in patients with coronary disease and left ventricular ejection fraction>35%. J Am Coll Cardiol. 2010;56:206–14.
28. Wieland DM, Brown LE, Rogers WL, Worthington KC, Wu JL, Clinthorne NH, et al. Myocardial imaging with a radioiodinated norepinephrine storage analog. J Nucl Med. 1981;22:22–31.
29. Valette H, Syrota A. Nuclear techniques in the assessment of myocardial innervation. In: IPC M, PJ E, editors. Nuclear

medicine in clinical diagnosis and treatment. Edinburgh, UK: Churchill Livininastone; 1998. p. 1525–9.

30. Sisson JC, Wieland DM, Sherman P, Mangner TJ, Tobes MC, Jacques Jr S. Metaiodobenzylguanidine as an index of the adrenergic nervous system integrity and function. J Nucl Med. 1987;28(10):1620–4.
31. Sisson JC, Lynch JJ, Johnson J, Jaques Jr S, Wu D, Bolgos G, et al. Scintigraphic detection of regional disruption of adrenergic neurons in the heart. Am Heart J. 1988;116:67–76.
32. Dae MW, De Marco T, Botvinick EH, O'Connell JW, Hattner RS, Huberty JP, et al. Scintigraphic assessment of MIBG uptake in globally denervated human and canine hearts--implications for clinical studies. J Nucl Med. 1992;33:1444–50.
33. Dae MW, O'Connell JW, Botvinick EH, Ahearn T, Yee E, Huberty JP, et al. Scintigraphic assessment of regional cardiac adrenergic innervation. Circulation. 1989;79:634–44.
34. Spyrou N, Rosen SD, Fath-Ordoubadi F, Jagathesan R, Foale R, Kooner JS, et al. Myocardial beta-adrenoceptor density one month after acute myocardial infarction predicts left ventricular volumes at six months. J Am Coll Cardiol. 2002;40:1216–24.
35. Merlet P, Delforge J, Syrota A, Angevin E, Maziere B, Crouzel C, et al. Positron emission tomography with 11C CGP-12177 to assess beta-adrenergic receptor concentration in idiopathic dilated cardiomyopathy. Circulation. 1993;87:1169–78.
36. Schofer J, Spielmann R, Schuchert A, Weber K, Schluter M. Iodine-123 meta-iodobenzylguanidine scintigraphy: a noninvasive method to demonstrate myocardial adrenergic nervous system disintegrity in patients with idiopathic dilated cardiomyopathy. J Am Coll Cardiol. 1988;12:1252–8.
37. Murata K, Kusachi S, Murakami T, Nogami K, Murakami M, Hirohata S, et al. Relation of iodine-123 metaiodobenzylguanidine myocardial scintigraphy to endomyocardial biopsy findings in patients with dilated cardiomyopathy. Clin Cardiol. 1997;20:61–6.
38. McGhie AI, Corbett JR, Akers MS, Kulkarni P, Sills MN, Kremers M, et al. Regional cardiac adrenergic function using I-123 meta-iodobenzylguanidine tomographic imaging after acute myocardial infarction. Am J Cardiol. 1991;67:236–42.
39. Tomoda H, Yoshioka K, Shiina Y, Tagawa R, Ide M, Suzuki Y. Regional sympathetic denervation detected by iodine 123 metaiodobenzylguanidine in non-Q-wave myocardial infarction and unstable angina. Am Heart J. 1994;128:452–8.
40. Stanton MS, Zipes DP. Modulation of drug effects by regional sympathetic denervation and supersensitivity. Circulation. 1991;84:1709–14.
41. Inoue H, Zipes DP. Results of sympathetic denervation in the canine heart: supersensitivity that may be arrhythmogenic. Circulation. 1987;75:877–87.
42. Gerson MC, Craft LL, McGuire N, Suresh DP, Abraham WT, Wagoner LE. Carvedilol improves left ventricular function in heart failure patients with idiopathic dilated cardiomyopathy and a wide range of sympathetic nervous system function as measured by iodine 123 metaiodobenzylguanidine. J Nucl Cardiol. 2002;9:608–15.
43. de Milliano PA, de Groot AC, Tijssen JG, van Eck-Smit BL, Van Zwieten PA, Lie KI. Beneficial effects of metoprolol on myocardial sympathetic function: Evidence from a randomized, placebo-controlled study in patients with congestive heart failure. Am Heart J. 2002;144, E3.
44. Naya M, Tsukamoto T, Morita K, Katoh C, Nishijima K, Komatsu H, et al. Myocardial beta-adrenergic receptor density assessed by 11C-CGP12177 PET predicts improvement of cardiac function after carvedilol treatment in patients with idiopathic dilated cardiomyopathy. J Nucl Med. 2009;50:220–5.
45. Tachikawa H, Kodama M, Watanabe K, Takahashi T, Ma M, Kashimura T, et al. Amiodarone improves cardiac sympathetic nerve function to hold norepinephrine in the heart, prevents left ventricular remodeling, and improves cardiac function in rat dilated cardiomyopathy. Circulation. 2005;111:894–9.
46. Toyama T, Hoshizaki H, Seki R, Isobe N, Adachi H, Naito S, et al. Efficacy of amiodarone treatment on cardiac symptom, function, and sympathetic nerve activity in patients with dilated cardiomyopathy: comparison with beta-blocker therapy. J Nucl Cardiol. 2004;11:134–41.
47. Toyama T, Hoshizaki H, Yoshimura Y, Kasama S, Isobe N, Adachi H, et al. Combined therapy with carvedilol and amiodarone is more effective in improving cardiac symptoms, function, and sympathetic nerve activity in patients with dilated cardiomyopathy: comparison with carvedilol therapy alone. J Nucl Cardiol. 2008;15:57–64.
48. Iuliano S, Fisher SG, Karasik PE, Fletcher RD, Singh SN. QRS duration and mortality in patients with congestive heart failure. Am Heart J. 2002;143:1085–91.
49. Cleland JG, Daubert JC, Erdmann E, Freemantle N, Gras D, Kappenberger L, et al. The effect of cardiac resynchronization on morbidity and mortality in heart failure. N Engl J Med. 2005;352:1539–49.
50. Nishioka SA, Martinelli Filho M, Brandao SC, Giorgi MC, Vieira ML, Costa R, et al. Cardiac sympathetic activity pre and post resynchronization therapy evaluated by 123I-MIBG myocardial scintigraphy. J Nucl Cardiol. 2007;14(6):852–9.
51. Jacobson AF, Senior R, Cerqueira MD, Wong ND, Thomas GS, Lopez VA, Agostini D, Weiland F, Chandna H, Narula J. ADMIRE-HF Investigators. Myocardial iodine-123 meta-iodobenzylguanidine imaging and cardiac events in heart failure. Results of the prospective ADMIRE-HF (Adre View myocardial imaging for risk evaluation in heart failure) study. J Am Coll Cardiol. 2010;55:2212–21.
52. Nakata T, Nakajima K, Yamashina S, Yamada T, Momose M, Kasama S, et al. A pooled analysis of multicenter cohort studies of (123)I-mIBG imaging of sympathetic innervation for assessment of long-term prognosis in heart failure. JACC Cardiovasc Imaging. 2013;6:772–84.
53. Tamaki S, Yamada T, Okuyama Y, Morita T, Sanada S, Tsukamoto Y, et al. Cardiac iodine-123 metaiodobenzylguanidine imaging predicts sudden cardiac death independently of left ventricular ejection fraction in patients with chronic heart failure and left ventricular systolic dysfunction: results from a comparative study with signal-averaged electrocardiogram, heart rate variability, and QT dispersion. J Am Coll Cardiol. 2009;53:426–35.
54. Fujimoto S, Inoue A, Hisatake S, Yamashina S, Yamashina H, Nakano H, et al. Usefulness of 123I-metaiodobenzylguanidine myocardial scintigraphy for predicting the effectiveness of beta-blockers in patients with dilated cardiomyopathy from the standpoint of long-term prognosis. Eur J Nucl Med Mol Imaging. 2004;31:1356–61.
55. Kuramoto Y, Yamada T, Tamaki S, Okuyama Y, Morita T, Furukawa Y, et al. Usefulness of cardiac iodine-123 meta-iodobenzylguanidine imaging to improve prognostic power of Seattle heart failure model in patients with chronic heart failure. Am J Cardiol. 2011;107(8):1185–90.
56. Kawai T, Yamada T, Tamaki S, Morita T, Furukawa Y, Iwasaki Y, Kawasaki M, Kikuchi A, Kondo T, Takahashi S, Ishimi M, Hakui H, Ozaki T, Sato Y, Seo M, Sakata Y, Fukunami M. Usefulness of cardiac meta-iodobenzylguanidine imaging to identify patients with chronic heart failure and left ventricular ejection fraction <35% at low risk for sudden cardiac death. Am J Cardiol. 2015;115:1549–54.
57. Shah AM, Bourgoun M, Narula J, Jacobson AF, Solomon SD. Influence of ejection fraction on the prognostic value of sympathetic innervation imaging with iodine-123 MIBG in heart failure. JACC Cardiovasc Imaging. 2012;5:1139–46.
58. Gemayel C, Pelliccia A, Thompson PD. Arrhythmogenic right ventricular cardiomyopathy. J Am Coll Cardiol. 2001;38:1773–81.
59. Corrado D, Basso C, Schiavon M, Thiene G. Screening for hypertrophic cardiomyopathy in young athletes. N Engl J Med. 1998;339:364–9.
60. Paul M, Wichter T, Kies P, Gerss J, Wollmann C, Rahbar K, et al. Cardiac sympathetic dysfunction in genotyped patients

with arrhythmogenic right ventricular cardiomyopathy and risk of recurrent ventricular tachyarrhythmias. J Nucl Med. 2011;52:1559–65.

61. Wichter T, Hindricks G, Lerch H, Bartenstein P, Borggrefe M, Schober O, et al. Regional myocardial sympathetic dysinnervation in arrhythmogenic right ventricular cardiomyopathy. An analysis using 123I-meta-iodobenzylguanidine scintigraphy. Circulation. 1994;89:667–83.

62. Wichter T, Schafers M, Rhodes CG, Borggrefe M, Lerch H, Lammertsma AA, Hermansen F, Schober O, Breithardt G, Camici PG. Abnormalities of cardiac sympathetic innervation in arrhythmogenic right ventricular cardiomyopathy. Quantitative assessment of presynaptic norepinephrine reuptake and postsynaptic β-adrenergic receptor density with positron emission tomography. Circulation. 2000;101:1552–8.

63. Wichter T, Matheja P, Eckardt L, Kies P, Schafers K, Schulze-Bahr E, et al. Cardiac autonomic dysfunction in brugada syndrome. Circulation. 2002;105(6):702–6.

64. Kies P, Wichter T, Schafers M, Paul M, Schafers KP, Eckardt L, Stegger L, Schulze-Bahr E, Rimoldi O, Breithardt G, Schober O, Camici PG. Abnormal myocardial presynaptic norepinephrine recycling in patients with brugada syndrome. Circulation. 2004;110:3017–22.

65. Kies P, Paul M, Gerss J, Stegger L, Monnig G, Schober O, et al. Impaired cardiac sympathetic innervation in symptomatic patients with long QT syndrome. Eur J Nucl Med Mol Imaging. 2011;38:1899–907.

66. Muller KD, Jakob H, Neuzner J, Grebe SF, Schlepper M, Pitschner HF. 123I-metaiodobenzylguanidine scintigraphy in the detection of irregular regional sympathetic innervation in long QT syndrome. Eur Heart J. 1993;14:316–25.

67. Mazzadi AN, Andre-Fouet X, Duisit J, Gebuhrer V, Costes N, Chevalier P, Rodriguez C, Schott J-J, Le Marec H, Guicheney P, Le Bars D, Janier M. Cardiac retention of [11C]HED in genotyped long QT patients: a potential amplifier role for severity of the disease. Am J Physiol Heart Circ Physiol. 2003;285:H1286–93.

68. Chevalier P, Rodriguez C, Bontemps L, Miquel M, Kirkorian G, Rousson R, Potet F, Schott J-J, Baro I, Touboul P. Non-invasive testing of acquired long QT syndrome: Evidence for multiple arrhythmogenic substrates. Cardiovasc Res. 2001;50:386–98.

69. Yamanari H, Nakayama K, Morita H, Miyazi K, Fukushima K, Matsubara H, Emori T, Ohe T. Effects of cardiac sympathetic innervation on regional wall motion abnormality in patients with long QT syndrome. Heart. 2000;83:295–300.

70. Calkins H, Lehmann MH, Allman K, Wieland D, Schwaiger M. Scintigraphic pattern of regional cardiac sympathetic innervation in patients with familial long QT syndrome using positron emission tomography. Circulation. 1993;87:1616–21.

71. Schäfers M, Wichter T, Lerch H, Matheja P, Kuwert T, Schafers K, et al. Cardiac 123I-MIBG uptake in idiopathic ventricular tachycardia and fibrillation. J Nucl Med. 1999;40:1–5.

72. Gill JS, Hunter GJ, Gane J, Ward DE, Camm AJ. Asymmetry of cardiac [123I] meta-iodobenzylguanidine scans in patients with ventricular tachycardia and a "clinically normal" heart. Br Heart J. 1993;69:6–13.

73. Schafers M, Lerch H, Wichter T, Rhodes CG, Lammertsma AA, Borggrefe M, Hermansen F, Schober O, Breithardt G, Camici PG. Cardiac sympathetic innervation in patients with idiopathic right ventricular outflow tract tachycardia. J Am Coll Cardiol. 1998;32:181–6.

74. Arora R, Ferrick KJ, Nakata T, Kaplan RC, Rozengarten M, Latif F, et al. I-123 MIBG imaging and heart rate variability analysis to predict the need for an implantable cardioverter defibrillator. J Nucl Cardiol. 2003;10:121–31.

75. Nagahara D, Nakata T, Hashimoto A, Wakabayashi T, Kyuma M, Noda R, et al. Predicting the need for an implantable cardioverter defibrillator using cardiac metaiodobenzylguanidine activity together with plasma natriuretic peptide concentration or left ventricular function. J Nucl Med. 2008;49:225–33.

76. Koutelou M, Katsikis A, Flevari P, Theodorakis G, Livanis E, Georgiadis M, et al. Predictive value of cardiac autonomic indexes and MIBG washout in ICD recipients with mild to moderate heart failure. Ann Nucl Med. 2009;23:677–84.

77. Boogers MJ, Borleffs CJ, Henneman MM, van Bommel RJ, van Ramshorst J, Boersma E, et al. Cardiac sympathetic denervation assessed with 123-iodine metaiodobenzylguanidine imaging predicts ventricular arrhythmias in implantable cardioverter-defibrillator patients. J Am Coll Cardiol. 2010;55:2769–77.

78. Nishisato K, Hashimoto A, Nakata T, Doi T, Yamamoto H, Nagahara D, et al. Impaired cardiac sympathetic innervation and myocardial perfusion are related to lethal arrhythmia: quantification of cardiac tracers in patients with ICDs. J Nucl Med. 2010;51:1241–9.

79. Sood N, Al Badarin F, Parker M, Pullatt R, Jacobson AF, Bateman TM, et al. Resting perfusion MPI-SPECT combined with cardiac 123I-mIBG sympathetic innervation imaging improves prediction of arrhythmic events in non-ischemic cardiomyopathy patients: sub-study from the ADMIRE-HF trial. J Nucl Cardiol. 2013;20:813–20.

80. Kramer CM, Nicol PD, Rogers WJ, Suzuki MM, Shaffer A, Theobald TM, et al. Reduced sympathetic innervation underlies adjacent noninfarcted region dysfunction during left ventricular remodeling. J Am Coll Cardiol. 1997;30(4):1079–85.

81. Matsunari I, Schricke U, Bengel FM, Haase HU, Barthel P, Schmidt G, et al. Extent of cardiac sympathetic neuronal damage is determined by the area of ischemia in patients with acute coronary syndromes. Circulation. 2000;101(22):2579–85.

82. Pettersen MD, Abe T, Morgan DA, Gutterman DD. Role of adenosine in postischemic dysfunction of coronary innervation. Circ Res. 1995;76(1):95–101.

83. Canty Jr JM, Suzuki G, Banas MD, Verheyen F, Borgers M, Fallavollita JA. Hibernating myocardium: chronically adapted to ischemia but vulnerable to sudden death. Circ Res. 2004;94:1142–9.

84. Luisi Jr AJ, Suzuki G, Dekemp R, Haka MS, Toorongian SA, Canty Jr JM, et al. Regional 11C-hydroxyephedrine retention in hibernating myocardium: chronic inhomogeneity of sympathetic innervation in the absence of infarction. J Nucl Med. 2005;46:1368–74.

85. Sasano T, Abraham MR, Chang KC, Ashikaga H, Mills KJ, Holt DP, et al. Abnormal sympathetic innervation of viable myocardium and the substrate of ventricular tachycardia after myocardial infarction. J Am Coll Cardiol. 2008;51:2266–75.

86. Fallavollita JA, Heavey BM, Luisi Jr AJ, Michalek SM, Baldwa S, Mashtare Jr TL, et al. Regional myocardial sympathetic denervation predicts the risk of sudden cardiac arrest in ischemic cardiomyopathy. J Am Coll Cardiol. 2014;63:141–9.

8 Cardiac Sympathetic Innervation and Ablation of Ventricular Tachycardia

John T. Duell, Thomas Klein, Mark F. Smith,
Wengen Chen, Vasken Dilsizian, and Timm Dickfeld

The cornerstone of current techniques for identifying successful ablation sites of ventricular tachyarrhythmias in patients with structural heart disease is the localization of abnormal or scarred myocardium. This tissue usually contains areas of slow conduction, which are critical for maintaining reentrant arrhythmias. Electroanatomic mapping performed in the electrophysiology laboratory identifies the presence of anatomic scar by decreased bipolar voltages measured with roving, steerable catheters. Given the inherent limitations of this technique, such as falsely low voltage recording due to poor catheter contact, the inability to detect intramural scar, and limited mapping density, imaging modalities such magnetic resonance imaging (MRI) [1], computed tomography (CT) [2], positron emission tomography (PET) [3], and single photon emission computed tomography [4] have been used to assess scar by demonstrating gadolinium enhancement, thinned walls, and perfusion/metabolic abnormalities. However, the recurrence rate in multicenter trials using state-of-the-art technology is close to 50% in the first 6 months after ventricular tachycardia (VT) ablation [5].

One possible explanation is that current ablation approaches focus primarily on anatomic substrate, which is necessary but not sufficient for the initiation of VT. The traditional paradigm of sustained VT also requires a substrate-modulating mechanism to trigger and maintain the arrhythmia. An example of such a triggering mechanism is innervation, which is known to modulate the incidence and prevalence of ventricular arrhythmias. Abnormal innervation has been correlated with increased arrhythmia risk and mortality for several decades [6, 7]. Recent studies in patients with cardiomyopathy have shown that damaged myocardial presynaptic nerve terminals lead to a reduced uptake of catecholamines via the uptake-1 mechanism [8]. This results in an accumulation of neurotransmitters in the synaptic cleft, with consequent downregulation of postsynaptic β-adrenergic receptors and an imbalance between pre- and postsynaptic signaling [9]. This disturbance is thought to lead to an increased risk of arrhythmias and contractile dysfunction. Indeed, pharmacologic sympathetic blockade resulted in a decreased risk for ventricular arrhythmias in this model [10]. Similarly, left and bilateral stellate ganglion block with resultant cardiac sympathetic denervation resulted in fewer implantable cardioverter–defibrillator (ICD) shocks [11]. In addition, sympathetic hypersensitivity, thought to be the result of nerve sprouting after myocardial injury, may lead to an increased risk of VT/ventricular fibrillation (VF) and sudden death [12, 13].

Cardiac innervation can be assessed by imaging the sympathetic and parasympathetic systems with a variety of radiotracers. Abnormalities in cardiac innervation have been demonstrated to correlate with an increased incidence of ICD shocks, VT inducibility, and mortality. In recent years, limited trials demonstrated the feasibility of image-guided therapeutic intervention, such as pharmacologic sympathetic blockade, which may be evaluated by using cardiac innervation tracers.

Advances in innervation imaging, as well the evolving understanding of the innervation–arrhythmia interplay, may allow for a novel paradigm of innervation-guided VT ablation that integrates possible triggering mechanisms and substrate modulators into ablation strategies.

V. Dilsizian, J. Narula (eds.), *Atlas of Cardiac Innervation*, DOI 10.1007/978-3-319-45800-7_8

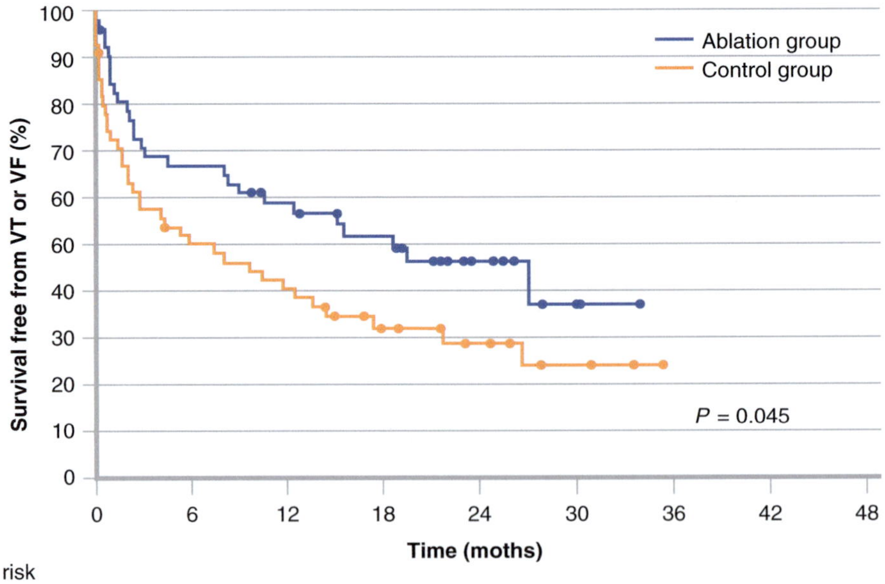

Number at risk

Ablation group	52	34	28	21	9	3	0
Control group	55	26	21	12	8	4	0

Figure 8-1. Success rates of VT ablation. The VTACH study [**14**] was a multicenter, open-label, randomized, controlled trial that enrolled patients with at least one prior VT episode and a history of coronary artery disease who were to undergo ICD implantation for secondary prevention. A total of 110 patients at 16 centers were randomly assigned to undergo either ICD implantation plus VT ablation, or ICD implantation alone. The primary end point was time from defibrillator implantation to recurrence of sustained ventricular arrhythmias. The protocol recommended traditional activation and entrainment mapping in conjunction with electroanatomic mapping used to identify substrate (discussed in subsequent figures). Additional imaging techniques to further refine targets for ablation were not part of the protocol. The primary end point of the study was positive (15.9 vs. 11.3 months to first recurrence; $P=0.045$), as the Kaplan–Meier curves demonstrate. However, even in the ablation group, a significant number of patients had recurrence of ventricular arrhythmias (41 % at 12 months, 53% at 24 months), demonstrating the need for further improvement to the procedure, possibly by including additional imaging modalities to define ablation targets. *VF* ventricular fibrillation.

Table 8-1. Traditional mapping methods.

Method	Description	Strengths	Weaknesses
Entrainment	Pacing during tachycardia, with responses indicating proximity of pacing catheter to tachycardia circuit	Localizes tachycardia Identifies different parts of tachycardia circuit (isthmus, exit site, outer loop)	Requires inducible, sustained, hemodynamically stable tachycardia
Activation	Sensing during tachycardia, with earlier signal demonstrating catheter is close to or within circuit	Localizes tachycardia Identifies different parts of tachycardia circuit (isthmus, exit site, outer loop)	Requires inducible, sustained, hemodynamically stable tachycardia
Pace match	Pacing during sinus rhythm with comparison of paced-beat QRS morphology with QRS morphology of tachycardia	Does not require sustained, hemodynamically stable tachycardia	Requires ECG of tachycardia Areas of functional block may vary
Electroanatomic	Measurement of voltage signal strength, with higher or normal voltage indicating healthy myocardium and lower voltage indicating areas of scar	Does not require ECG of tachycardia	Cannot identify tachycardia circuit, only areas of substrate at risk for causing tachycardia
Signal analysis	Assessment of signal characteristics in addition to voltage, such as electrogram fractionation, local abnormal ventricular activity, and diastolic potentials	In conjunction with electroanatomic mapping, can identify areas likely to be part of tachycardia circuit	Abnormal signals also may be found in areas of scar not in clinical tachycardia circuit

Several methods exist for mapping the location of the VT circuit; the table describes five of the most commonly used methods. Entrainment and activation mapping are considered the traditional gold standard of mapping. By moving the catheter around the ventricle while either pacing (entrainment) or sensing (activation) during tachycardia, it is possible to identify not only the points distant from, close to, and within the circuit, but also the critical isthmus of the circuit. Ablation at that point will break the circuit and render the tachycardia noninducible. However, these maneuvers must be performed during the tachycardia. In up to 90% of cases, the tachycardia cannot be induced, is not sustained, or is not tolerated by the patient for prolonged periods [**15**]. Under these circumstances, entrainment and activation mapping cannot be used

Pace match mapping overcomes some of these limitations because it can be performed during sinus rhythm. The QRS morphology during pacing is compared with the morphology of the tachycardia. When pacing demonstrates an identical match, this indicates that the catheter should be within the tachycardia circuit. Additional features, such as delay from pacing stimulation to QRS onset, may provide further help in identifying which part of the tachycardia circuit the catheter is in. One drawback to pace match mapping is that some areas of myocardium near the circuit may conduct differently in sinus rhythm than in VT, leading to differences in QRS morphologies even if the catheter is in the appropriate location. Additionally, it requires an ECG of the tachycardia for comparison with the paced QRS

Electroanatomic mapping, which uses the voltage strength of sensed signals to identify presumed areas of scar tissue, frequently is used as an adjunct to the previously described methods. During a VT ablation, a roving bipolar catheter is moved along the endocardial surface of the left ventricle. Position and bipolar signal are recorded every few millimeters along the left ventricular (LV) surface. Normal myocardium displays a bipolar voltage >1.5 mV, whereas a continuously decreasing voltage is found with increasing scar transmurality [**16**], allowing differentiation between the voltage-defined border zone (0.5–1.5 mV) and scar (<0.5 mV). Tachycardia circuits involve areas of scar, and identifying these areas during the procedure may help localize areas to target for ablation. Signal analysis during electroanatomic mapping can help identify other electrophysiologic markers of abnormal tissue, such as fractionated signals [**17**], diastolic potentials [**18**], and local abnormal ventricular activity [**19**]. If, because of an unstable or noninducible arrhythmia, the tachycardia cannot be mapped by entrainment, activation, or pace matching, electroanatomic mapping and signal analysis can identify areas for substrate modification via ablation (e.g., transecting across or ablating along a scar border) [**16**]

Even when taken together, these mapping methods have some significant drawbacks. All are performed with catheters in the heart, increasing procedure time and, therefore, complication risk. They may not identify scar that is not endocardial in location. Lastly, because of the focus on the anatomic substrate, potential triggering/substrate-modulating mechanisms required for arrhythmia initiation cannot be taken into consideration

Table 8-2. Imaging for VT ablation guidance.

Method	Possible benefits
CT	Assesses segmental anatomic (wall thickness), dynamic (wall thickening and motion), and perfusion (hypo/ hyperenhancement) abnormalities, which can predict electroanatomic abnormalities
MRI	Assesses areas of scar via late gadolinium enhancement
SPECT	Assesses regional myocardial perfusion and sarcolemmal or mitochondrial integrity, thereby differentiating viable from scarred myocardium
FDG-PET	Assesses metabolically abnormal myocardium
MIBG	Assesses areas of abnormal cardiac sympathetic innervation

Mapping ventricular tachycardia often is complicated by the fact that in 70–90% of cases, these rhythms are not hemodynamically tolerated or multiple VT morphologies are induced in the electrophysiology laboratory, making certain mapping techniques impossible [**5**, **15**, **16**]. Substrate-guided ablation of VT in structurally abnormal hearts via electroanatomic mapping involves placing ablation lesions in regions of scar (bipolar voltage <0.5 mV) or the border zone (bipolar voltage between 0.5 and 1.5 mV). As previously mentioned, electroanatomic mapping adds significant time to the procedure, averaging almost 2.5 h in one study [**20**]. Furthermore, a single endocardial voltage measurement only incompletely describes a complex intramural scar anatomy, and falsely low-voltage measurements due to suboptimal catheter contact may lead to incorrect scar definition

In the past several years, additional imaging modalities have been explored to compensate for the weakness of traditional mapping methods. Both cardiac CT and MRI may be used to assess for areas of scar before the procedure, potentially reducing procedure time by decreasing reliance on electroanatomic mapping. SPECT myocardial perfusion tracers are used to assess sarcolemmal or mitochondrial membrane integrity, beyond regional perfusion, thereby differentiating viable from scarred myocardium. Fludeoxyglucose (FDG)-PET and iodine-123 metaiodobenzylguanidine (^{123}I-MIBG) are used to evaluate metabolism and cardiac sympathetic innervation, respectively, revealing myocardial scar as well as possible trigger mechanisms contributing to ventricular arrhythmias in addition to anatomic substrate

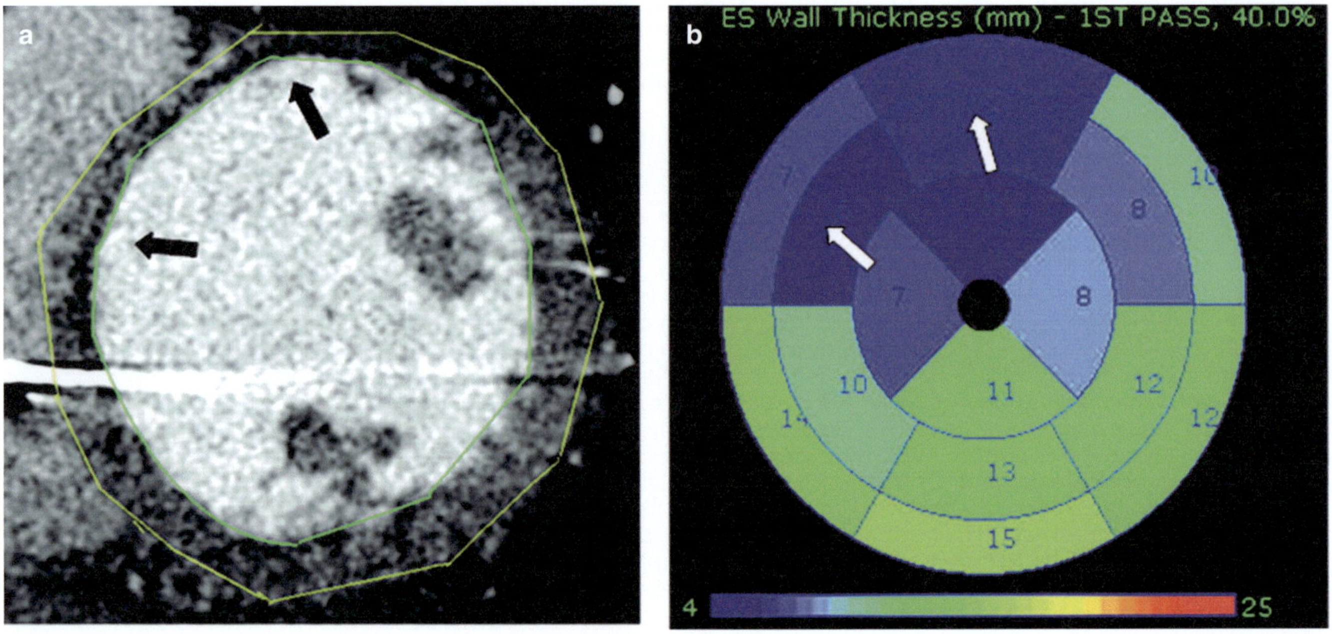

Figure 8-2. Contrast-enhanced CT. Contrast-enhanced CT may help in locating regions of scar exhibiting low voltage on electroanatomic mapping by incorporating perfusion (first-pass hypoperfusion or delayed enhancement), dynamic (wall motion, wall thickening), and anatomic (wall thinning) characteristics. (**a**), the anterior septum is thinned (*arrows*) compared with other myocardial segments, consistent with scar. Endocardium and epicardium are delineated with green and yellow lines, respectively. ICD metal streak artifact is noted in the septal and lateral walls. (**b**), Polar plot analysis of the ventricle based on end-systolic wall thickness. The wall thickness is assessed for each of the 17 segments, and the corresponding thickness (in millimeters) is shown for each segment. Note the color scale from green (normal thickness) to purple (abnormally thin), demonstrating the corresponding wall thinning in the anteroseptal wall segments (*arrows*). (**c**), three-dimensional (3D) reconstruction in short axis; *arrows* mark the scar region with visible wall thinning. (**d**), 17-segment analysis of the corresponding endocardial voltage map. Voltage-defined scar (red) is displayed in the same anteroseptal wall segments (*arrows*) as wall thinning in **b**, **c** (From Tian et al. [**2**]).

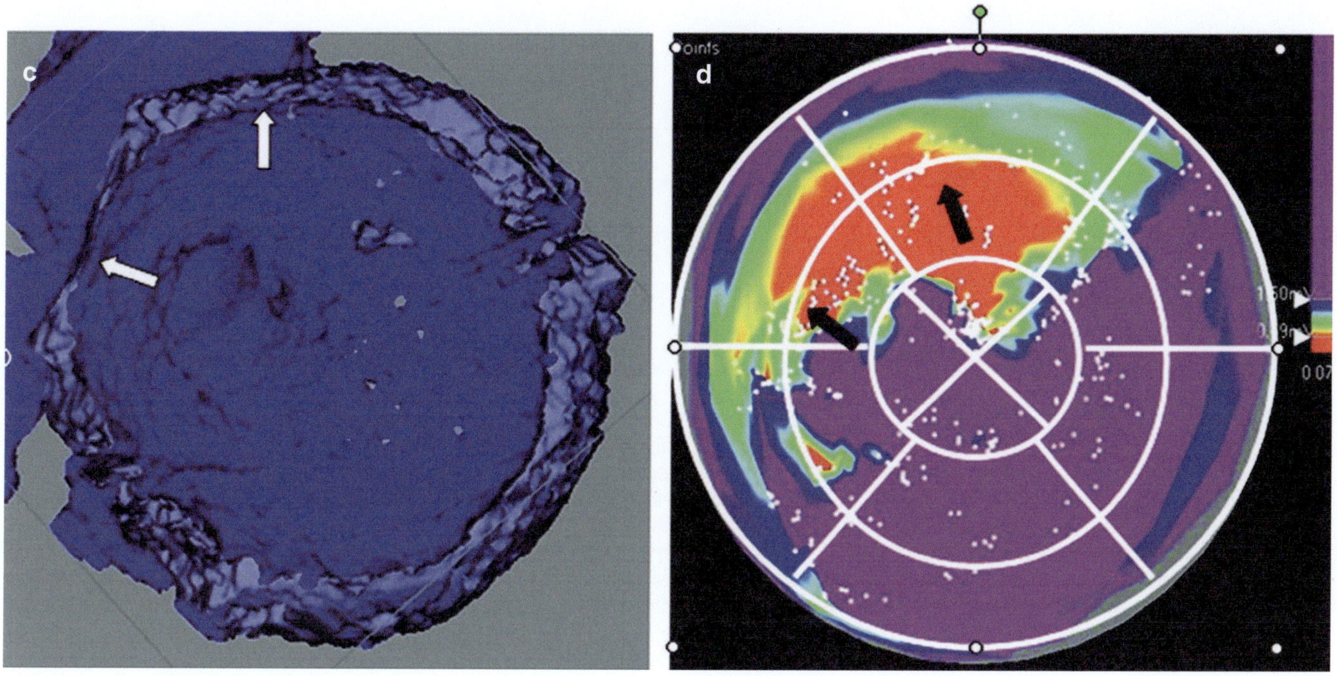

Figure 8-2. (continued)

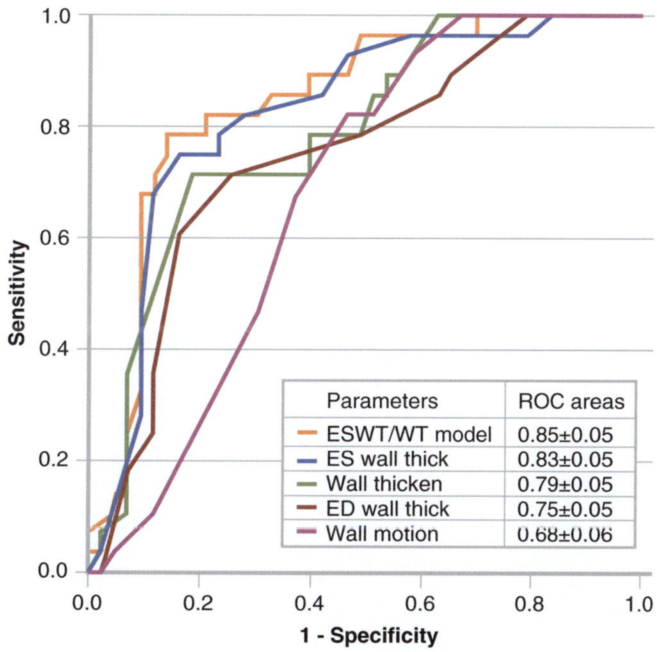

Figure 8-3. CT parameters to predict scar. Multiple parameters from contrast-enhanced cardiac CT were evaluated, including end-systolic (*ES*) wall thickness (*ESWT*), end-diastolic (*ED*) wall thickness, wall thickening (*WT*), and wall motion. ESWT and WT also were analyzed together, and this combination was best at predicting ventricular scar based on electroanatomic mapping, with ESWT being the best single parameter. Both these parameters were statistically better than wall motion. The combination correctly classified 81.7% of voltage segments into the appropriate category. The discrepancy between electroanatomic mapping and cardiac CT may the result of several factors. Small amounts of endocardial scar may result in decreased bipolar voltage, but may not yet result in significant anatomic and dynamic CT parameter changes. On the other hand, CT may be more sensitive at locating nonendocardial scar. Low-voltage areas on electroanatomic mapping that correspond to normal myocardium on cardiac CT may the result of poor catheter contact and falsely low voltage readings during mapping. *ROC* receiver operating characteristic (Adapted from Tian et al. [**2**]).

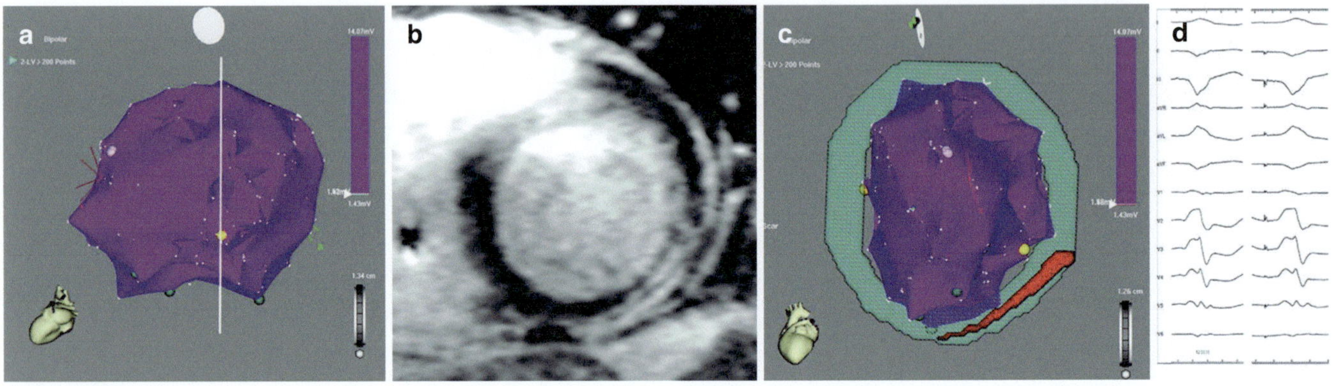

Figure 8-4. Cardiac MRI. Gadolinium-enhanced cardiac MRI can identify scar substrate for VT before ablation, potentially shortening procedure times and increasing success rates. This figure shows MRI-guided detection and ablation of mid-myocardial scar using traditional MRI sequences. (**a**), 3D electroanatomic map showing normal endocardial voltage, with the lowest bipolar voltage of 1.56 mV (categorized as normal myocardium) seen at the lateral left LV wall (*yellow point*). Based only on these data, there is little information available to guide pace match mapping or substrate modification. (**b**), however, the patient's corresponding gadolinium-enhanced cardiac MRI scan (in location of the white slice in **a**) demonstrates mid-myocardial scar with epicardial extension. (**c**), the image is reconstructed and registered to the endocardial voltage map, and is used to guide successful ablation. (**d**), comparison of the clinical VT (*left*) with the pace map match at the yellow point demonstrates a close similarity (>11/12 pace match; *right*), suggesting an endocardial exit site of the VT. Ablation at this site eliminated the VT (From Dickfeld et al. [**1**]).

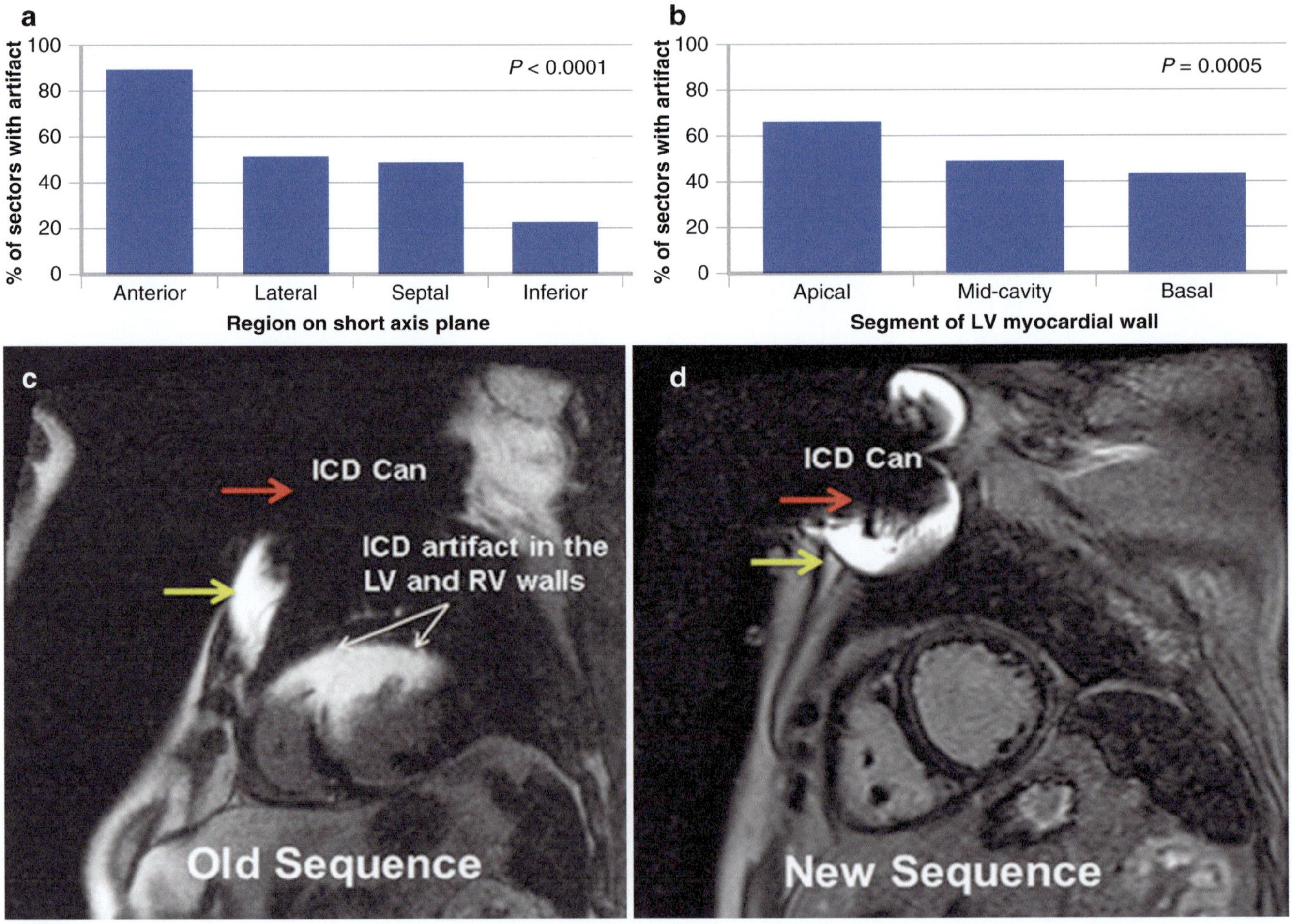

Figure 8-5. ICD artifact on MRI. Although gadolinium-enhanced cardiac MRI can assess myocardial scar in patients with VT before they undergo ablation, a potential drawback is the risk of device-associated artifact limiting MRI interpretation. In traditional late gadolinium MRI sequences, central signal void and peripheral increased signal intensity may be seen as a result of full and partial voxel dephasing. Although artifact often is present in the anterior wall, full or partial scar assessment is still possible in the rest of the myocardial segments. Additionally, new MRI sequences for scar characterization using bandwidth modulation significantly reduce ICD-induced artifact and are undergoing clinical testing. Successful ablation sites display late gadolinium enhancement (LGE) in nearly all cases, and can be registered to clinical mapping systems to guide VT ablation. This figure shows the areas of greatest impact of device-related artifact on evaluating cardiac fibrosis as assessed by LGE. (**a**, **b**), as seen here, the anterior and apical regions are most affected. In a series of 31 patients imaged with the traditional LGE protocol [**21**], at least some artifact was present in all patients. As a total proportion of LV myocardial area determined on short axis imaging, 54% of the myocardium was affected. Nevertheless, in all but one patient, a sufficient number of the LGE sequences were still interpretable, allowing for meaningful clinical utility in planning for VT ablation. (**c**, **d**), images exemplifying newer techniques for artifact suppression. (**c**), short axis slice at the mid-myocardium level using the standard LGE protocol. The black center correlates with the location of the ICD can (*red arrow*), leading to complete dephasing of the MRI voxel, resulting in a signal void. Surrounding this area is a "white halo" of high signal intensity, corresponding to partial MRI voxel dephasing (*yellow arrow*). Significant artifact is seen, affecting the assessment of LGE in the anterior and anteroseptal walls. (**d**), short axis image at the same level in the same patient, obtained by using a novel inversion sequence. No significant artifact involving the LV myocardium is noted, allowing complete assessment of myocardial scar. *RV* right ventricular (**a**, **b** adapted from Mesubi et al. [**21**]).

Table 8-3. Safety of cardiac MRI in patients with an ICD.

Parameter[a]	Pre-MRI	Post-MRI	Follow-up	P (pre/post)[b]
P-wave amplitude, *mV*	3.3±2.1	3.0±1.4	3.1±1.6	0.35
R-wave amplitude, *mV*	9.9±5.2	10.2±5.4	10.1±5.9	0.09
Atrial lead impedance, Ω	475±78	476±69	462±83	0.51
Ventricular lead impedance, Ω	461±97	451±89	450±95	0.82
Shock impedance, Ω	45±8	45±8	44±7	0.34
Atrial capture, *V*	1.5±0.9	1.4±0.9	1.5±1.0	0.32
V×ms	0.41±0.23	0.41±0.22	0.41±0.28	0.66
Ventricular capture, *V*	1.6±0.7	1.6±0.7	1.5±0.7	0.32
V×ms	0.43±0.18	0.44±0.16	0.44±0.15	0.79
Battery, *V*	2.97±0.21	2.97±0.21	2.95±0.22	0.08

[a]ICD parameters measured before and after MRI as well as after 68±21 days of follow-up summarize ventricular ($n=22$) and atrial ($n=13$) lead measurements. To account for devices allowing only pulse-width decrements, thresholds also are displayed as volts times milliseconds (V × ms)

[b]Significance was evaluated with Wilcoxon signed-rank tests

The safety of using cardiac MRI to assess myocardial scar burden in patients with defibrillators is of paramount importance. Historically, MRI was contraindicated in patients with implanted cardiac devices because of concerns regarding interactions between the magnetic field and the hardware and software of the device and leads, resulting in possible battery depletion, reprogramming, lead heating, or inappropriate shocks. The practical significance of these interactions has been brought into question, and more recent data indicate that MRI can be performed safely with the appropriate patient selection and safeguards. Several studies demonstrated the safety of using MRI to provide improved substrate evaluation and to facilitate VT ablation. The data from one such study [1] are summarized in the table. In this series of 22 patients, each patient's device was interrogated before, immediately after, and an average of 68 days after cardiac MRI was performed. The patients had a variety of devices, including single-chamber, dual chamber, and biventricular ICDs, as well as devices with wireless communication capacity. Furthermore, two patients were pacemaker dependent, with escape rhythms <30 bpm. As the data show, there were no significant changes in device battery status, lead parameters, or device programming. Importantly, there were no complications during MRI scan acquisition, including no inappropriate or inhibited pacing or tachytherapies

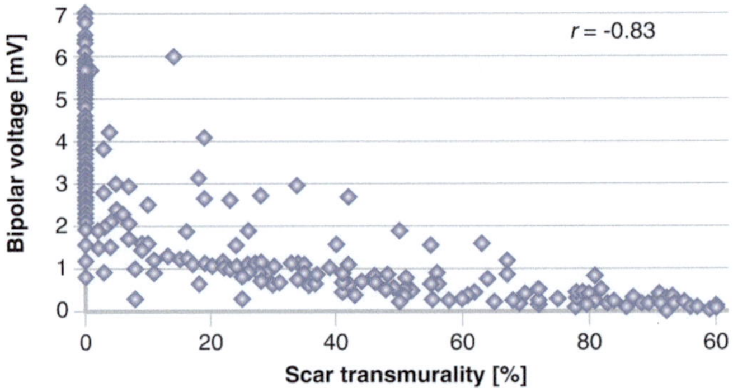

Figure 8-6. Correlation between MRI and voltage mapping. Cardiac MRI data from the same series of 22 patients were integrated with voltage mapping during VT ablation [**1**]. As seen here, there was a good correlation between scar transmurality, as assessed on cardiac MRI, and decreasing voltage. Additionally, cardiac MRI was helpful in determining false positive and false negative results when assessing scar by voltage. Areas without scar on MRI imaging with low voltage (<1.5 mV) suggested imperfect contact between the catheter and myocardium. After repeat mapping using echocardiography to confirm adequate contact, 78% of such points were shown to have normal voltage (>1.5 mV). Additionally, there were points at which nontransmural scar, identified on cardiac MRI, was not evident based on voltage mapping, presumably because of sparing of the endocardium or insufficient scar burden to diminish the voltage of that point (Adapted from Dickfeld et al. [**1**]).

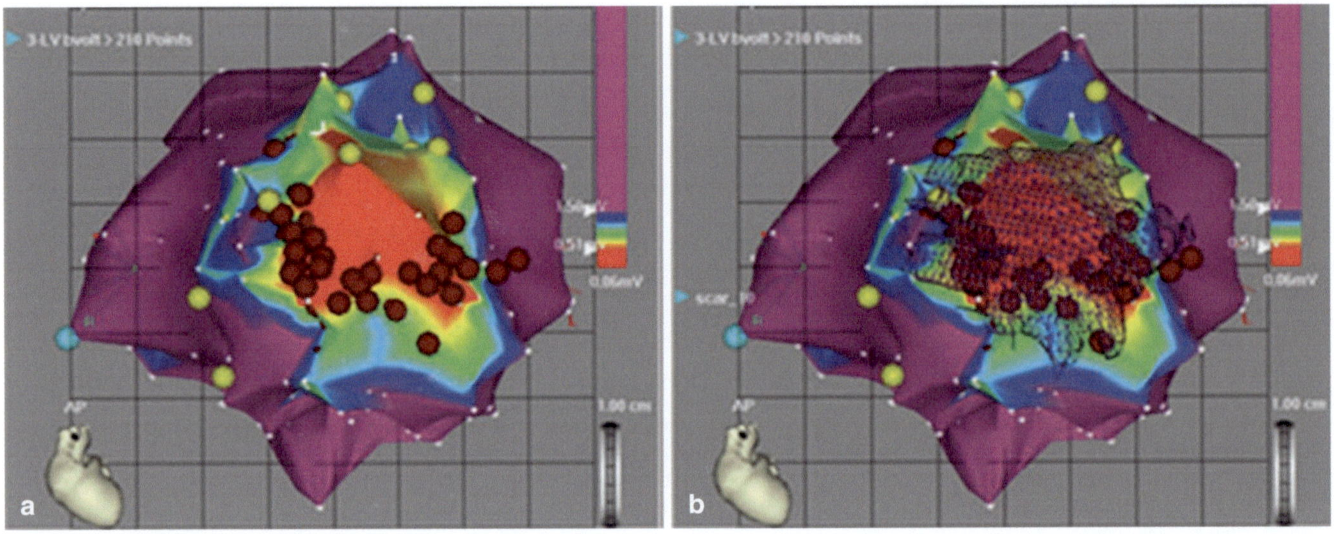

Figure 8-7. FDG-PET complements voltage mapping. FDG-PET imaging may be used to localize ablation sites for VT in structural heart disease. (**a**) left lateral view of the left ventricle with an apical scar (red: <0.5 mV). Surrounding areas demonstrate an adjacent border zone (yellow to blue: 0.5–1.5 mV) with preserved voltage in the remaining LV myocardium (purple >1.5 mV). Metabolic imaging with PET provides functional imaging data on the viability of myocardium and allows characterization of metabolically inactive, transmural LV scar (<50% tracer uptake) and border zone with only partial transmurality or residual metabolic activity (50–70% tracer uptake), as well as normal myocardium (70–100% tracer uptake). Reconstructions from serial short axis two-dimensional (2D) images can be reconstructed to 3D datasets, allowing detection of areas of scar. (**b**), the FDG-PET data are represented by a mesh network overlain on the voltage map. This may reveal intra-myocardial scar that is otherwise difficult to detect with either endo- or epicardial mapping. Importantly, it allows identification of areas within voltage-defined scar that represent possible channels of surviving myocardium and potential ablation targets. Registration of the metabolic PET reconstruction with the 3D electroanatomic map allows visualization of channels of alive myocardium otherwise thought to represent solely scar by voltage mapping traversing the "red" scar area. Brown "dots" mark areas of radiofrequency ablation to destroy surviving myocardium and cure the VT [**3**].

Table 8-4. Scar location according to the 17-segment American Heart Association model.

	Scar only		Partial scar	
Patient	Voltage map	3D PET	Voltage map	3D PET
1	4, 12	4, 12	3	3
2	4, 10	4, 10	3	3
3	10	9, 10	None	None
4	7, 13	7, 13	6, 8, 12, 16	6, 8, 12, 16
5	7, 8	7, 8	2, 13	2, 13
6	3, 14	3, 14	None	None
7	3, 5, 11, 12, 16	3, 5, 11, 12, 16	4, 10, 15	2, 10, 15
8	14	None	7, 10, 16	7, 10, 13
9	4	4	None	None
10	5	5	6, 11, 12	6, 11, 12

Tian et al. [**22**] reported a series of 10 patients who underwent FDG-PET before voltage mapping during VT ablation. Scar location based on both methods was assessed for each segment of the standard 17-segment model. Each segment was evaluated for no scar, partial scar, or complete scar; the table summarizes the findings. Fourteen of 15 segments (93.3%) identified as complete scar on FDG-PET matched the voltage map. Fifteen of 17 segments (88.2%) with metabolically defined partial scar matched the voltage map segments

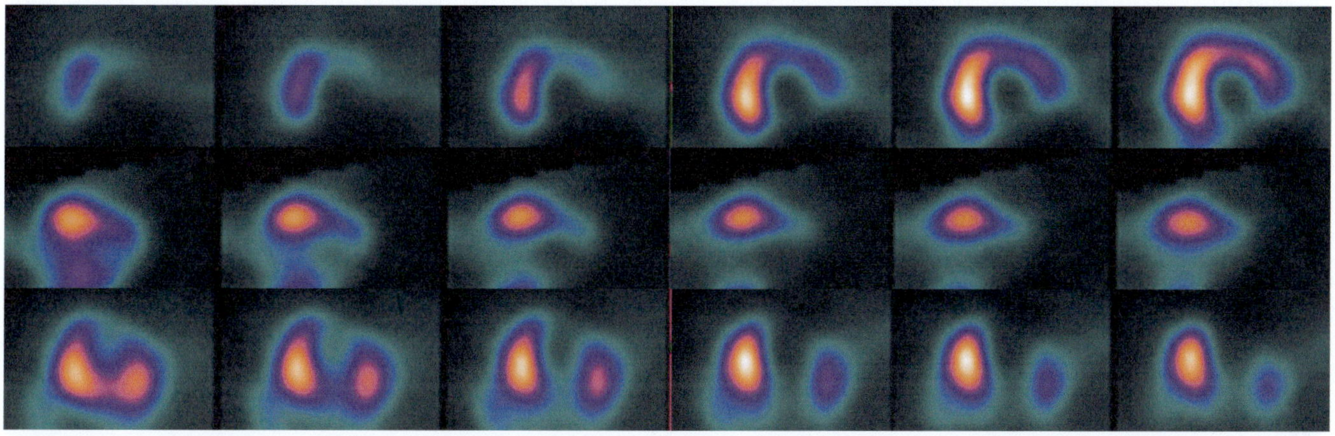

Figure 8-8. ^{123}I-MIBG SPECT imaging. Assessment of cardiac sympathetic innervation is another important imaging modality that may contribute to an understanding of the arrhythmia substrate and areas of abnormal innervation representing possible triggers for VT. The most studied radiotracer for imaging the cardiac sympathetic nervous system is ^{123}I-MIBG, which does not require an on-site cyclotron for preparation and is commercially available throughout the United States. ^{123}I-MIBG is a physiologic analogue of norepinephrine that is released into the synaptic cleft from presynaptic neurons in response to a sympathetic surge. In addition to global parameters of innervation, such as heart-to-mediastinum ratio and washout rate, which have been shown to correlate with heart failure outcomes [**23**], ^{123}I-MIBG SPECT imaging may be performed. This technique produces sequential short axis 2D slices, allowing a comprehensive 3D evaluation of the sympathetic LV innervation. Shown here is an example of ^{123}I-MIBG SPECT imaging, demonstrating significantly reduced ^{123}I-MIBG uptake, most notably in the inferior and inferolateral mid- to apical region.

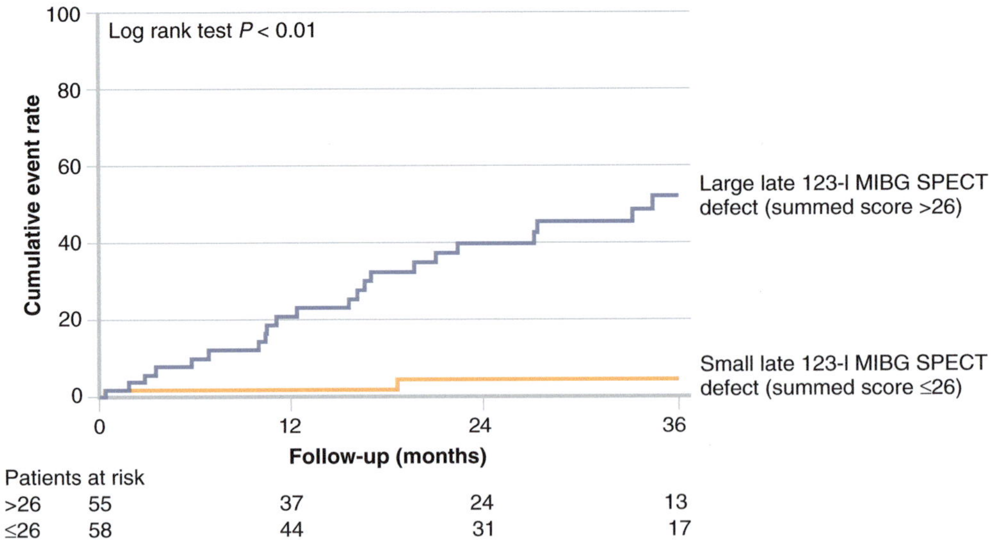

Figure 8-9. ^{123}I-MIBG SPECT imaging and ventricular arrhythmias. A series of 116 consecutive patients with heart failure who underwent ^{123}I-MIBG scanning before ICD placement looked at the association between defects seen on ^{123}I-MIBG imaging and appropriate ICD therapies. A summed defect score, calculated by assigning each segment within a 17-segment model a score between 0 and 4, was determined for each patient. Using a cut-off value of 26 to contrast large versus small/no defects, the authors demonstrated that larger defects predicted an increased risk for ventricular arrhythmias and ICD therapy [**24**] (Adapted from Boogers et al. [**24**]).

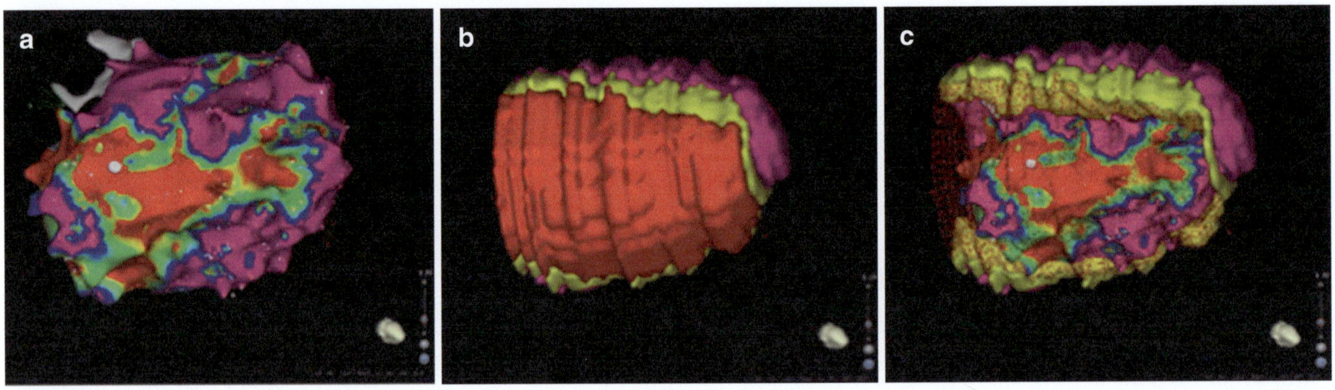

Figure 8-10. Cardiac sympathetic innervation and voltage map integration. Current approaches to ablation of VT in the setting of structural heart disease involve ablation of slowly conducting bundles of surviving cardiomyocytes within areas of scar that allow the propagation of reentrant arrhythmias. Although these bundles provide the substrate for reentrant arrhythmias, the current VT model also postulates a trigger initiating the arrhythmia. Because input from the sympathetic nervous system is thought to represent such a trigger, targeting abnormal sympathetic innervation to the heart may improve the current suboptimal success rate for VT ablation. Image integration has made guidance of VT ablation with innervation mapping possible. Three-dimensional reconstructions of ^{123}I-MIBG SPECT images can be created from sequential 2D short axis series and registered to electroanatomic maps obtained in the electrophysiology laboratory. This process allows innervation to be correlated with catheter-based electrophysiologic data during procedural planning and in laboratory. Abnormally innervated myocardium may be proarrhythmic, and successful ablation sites often are found in these regions [**25**]. With multimodality imaging, further characterization of the denervated substrate into, for example, denervated but viable myocardium (shown to be especially proarrhythmic in some studies [**25**]) is feasible even during the electrophysiologic procedure. (**a**) Inferior right anterior oblique view of a CARTO 3D electroanatomic endocardial map (Biosense-Webster, South Diamond Bar, CA) of the left ventricle. Purple endocardium represents normal voltage (bipolar voltage >1.5 mV). Blue, green, and yellow represent abnormal myocardium or scar border zone (bipolar voltage between 0.5 and 1.5 mV). Red represents scar (bipolar voltage <0.5 mV). The white dot represents a successful ablation site within scar. (**b**) Inferior right anterior oblique view of the corresponding 3D reconstructed ^{123}I-MIBG SPECT images. Denervated myocardium is represented by red (<50% tracer activity). Innervation transition zone (50–70% tracer activity) is represented by yellow. Normal innervation (>70% tracer uptake) is represented by purple. (**c**) Inferior right anterior oblique view of the reconstructed ^{123}I-MIBG innervation map registered to the endocardial voltage map. Denervated myocardium is shown in overlying red mesh, with the successful ablation point (white dot) within both endocardial scar and denervated myocardium (concordance of voltage-based scar and innervation defect).

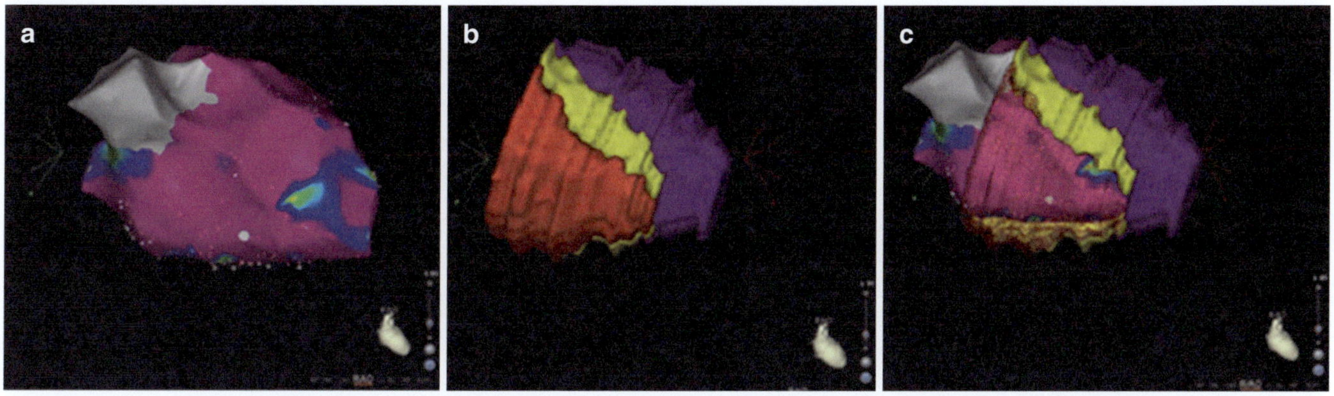

Figure 8-11. Innervation maps to guide VT ablation [**25**]. In an important subset of patients, successful ablation sites may be found in an area of normal voltage, without evidence of abnormal myocardium with decreased signal amplitude. This can make identifying and localizing successful sites of VT ablation challenging if using electroanatomic mapping alone. Cardiac innervation maps may provide additional information about the VT substrate not detected by electroanatomic voltage maps and help determine successful sites for VT. (**a**) Right anterior oblique view of an electroanatomic map of the left ventricle of a different patient, demonstrating a successful ablation site for VT (white dot) in an area of normal endocardial voltage (purple: >1.5 mV) on the interventricular septum. (**b**) Right anterior oblique view of a reconstructed ^{123}I-MIBG SPECT image demonstrating a large area of denervated myocardium (in red) on the interventricular septum extending to the inferior wall, surrounded by a rim of intermediate innervation. (**c**), the reconstructed ^{123}I-MIBG mage is registered to the endocardial voltage map in right anterior oblique view, and the successful ablation site again is seen in normal endocardial voltage; however, the ablation site is in an area of denervated myocardium (discordance of voltage-based scar and innervation defect).

Table 8-5. Localization of successful ablation sites by innervation and voltage status [**25**].

		Voltage map, sites, n		
		Scar	Border zone	Normal voltage
Innervation map, sites, *n*	Denervated	1	4	2
	Transition zone	1	3	3
	Normal myocardium	0	0	0

In a series of 15 patients with ischemic cardiomyopathy who underwent ^{123}I-MIBG imaging before VT ablation for drug-refractory VT, a total of 14 clinical VT sites were successfully mapped and ablated [**25**]. When considering abnormal myocardium as defined by voltage-based scar alone, fully 36% of these sites were in normal myocardium. However, 100% of the successful ablation sites were within areas of abnormal innervation, demonstrating the value of this imaging modality in helping to localize areas for successful ablation. This finding also suggests that innervation abnormalities may play a critical role as a trigger and substrate modulator responsible for ventricular arrhythmogenesis. In this study, traditional voltage mapping could not predict denervation reliably. Therefore, molecular innervation tracers, such as ^{123}I-MIBG have an important role in identifying areas of abnormal sympathetic innervation. Indeed, consistent with previous animal studies [**8**], areas of denervation were more than twice the size of voltage-defined scar

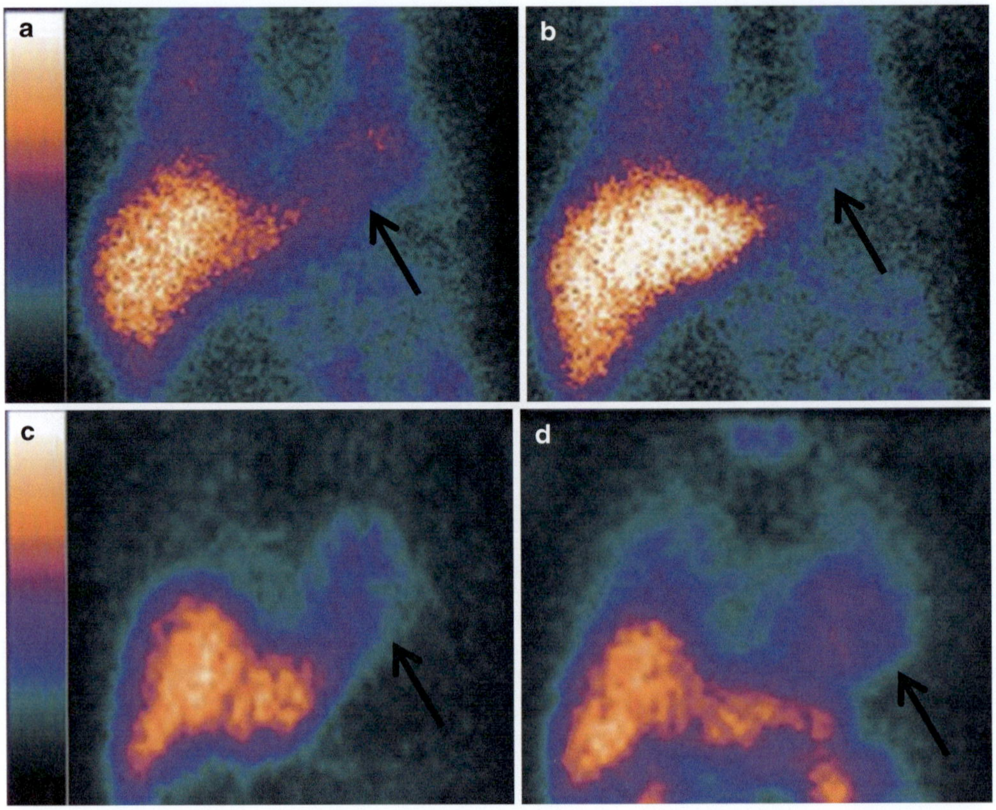

Figure 8-12. Change in cardiac sympathetic innervation as measured by ^{123}I-MIBG. Pharmacologic β-blockade, as well as modulation of the renin–angiotensin–aldosterone system and cardiac resynchronization therapy, has been shown to improve cardiac sympathetic innervation as assessed with ^{123}I-MIBG. Similarly, ablation of VT can also modify global cardiac sympathetic innervation. This image demonstrates changes in cardiac innervation after VT ablation in two patients, as assessed by 4-h delayed ^{123}I-MIBG images before and 6 months after the procedure. (**a**, **b**), in the first patient, there is a significant decrease in myocardial uptake (*arrows*). (**c**, **d**), in the second patient, there is a significant increase in myocardial uptake after the ablation (*arrows*). (**a**, **c**: before ablation; **b**, **d**: after ablation) (From Klein et al. [**26**]).

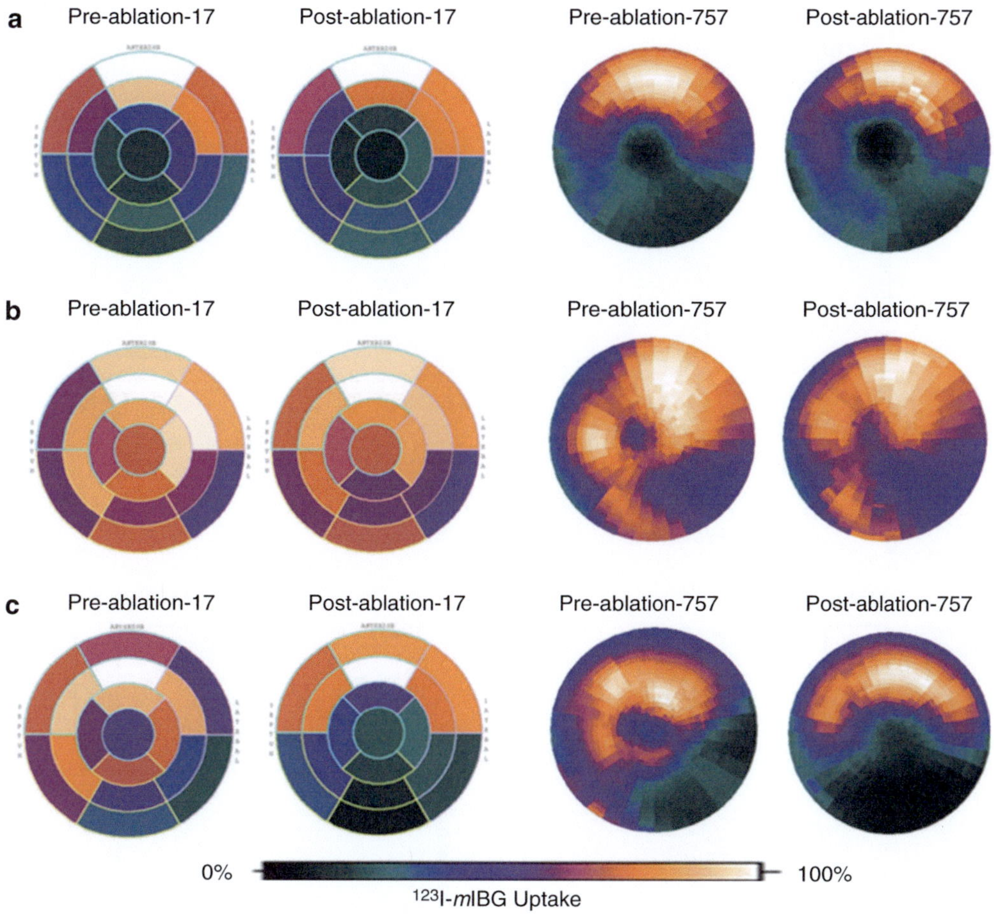

Figure 8-13. High-resolution, 757-segment model for innervation. Current assessments of cardiac sympathetic innervation using global parameters and the 17-segment model have several shortcomings. Loss of sympathetic innervation is regional and heterogeneous, limiting the utility of global parameters. The current 17-segment model was designed with consideration of coronary artery distribution, in which localizing perfusion to portions of the three major coronary arteries is needed [**27**]. Importantly, segment sizes of the 17-segment model do not have the resolution to identify small regional innervation changes relevant for possible proarrhythmicity or to analyze the effects of ablation with catheter tips as small as 3.5 mm. To overcome these obstacles, a novel arrhythmia-specific 757-segment model of cardiac sympathetic innervation was applied in a series of patients who underwent ^{123}I-MIBG imaging before and 6 months after VT ablation [**28**]. Polar plots of the standard 17-segment and 757-segment ^{123}I-MIBG uptake at baseline and after VT ablation are shown here. The three panels show the 17-segment polar plots (*left*) and corresponding 757-segment plots (*right*) from three patients, contrasting baseline ^{123}I-MIBG scans with those done 6 months after ablation. (**a**), images from a patient with ischemic cardiomyopathy; no significant changes are seen after VT ablation. (**b**), images from a patient with nonischemic cardiomyopathy; again, no significant changes are seen after VT ablation. (**c**), images from a different patient with ischemic cardiomyopathy; ^{123}I-MIBG uptake is reduced after VT ablation, indicating diminished cardiac sympathetic innervation (From Abdulghani et al. [**28**]).

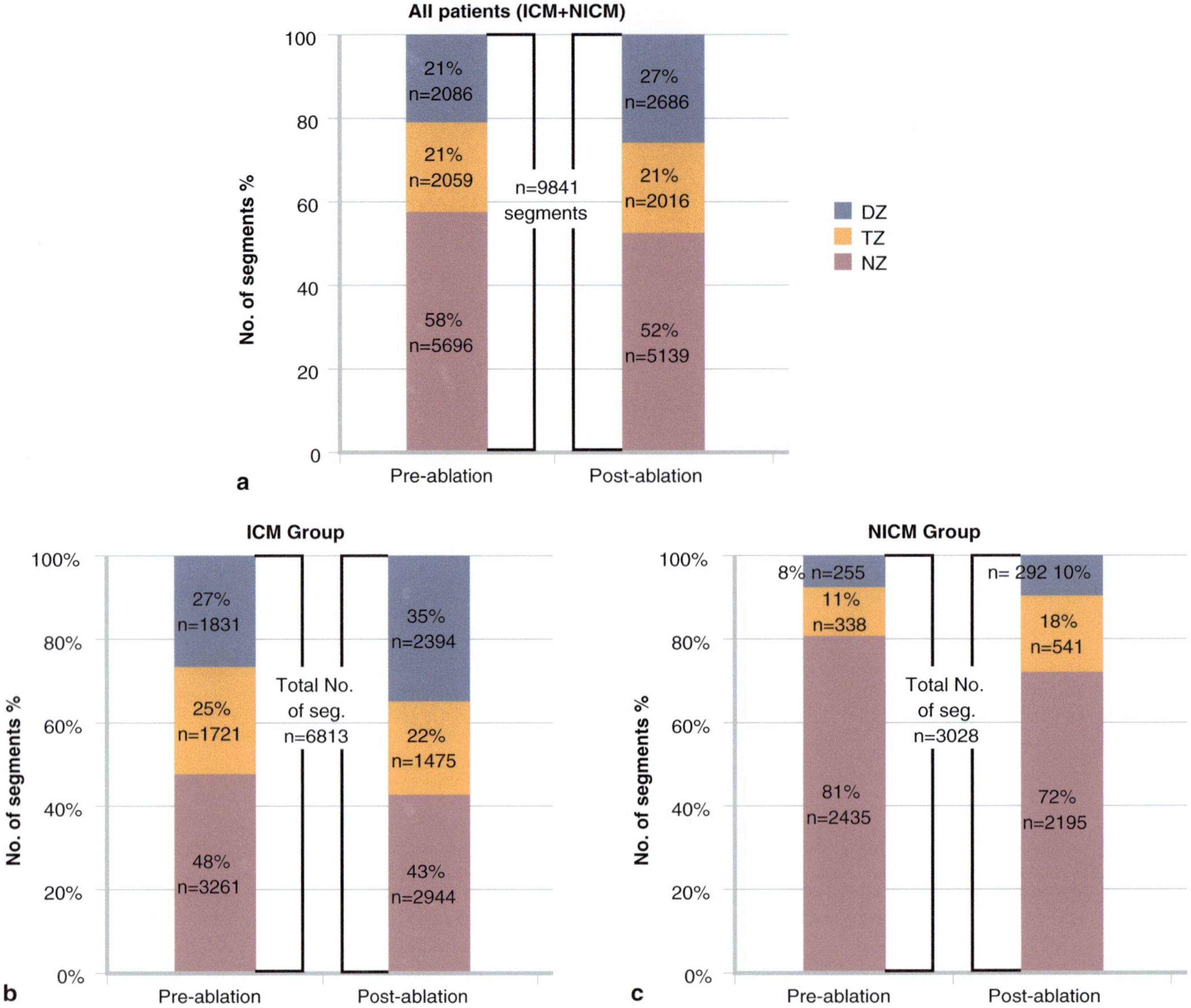

Figure 8-14. Changes in cardiac sympathetic innervation by segment type. Innervation on SPECT ^{123}I-MIBG imaging may be divided into three zones by comparing a particular segment's signal strength with the segment that has the greatest signal strength. The following threshold values were derived from ROC curves in a recent study: normal innervation (uptake >47%), denervated myocardium (<30%), and a transition zone (TZ; 30–47%) [**28**]. From the previously mentioned series, the percentage of segments from the 757-segment model in each of the three categories is shown before and after VT ablation. (**a**), summary of all patients (ischemic [ICM] and nonischemic cardiomyopathy [NICM]). (**b**, **c**) comparison of patients with ICM (**b**) with those with NICM (**c**). The patients with ICM had a significantly higher percentage of abnormally innervated myocardium (denervated zone [DZ] or TZ) compared with those with NICM, both before and after ablation. Although global cardiac sympathetic innervation did not change significantly after VT ablation, dynamic changes from before to after ablation were seen at the segmental level in all patients, supporting the importance of a high-resolution segmental analytic approach. Changes predominantly occurred at areas that did not undergo ablation themselves. Changes distant from points of ablation may be the result of a variety of causes, including downstream effects of ablation on proximal nerve sites, changes in the ventricular milieu due to decreased arrhythmia burden, or other unknown feedback mechanisms that contribute to the regulation of cardiac sympathetic innervation. Regional changes affected all three innervation categories, but were proportionally highest in the TZ, possibly indicating an area with increased innervation instability. *NZ* normally innervated zone (Adapted from Abdulghani et al. [**28**]).

References

1. Dickfeld T, Tian J, Ahmad G, et al. MRI-Guided ventricular tachycardia ablation: integration of late gadolinium-enhanced 3D scar in patients with implantable cardioverter-defibrillators. Circ Arrhythm Electrophysiol. 2011;4:172–84.
2. Tian J, Jeudy J, Smith MF, et al. Three-dimensional contrast-enhanced multidetector CT for anatomic, dynamic, and perfusion characterization of abnormal myocardium to guide ventricular tachycardia ablations. Circ Arrhythm Electrophysiol. 2010;3:496–504.
3. Dickfeld T, Lei P, Dilsizian V, et al. Integration of three-dimensional scar maps for ventricular tachycardia ablation with positron emission tomography-computed tomography. JACC Cardiovasc Imaging. 2008;1:73–82.
4. Tian J, Smith M, Ahmad G, Dilsizian V, Jimenez A, Dickfeld T. Integration of three dimensional scar maps using single photon emission computed tomography to guide ventricular tachycardia ablation. J Nucl Med. 2012;53:894–901.
5. Stevenson WG, Wilber DJ, Natale A, et al. Irrigated radiofrequency catheter ablation guided by electroanatomic mapping for recurrent ventricular tachycardia after myocardial infarction: the multicenter thermocool ventricular tachycardia ablation trial. Circulation. 2008;118:2773–82.
6. Cohn JN, Levine TB, Olivari MT, et al. Plasma norepinephrine as a guide to prognosis in patients with chronic congestive heart failure. N Engl J Med. 1984;311:819–23.
7. Merlet P, Valette H, Dubois-Rande JL, et al. Prognostic value of cardiac metaiodobenzylguanidine imaging in patients with heart failure. J Nucl Med. 1992;33:471–7.
8. Sasano T, Abraham MR, Chang KC, et al. Abnormal sympathetic innervation of viable myocardium and the substrate of ventricular tachycardia after myocardial infarction. J Am Coll Cardiol. 2008;51:2266–75.
9. Caldwell JH, Link JM, Levy WC, Poole JE, Stratton JR. Evidence for pre- to postsynaptic mismatch of the cardiac sympathetic nervous system in ischemic congestive heart failure. J Nucl Med. 2008;49:234–41.
10. Packer M, Bristow MR, Cohn JN, et al. The effect of carvedilol on morbidity and mortality in patients with chronic heart failure. U.S. Carvedilol Heart Failure Study Group. N Engl J Med. 1996;334:1349–55.
11. Vaseghi M, Gima J, Kanaan C, et al. Cardiac sympathetic denervation in patients with refractory ventricular arrhythmias or electrical storm: intermediate and long-term follow-up. Heart Rhythm. 2014;11:360–6.
12. Chen PS, Chen LS, Cao JM, Sharifi B, Karagueuzian HS, Fishbein MC. Sympathetic nerve sprouting, electrical remodeling and the mechanisms of sudden cardiac death. Cardiovasc Res. 2001;50:409–16.
13. Cao JM, Fishbein MC, Han JB, et al. Relationship between regional cardiac hyperinnervation and ventricular arrhythmia. Circulation. 2000;101:1960–9.
14. Kuck KH, Schaumann A, Eckardt L, et al. Catheter ablation of stable ventricular tachycardia before defibrillator implantation in patients with coronary heart disease (VTACH): a multicentre randomised controlled trial. Lancet. 2010;375:31–40.
15. Morady F, Harvey M, Kalbfleisch SJ, el-Atassi R, Calkins H, Langberg JJ. Radiofrequency catheter ablation of ventricular tachycardia in patients with coronary artery disease. Circulation. 1993;87:363–72.
16. Marchlinski FE, Callans DJ, Gottlieb CD, Zado E. Linear ablation lesions for control of unmappable ventricular tachycardia in patients with ischemic and nonischemic cardiomyopathy. Circulation. 2000;101:1288–96.
17. Haqqani HM, Marchlinski FE. Electrophysiologic substrate underlying postinfarction ventricular tachycardia: characterization and role in catheter ablation. Heart Rhythm. 2009;6:S70–6.
18. Cabo C, Schmitt H, Masters G, Coromilas J, Wit AL, Scheinman MM. Location of diastolic potentials in reentrant circuits causing sustained ventricular tachycardia in the infarcted canine heart: relationship to predicted critical ablation sites. Circulation. 1998;98:2598–607.
19. Jais P, Maury P, Khairy P, et al. Elimination of local abnormal ventricular activities: a new end point for substrate modification in patients with scar-related ventricular tachycardia. Circulation. 2012;125:2184–96.
20. Fahmy TS, Wazni OM, Jaber WA, et al. Integration of positron emission tomography/computed tomography with electroanatomical mapping: a novel approach for ablation of scar-related ventricular tachycardia. Heart Rhythm. 2008;5:1538–45.
21. Mesubi O, Ahmad G, Jeudy J, et al. Impact of ICD artifact burden on late gadolinium enhancement cardiac MR imaging in patients undergoing ventricular tachycardia ablation. Pacing Clin Electrophysiol. 2014;37:1274–83.
22. Tian J, Smith MF, Chinnadurai P, et al. Clinical application of PET/CT fusion imaging for three-dimensional myocardial scar and left ventricular anatomy during ventricular tachycardia ablation. J Cardiovasc Electrophysiol. 2009;20:597–604.
23. Jacobson AF, Senior R, Cerqueira MD, et al. Myocardial iodine-123 meta-iodobenzylguanidine imaging and cardiac events in heart failure. Results of the prospective ADMIRE-HF (AdreView Myocardial Imaging for Risk Evaluation in Heart Failure) study. J Am Coll Cardiol. 2010;55:2212–21.
24. Boogers MJ, Borleffs CJ, Henneman MM, et al. Cardiac sympathetic denervation assessed with 123-iodine metaiodobenzylguanidine imaging predicts ventricular arrhythmias in implantable cardioverter-defibrillator patients. J Am Coll Cardiol. 2010;55:2769–77.
25. Klein T, Abdulghani M, Smith M, et al. Three-dimensional 123I-meta-iodobenzylguanidine cardiac innervation maps to assess substrate and successful ablation sites for ventricular tachycardia: a feasibility study for a novel paradigm of innervation imaging. Circ Arrhythm Electrophysiol. 2015;8:583–91.
26. Klein T, Dilsizian V, Cao Q, Chen W, Dickfeld TM. The potential role of iodine-123 metaiodobenzylguanidine imaging for identifying sustained ventricular tachycardia in patients with cardiomyopathy. Curr Cardiol Rep. 2013;15:359.
27. Cerqueira MD, Weissman NJ, Dilsizian V, et al. Standardized myocardial segmentation and nomenclature for tomographic imaging of the heart. A statement for healthcare professionals from the Cardiac Imaging Committee of the Council on Clinical Cardiology of the American Heart Association. Circulation. 2002;105:539–42.
28. Abdulghani M, Duell J, Smith M, et al. Global and regional myocardial innervation before and after ablation of drug-refractory ventricular tachycardia assessed with 123I-MIBG. J Nucl Med. 2015;56 Suppl 4:52s–8.

9 Dysautonomia: From the Brain Disorders to Neuropathies and Including Diabetes

Albert Flotats and Ignasi Carrió

Introduction

Table 9-1. Common causes of dysautonomia.

Synucleinopathies
Lewy body disorders
Parkinson disease
Primary motor disease with parkinsonism and frequent peripheral autonomic neuropathy, orthostatic hypotension, and dementia
Dementia with Lewy bodies
Rapidly progressive dementia with frequent peripheral autonomic neuropathy, orthostatic hypotension, and parkinsonism
Pure autonomic failure (idiopathic orthostatic hypotension)
Sporadic, primary peripheral (postganglionic) autonomic neuropathy that occurs isolated from other neurologic disorders
Multiple system atrophy (MSA)
Sporadic, central (preganglionic) autonomic neuropathy with orthostatic hypotension, parkinsonism, and cerebellar ataxia in any combination
MSA–parkinsonian
Formerly designated striatonigral degeneration. The striatum and mesencephalon are especially vulnerable and dysfunctional, and parkinsonism dominates the clinical picture.
MSA–cerebellar
Formerly designated olivopontocerebellar atrophy. The brainstem and cerebellum are especially vulnerable and dysfunctional, and cerebellar features dominate the clinical picture.
Shy–Drager syndrome
Autonomic failure dominates the clinical picture.

V. Dilsizian, J. Narula (eds.), *Atlas of Cardiac Innervation*, DOI 10.1007/978-3-319-45800-7_9

Table 9-1. (continued)

Diabetes mellitus
Peripheral autonomic neuropathy with frequent orthostatic hypotension
Toxicity
Peripheral autonomic neuropathy caused by alcohol, chemotherapy drugs, metal poisoning, or ganglionic blockers
Amyloidosis
Autonomic neuropathy caused by neuronal amyloid protein deposition
Autoimmune ganglionic neuropathy
Peripheral autonomic neuropathy caused by antibody targeting of the a3 subunit of the acetylcholine receptor at the autonomic ganglia level
Familial dysautonomia (Riley–Day syndrome)
Autosomal recessive disease of the autonomic nervous system with loss of neuronal fibers (most commonly seen in Ashkenazi Jews)

Rapid adjustments in blood pressure, temperature, and countless other vital physiologic processes are accomplished by the autonomic nervous system. *Dysautonomia* refers to dysfunction of the autonomic nervous system, which may occur as a primary disorder or secondary to other pathologic conditions causing damage to the central or peripheral nervous system. Some of the common causes of dysautonomia, along with their main features, are listed in the table

When severe autonomic failure occurs, there are striking and sometimes paradoxic responses to a variety of physiologic and pharmacologic stimuli with common clinical features. However, initial symptoms may be difficult to identify

Radionuclide techniques for cardiac neurotransmission imaging allow in vivo noninvasive assessment of cardiac sympathetic innervation, which provides an important supplement to physiologic, neurochemical, and neuropharmacologic methods for evaluating patients with dysautonomia. Most sympathetic neuroimaging to date has involved visualization of noradrenergic innervation in the left ventricle, mainly by means of cardiac iodine-123 metaiodobenzylguanidine (^{123}I-MIBG) imaging. Decreased ^{123}I-MIBG uptake, as reflected by heart-to-mediastinum ratio (H/M), increased washout rate (WR), or both have been reported in some patients with dysautonomia. The assessment of these scintigraphic parameters has several advantages for the study of such patients, including its simplicity and reproducibility [1]

Neurodegenerative Diseases

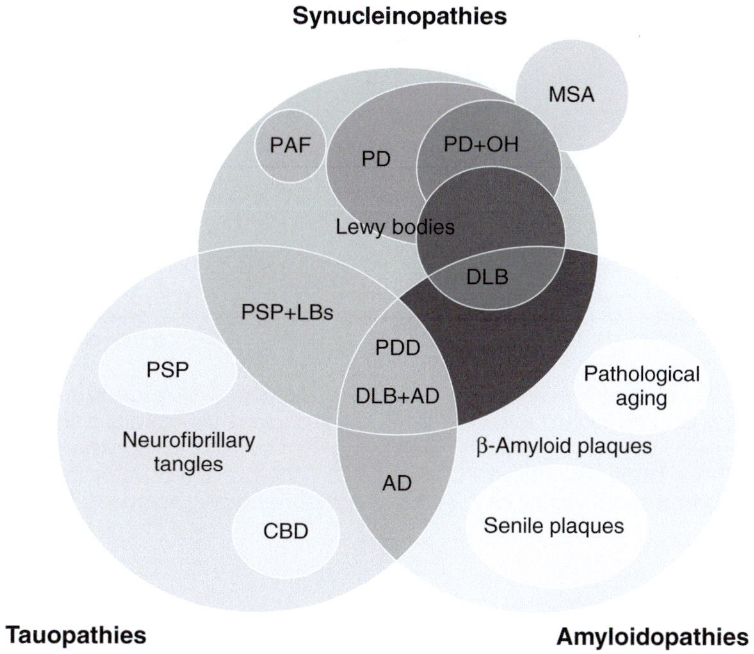

Figure 9-1. Some of the most severe forms of dysautonomia appear in neurodegenerative diseases. Aggregation of misfolded protein is a common characteristic of many neurodegenerative disorders, with considerable interaction between pathologic/toxic proteins and neurodegeneration. Dysautonomia is common in the synucleinopathies, a group of disorders characterized by intracellular cytoplasmic inclusions of abnormal accumulation of misfolded α-synuclein protein. Synucleinopathies include Lewy body disorders (Parkinson disease [*PD*], dementia with Lewy bodies [*DLB*], and pure autonomic failure [*PAF*]), as well as multiple system atrophy (*MSA*). Lewy body disorders are characterized by Lewy bodies and Lewy neurite aggregates, which mainly consist of α-synuclein assembled into fibrillar inclusions that stain with periodic acid–Schiff and ubiquitin [2, 3]. In addition, most of these neurodegenerative diseases, as well as others such as some tauopathies (characterized by accumulation of tau protein as a major constituent of neurofibrillary tangles, e.g. corticobasal degeneration [*CBD*] and progressive supranuclear palsy [*PSP*]), present with parkinsonian movement disorders, and some also present with dementia. The pathologic interaction among different neurodegenerative processes also includes the amyloidopathies, which also may present with dementia (e.g., Alzheimer disease [AD]). *LBs* Lewy bodies, *OH* orthostatic hypotension, *PDD* Parkinson disease dementia.

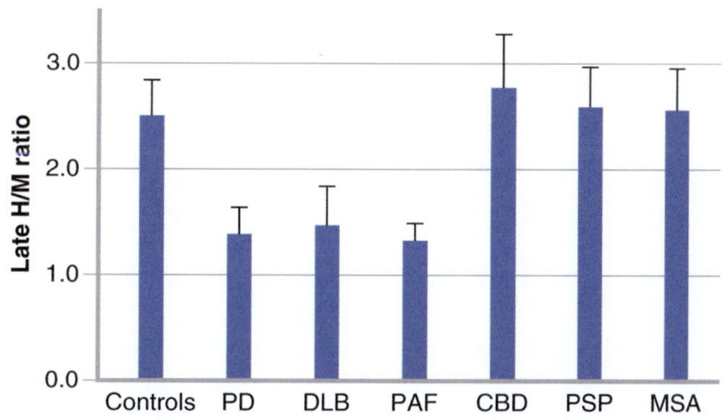

Figure 9-2. The overlapping of pathophysiologic and clinical features among different neurodegenerative diseases often makes the differential diagnosis difficult, especially in the early stages or in patients with atypical symptoms, resulting in an initial misdiagnosis in nearly 25% of patients with parkinsonism. Cardiac sympathetic imaging helps in this differential diagnosis, as can be seen here. The decreased cardiac ^{123}I-MIBG uptake reflects the extensive distribution of Lewy aggregates through the nervous system (in both the central and peripheral nervous systems in PD and DLB, and in the peripheral nervous system in PAF), including the postganglionic sympathetic and intrinsic neurons in the heart (Adapted from Kashihara et al. [4]).

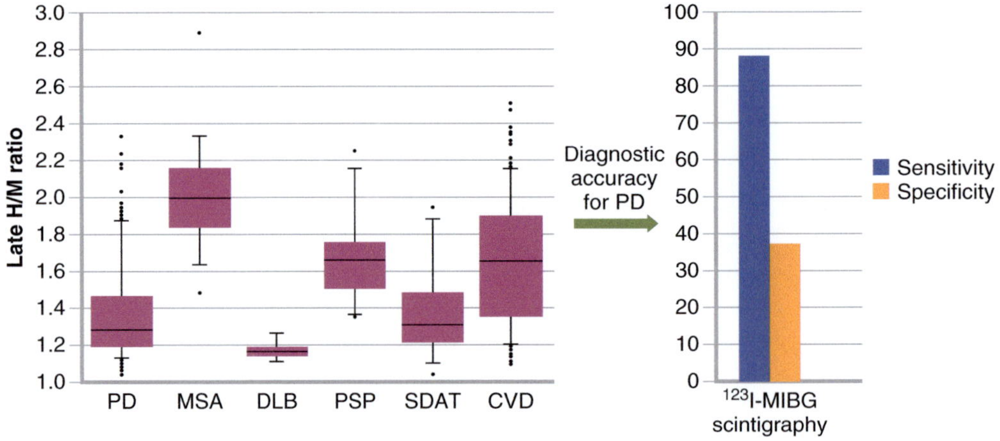

Figure 9-3. In a study including 391 outpatients with parkinsonian symptoms and 10 healthy control individuals of similar age, ^{123}I-MIBG was decreased in most patients with PD. However, more than half the patients without PD also exhibited low uptake, resulting in a sensitivity of 87.7% and specificity of 37.4% for detecting PD (H/M ratio cutoff value >2 standard deviations below the control mean), indicating that cardiac sympathetic denervation is not specific for PD. *CVD* cardiovascular disease, *SDAT* senile dementia of Alzheimer type (Adapted from Nagayama et al. [5]).

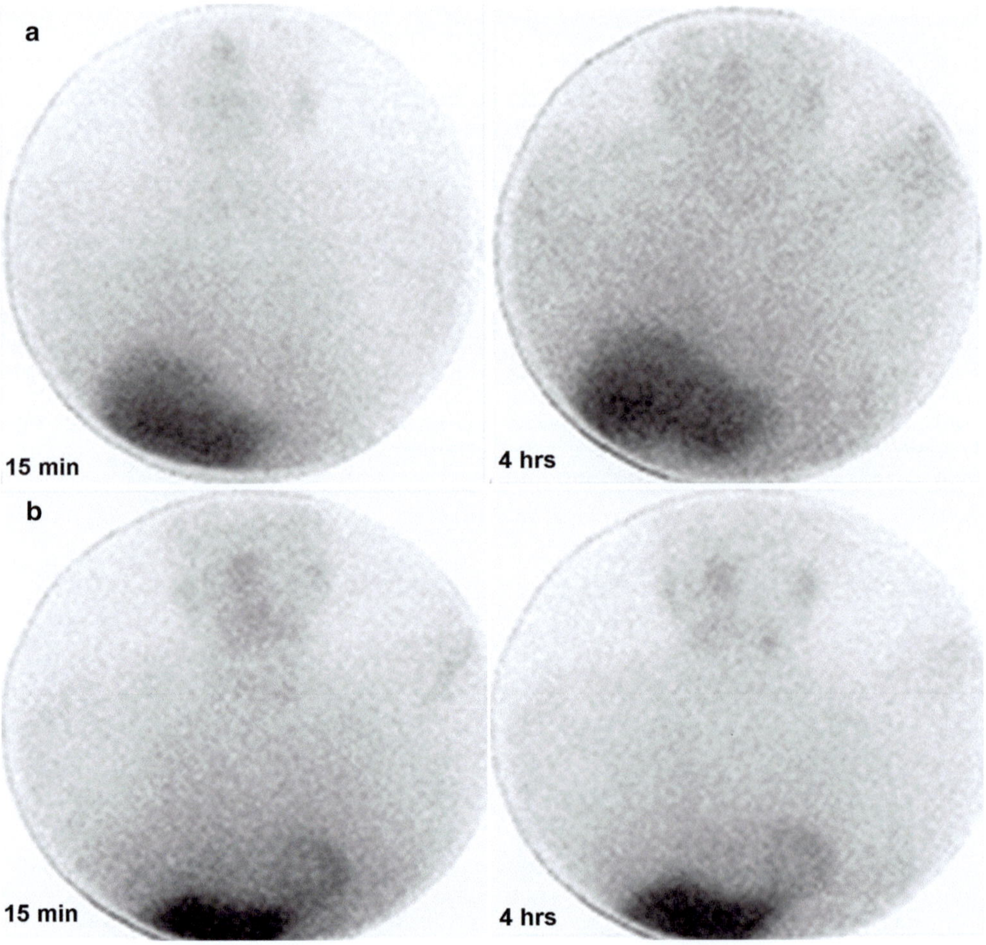

Figure 9-4. Planar images of the thorax in the anterior view acquired at 15 minutes and 4 h after ^{123}I-MIBG injection in a patient with PD (**a**) and a patient with MSA (**b**). Cardiac ^{123}I-MIBG uptake is extremely reduced in the patient with PD, but only mildly reduced in the patient with MSA.

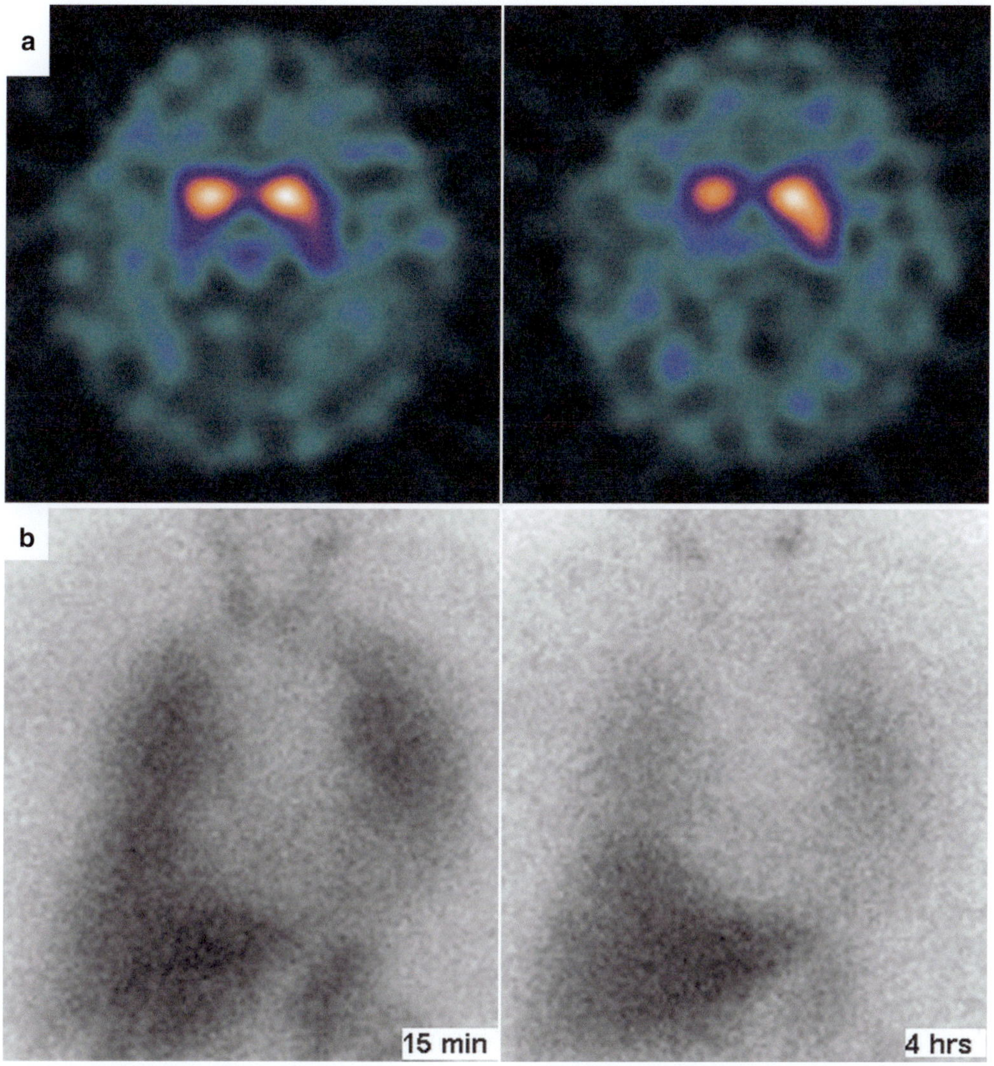

Figure 9-5. Dopamine transporter (DAT) imaging by means of brain single-photon emission computed tomography (SPECT) with [123]I- fluoropropyl (FP)-β-carbomethoxy-3 β-(4-iodophenyltropane) (CIT) usually is abnormal in patients with parkinsonian movement disorders, who show reduced striatal ^{123}I-FP-CIT uptake. (**a**), This abnormality is seen in this patient with DLB, who also shows impairment of cardiac sympathetic innervation, as reflected by extremely reduced cardiac ^{123}I-MIBG uptake. (**b**), Planar images of the thorax at 15 min and 4 h of ^{123}I-MIBG injection.

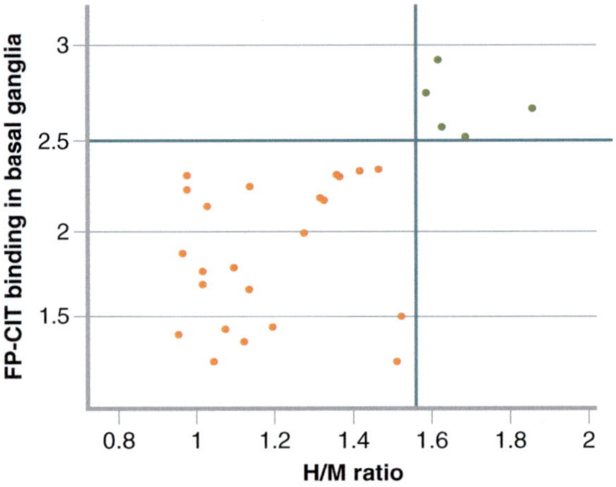

Figure 9-6. In patients older than 65 years with cognitive decline, DLB is the second most common neurodegenerative dementia after AD, accounting for 10% of all dementias [6–8]. Differential diagnosis between DLB and AD has important therapy implications, as DLB may benefit from treatment with cholinesterase inhibitors and carbidopa–levodopa, whereas it may worsen from treatment with anticholinergics and certain neuroleptic medications. Predominance of deficits in attention and visual perception over deterioration of memory and naming; psychiatric features, such as fluctuating cognition and recurrent visual hallucinations; parkinsonism; REM sleep behavior disorder; and dysautonomia are more common in DLB, but distinguishing DLB from AD is clinically challenging, especially in the early disease stages [6]. Among the different imaging techniques used in the diagnosis of DLB, DAT imaging has had the greatest effect so far. Exhibition of reduced DAT uptake in the basal ganglia is listed as one of the suggestive features of DLB [9]. However, cardiac ^{123}I-MIBG imaging also has been advocated as useful in this setting because of the similarities between PD and DLB (Fig. 9.1) [10, 11]. Decreased cardiac ^{123}I-MIBG uptake in DLB has been reported, whereas uptake is normal or near normal in AD. In a direct comparison between cardiac ^{123}I-MIBG imaging and ^{123}I-FP-CIT SPECT in the same cohort of DLB patients, Camacho et al. [12] found that all patients with reduced cardiac ^{123}I-MIBG uptake (23 of 28 patients with a clinical diagnosis of DLB) also showed reduced striatal ^{123}I-FP-CIT uptake (orange dots in the figure). Interestingly, the five patients with normal cardiac ^{123}I-MIBG uptake (green dots in the figure) also showed normal striatal ^{123}I-FP-CIT uptake. In addition, H/M ratio correlated positively with striatal ^{123}I-FP-CIT uptake ratios ($R=0.6$; $P<0.05$). Horizontal and vertical lines in the figure reflect normal values for H/M ratio (1.56) and ^{123}I-FP-CIT binding in basal ganglia (2.51). The severity of parkinsonism was highly correlated with striatal ^{123}I-FP-CIT uptake but not with cardiac ^{123}I-MIBG uptake. Other studies have shown that reduced cardiac ^{123}I-MIBG uptake in DLB is not related to autonomic failure or parkinsonism [4, 11], but patients with DLB and orthostatic hypotension (OI) have lower ^{123}I-MIBG uptake than patients with DLB without OI [13]. An advantage of cardiac ^{123}I-MIBG over DAT imaging is the short acquisition time and comfortable planar imaging, which is appreciated by patients and their caregivers [14]. Current guidelines include abnormal cardiac ^{123}I-MIBG imaging as one of the supportive features commonly present in DLB but not proven to have diagnostic specificity [9]. Debate is ongoing regarding whether abnormal cardiac ^{123}I-MIBG scintigraphy should be upgraded in the guidelines as a feature suggestive of DLB, but evidence is still lacking and further studies are warranted [15] (Adapted from Camacho et al. [12]).

Figure 9-7. Diabetes mellitus (DM) is the most common identifiable cause of neuropathy. Approximately 50% of patients with type 1 (T1DM) or type 2 DM (T2DM) will develop diabetic neuropathy, which is a serious complication involving variable multiple organ involvement, principally of the cardiovascular system but also of the gastrointestinal and urogenital tracts. Cardiovascular autonomic diabetic neuropathy (CADN) is the primary disorder of diabetic neuropathy, and it is defined as the impairment of cardiovascular autonomic control in patients with established DM after the exclusion of other causes [16]. CADN likely has a multifactorial pathogenesis, as shown here, leading to neuronal ischemia and/or direct neuronal death or dysfunction, as well as left ventricular (LV) dysfunction. It probably is the most common form of autonomic dysfunction worldwide, and its prevalence varies between 1 and 90% in patients with T1DM and 20 and 73% in those with T2DM. Such wide variation is a result of the discrepancy in the criteria used to diagnose CADN and differences in the study populations in relation to CADN risk factors (conventional cardiovascular risk factors, glycemic control, and DM duration) [17]. *AGE* advanced glycation end products, *BP* blood pressure, *Catechol* catecholamine, *FFA* free fatty acids, *Glu* glucose, *PARP* poly (ADP-ribose) polymerase; *PKC* protein kinase C, *RAAS* renin–angiotensin–aldosterone system, *RAGE* receptor for advanced glycation end products, *ROS* reactive oxygen species, *SNS* sympathetic nervous system, *Vc* vasoconstriction.

Cardiovascular Autonomic Diabetic Neuropathy

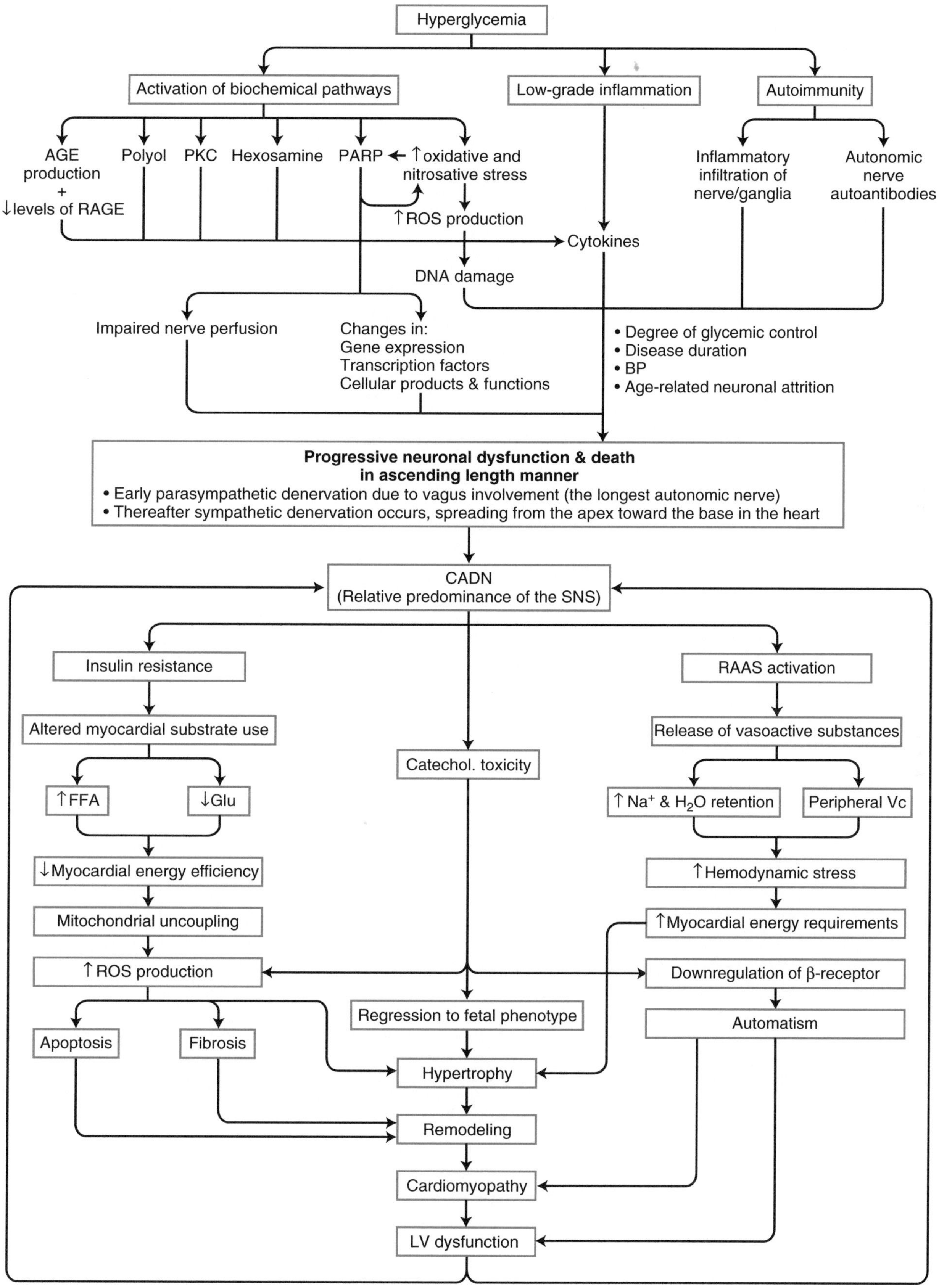

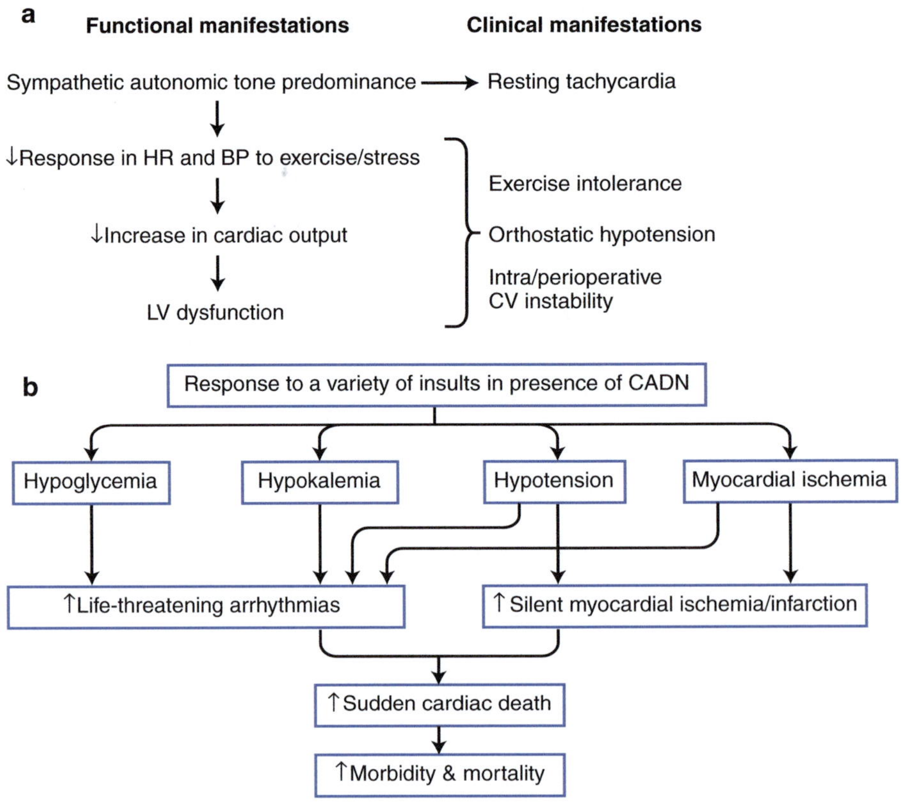

Figure 9-8. (**a**), CADN may result in disabling clinical and functional manifestations, with an associated increased mortality risk. A meta-analysis showed that the pooled estimated relative mortality risk for DM patients with CADN was 2.14 (95% CI, 1.83–2.51) [18]. In addition, among other risk factors, CADN has the strongest association with mortality [19]. (**b**), CADN remains a significant predictor of death after adjustment for conventional cardiovascular risk factors [20, 21], and CADN appears to be associated with major cardiovascular events [22]. Despite normal myocardial perfusion imaging in DM patients predicting an improved prognosis [23], the presence of CADN increases cardiovascular risk by mechanisms that are not fully understood [21]. CADN also is associated with a higher mortality risk in DM patients after a first myocardial infarction, which suggests that screening for CADN in these patients might be used for risk stratification [24].

Table 9-2. Recommendations on screening for CADN in patients with DM.

T2DM at time of diagnosis; T1DM within 5 years of diagnosis, especially recommended in patients with other macro- and/or microvascular complications
History of poor glycemic control
Candidates to begin a new exercise program
Perioperative assessment in patients with poor glycemic control and CAD
After a first MI

Screening for early CADN is recommended for both risk stratification of DM patients and early management of the disorder. CADN is commonly asymptomatic or subclinical, but when it becomes clinically evident, it is more difficult to manage. Improvement in glycemic control, lifestyle changes, cardioactive drugs, and cardiovascular risk factor management are the mainstay of treatment and generally slow rather than reverse CADN progression, highlighting the importance of screening for this disorder. *CAD* coronary artery disease, *MI* myocardial infarction

Table 9-3. Cardiac autonomic reflex tests.

Standard CART (SCART): measures HR and BP response to certain physiologic maneuvers
HR response to deep breathing[a]
Assessment of beat-to-beat HR variation (R-R variation) during paced breathing (expiration-to-inspiration ratio [E:I])
HR response to standing[a]
Expressed as the 30:15 ratio, which is the ratio of the longest R-R interval (between the 20th and 40th beats) to the shortest R-R interval (between beats 5 and 25) elicited by a change from horizontal to vertical position
HR response to Valsalva maneuver[b]
BP response to standing
BP response to sustained hand grip
HRV test: measures R-R interval
RR interval frequency- or spectral-domain analysis[c]
RR interval time- or statistical-domain analysis
Baroreflex sensitivity (BRS) test: measures changes in HR in response to changes in (systolic) BP[d]
Intravenous bolus injection of epinephrine/phenylephrine
Physical maneuvers, such as postural change
Criteria for diagnosis and staging of CADN
Possible or early CADN: presence of a single abnormal CART result
Definite or confirmed CADN: presence of two or three abnormal tests among the SCART and HRV tests
Severe or advanced CADN: presence of orthostatic hypotension in addition to the criteria for definite or confirmed CADN

Several cardiac autonomic reflex tests (CARTs) are available to measure cardiac autonomic function and diagnose CADN, but numerous factors may influence their results. In addition, heart rate variability (HRV) tests remain time consuming. Positron emission tomography (PET) and SPECT are the only imaging techniques sensitive enough to assess processes such as neurotransmission, which occurs at picomolar concentrations in the human heart [25–27]. The sensitivity of these techniques for detecting mild degrees of CADN may be superior to that of CART, thus potentially emerging as useful tools to characterize the effects of DM on myocardial sympathetic innervation. *BP* blood pressure, *HR* heart rate

[a]Reflects defects in parasympathetic activity

[b]Involves both the sympathetic and parasympathetic systems, although the Valsalva ratio mostly represents parasympathetic activity

[c]Low frequency represents sympathetic activity, and high frequency represents parasympathetic activity

[d]BRS in practice normally applies to parasympathetic activity

^{123}I-MIBG Imaging in CADN

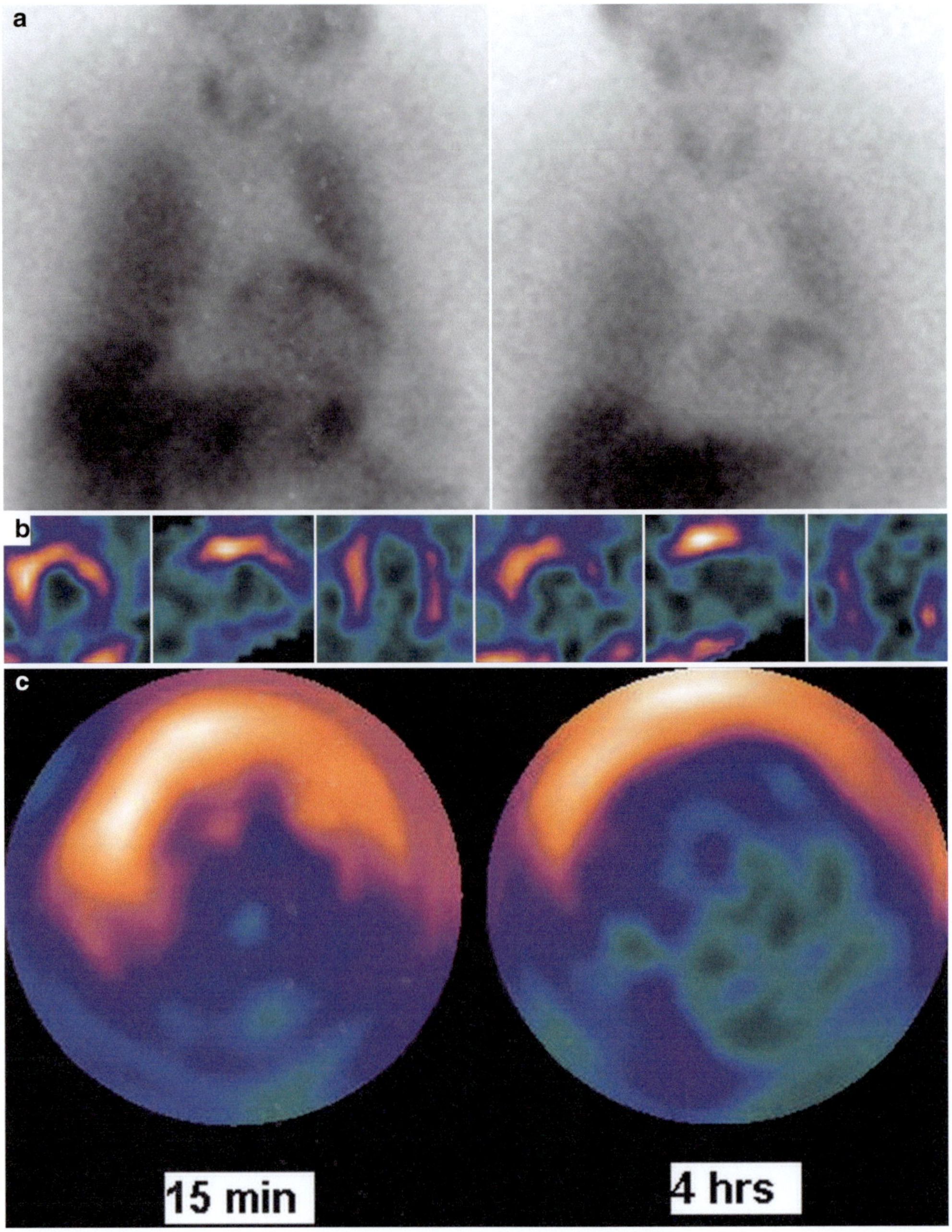

Figure 9-9. In patients with CADN, myocardial ^{123}I-MIBG uptake is decreased and heterogeneous [28]. Furthermore, some scintigraphic investigations have shown that in both T1DM and T2DM, cardiac sympathetic disturbances are more frequent than when assessed by CART. Myocardial sympathetic derangement is related to the severity of CADN. ^{123}I-MIBG defects initially are predominant in the LV inferior wall [28, 29] but may be complete in advanced CADN. This figure corresponds to cardiac ^{123}I-MIBG imaging of a patient with T2DM, at 15 min and 4 h of tracer injection: (**a**) anterior planar images, (**b**) mid-LV axial SPECT slices, and (**c**) SPECT polar maps, showing ^{123}I-MIBG defects mainly in the apical and inferior LV walls.

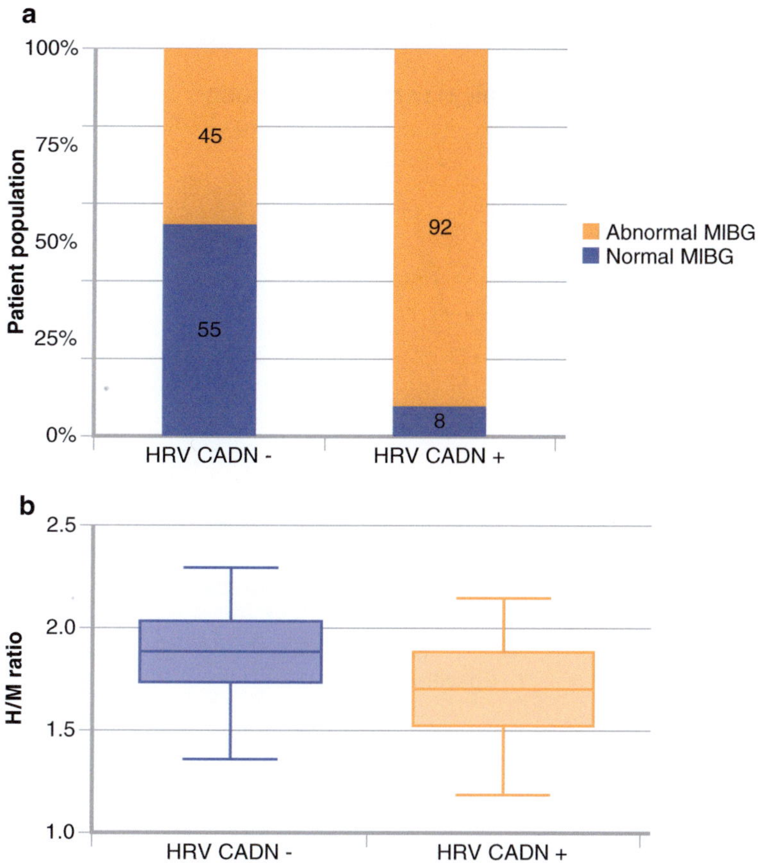

FIGURE 9-10. (**a**, **b**). Various studies have shown cardiac sympathetic dysinnervation both in patients with and in those without CART indicative of CADN, suggesting that cardiac ^{123}I-MIBG imaging is a more sensitive means to detect CADN, particularly in its early stages [30, 31]. Atherosclerosis of the large coronary arteries is not a prerequisite for these findings because ^{123}I-MIBG defects are present even in the absence of CAD; however, the role of microvascular disease has not been well defined (Adapted from Scholte et al. [31]).

^{123}I-MIBG Imaging in the Assessment of Prognosis

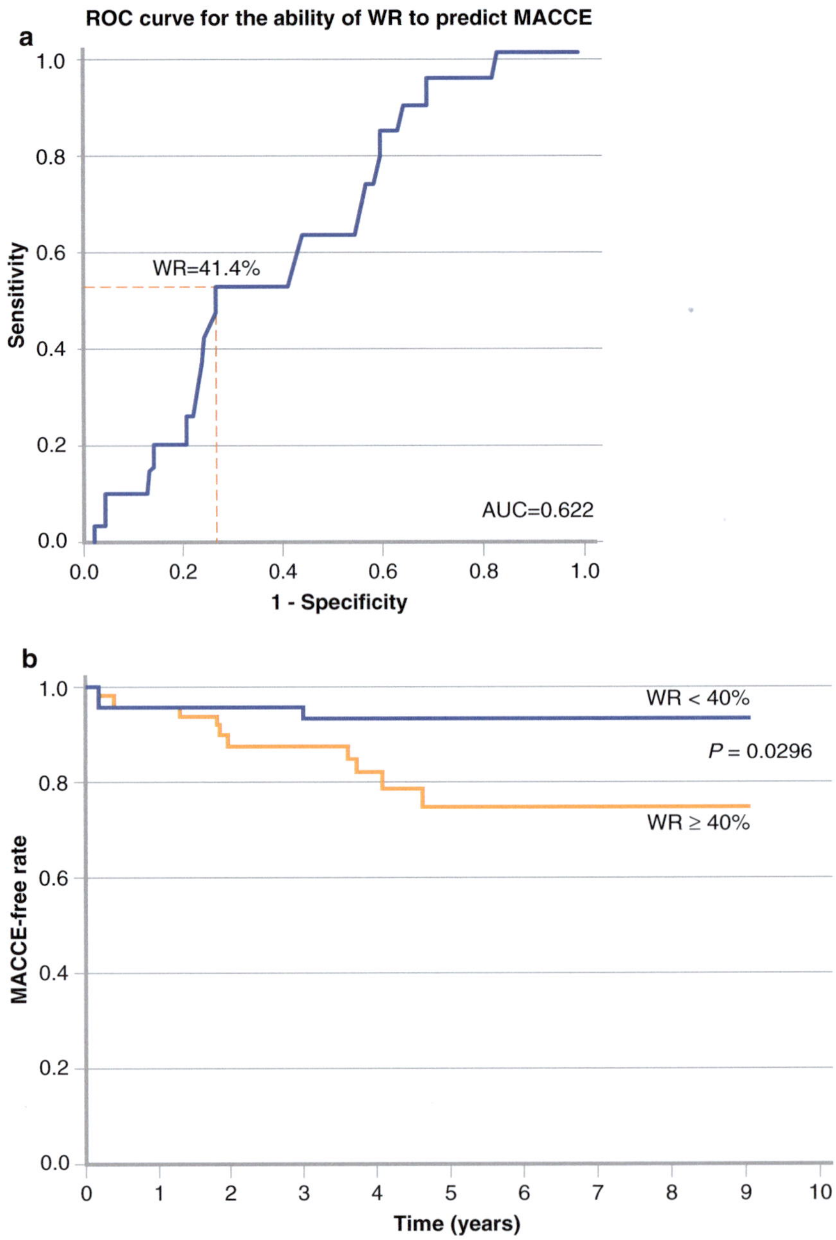

FIGURE 9-11. Several studies associated decreased and heterogeneous myocardial ^{123}I-MIBG uptake with increased mortality or other markers of adverse prognosis in patients with DM. Yufu et al. [32] reported that an abnormal WR of cardiac ^{123}I-MIBG at baseline had long-term cardiovascular predictive value in Japanese T2DM patients without structural heart disease or severe DM complications. The incidence of major adverse cerebral and cardiovascular events (MACCE), including cardiac death, coronary revascularization, stroke, and heart failure (HF) requiring admission, was significantly higher in patients with an abnormal WR than in those with a preserved WR during a follow-up of 4.6 years. Cox proportional hazards regression analysis showed that age and abnormal WR (defined by the receiver-operating characteristic [ROC] curve in panel **a**) were significantly and independently associated with the incidence of MACCE (panel **b**; HR, 4.06; 95% CI, 1.194–18.76) (Adapted from Yufu et al. [32]).

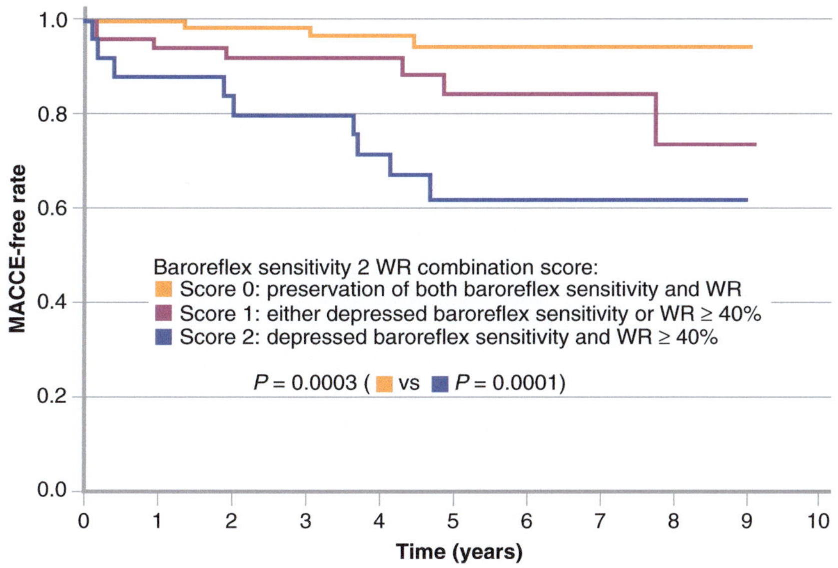

Figure 9-12. Recently, Murozono et al. [33] reported that the combination of baroreflex sensitivity and WR of ^{123}I-MIBG strengthened the power for predicting MACCE in T2DM patients without structural heart disease or severe DM complications during a mean follow-up period of 4.7 years. The MACCE-free ratio as evaluated by Kaplan–Meier analysis was significantly higher in patients with a lower baroreflex sensitivity–WR combination score. Likewise, Nagamachi et al. [34] reported on the prognostic value of ^{123}I-MIBG cardiac imaging and HRV in a retrospective study with a follow-up of 7.2 years in 144 patients with T2DM, normal myocardial perfusion imaging, and no other cardiac disease. Univariate and multivariate analysis showed that the combination of an abnormal late H/M ratio and coefficient of variance of the RR interval predicted the cardiac events (11.8%). In addition, an abnormal late H/M ratio independently predicted all-cause mortality (11.1%). It is noteworthy that ^{123}I-MIBG findings added prognostic value even with normal exercise myocardial perfusion testing. Several parameters associated with a high mortality in T2DM patients, such as elevated plasma levels of total homocysteine, microalbuminuria, and hepatocyte growth factor, were associated with CADN and insulin resistance and independently predicted by late ^{123}I-MIBG cardiac uptake in multiple regression analyses [35–37] (Adapted from Murozono et al. [33]).

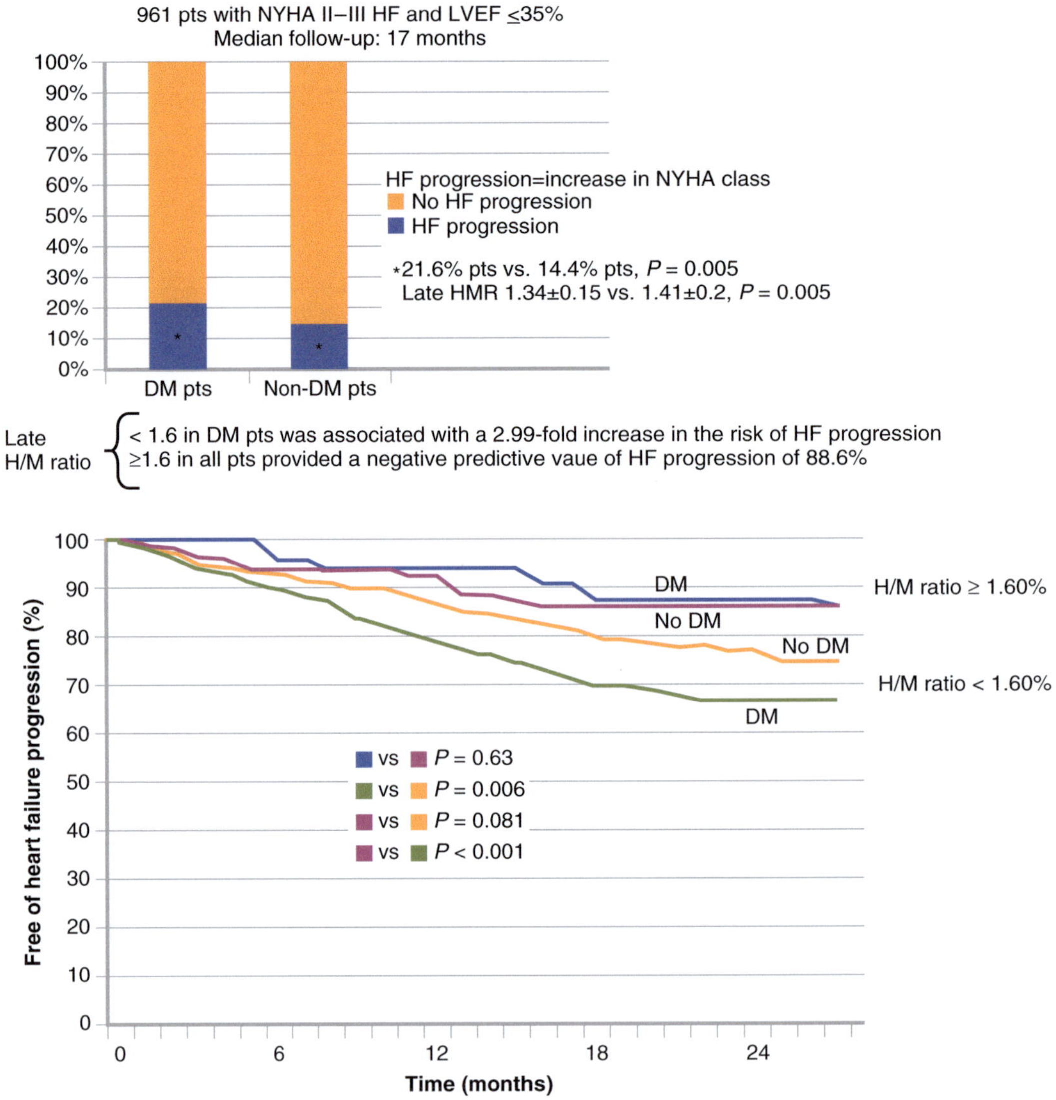

Figure 9-13. HF mortality is particularly high in patients with DM [38], in whom cardiac sympathetic nerve dysfunction increases the risk for HF progression, as shown by Gerson et al. [39]. In their substudy of the ADMIRE-HF trial, they found no difference in the risk of HF progression between patients with and those without DM if cardiac sympathetic innervation was relatively preserved, as revealed by a late H/M ratio ≥1.6, which suggests that the presence of DM has no influence on risk for HF progression. The variables significantly associated with time to an HF progression event were brain natriuretic peptide, LV ejection fraction (*LVEF*), late H/M ratio, the interaction term DM with late H/M ratio, early H/M ratio, and New York Heart Association (*NYHA*) class. The study did not include measures of myocardial ischemia; therefore, the role of ischemia in HF progression could not be compared with the contribution of sympathetic nerve dysfunction. Noteworthy, however, is that the presence of ischemic compared with nonischemic HF etiology was not an independent predictor of time to HF progression and did not alter the association between late H/M ratio and HF events. CADN also has been associated with an increased risk for sudden cardiac death (SCD) [17], and although the mechanisms are not fully understood, some experts suggest an increased rate of fatal cardiac arrhythmias due to the imbalance between the sympathetic and parasympathetic functions, as well as cardiac sympathetic denervation. QT-interval prolongation and QT dispersion, which indicate heterogeneous myocardial repolarization, have been associated with autonomic neuropathy in several studies [40, 41], and may provide an alternative explanation for the increased risk of SCD, rendering patients with CADN more susceptible to life-threatening cardiac arrhythmias. DM patients with QT prolongation have a 2.3-fold increased risk for CADN [42]. However, although such abnormalities are more pronounced in DM patients with CADN than in healthy control individuals, no consistent differences have been observed between DM patients with and those without CADN [43, 44]. In addition, most studies have failed to show a relationship between cardiac ^{123}I-MIBG uptake and the presence or absence of QT abnormalities [28, 45–47]. Therefore, the significance of CADN as an independent cause of SCD has been questioned, suggesting it is merely a contributing factor along with severe CAD or LV dysfunction [48]. It is possible that QT dispersion is based on more complex electrophysiologic mechanisms that remain to be elucidated.

^{123}I-MIBG Imaging in the Assessment of Treatment

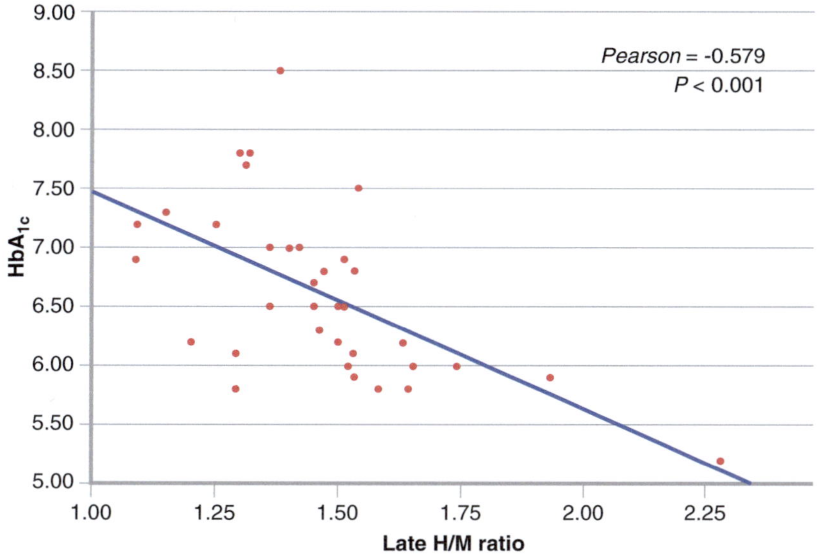

Figure 9-14. Long-term poor glycemic control is strongly related to the process of cardiac adrenergic denervation. Several studies investigated whether CADN may be reversed by improved glycemic control. Muhr-Becker et al. [49] reported that cardiac sympathetic dysinnervation in patients with poorly controlled, longer-term T1DM is dominated by irreversible neuronal abnormalities, as revealed by ^{123}I-MIBG cardiac scintigraphy. However, substantial metabolic improvement after 1 year of intensive insulin therapy partially restores cardiac sympathetic dysinnervation, indicating the presence of a reversible component of cardiac sympathetic dysfunction. Ziegler et al. [50] observed that global and regional ^{123}I-MIBG defect scores were increased in the inferior, posterior, and apical walls of patients with poorly controlled DM. After 4 years, patients with well-controlled DM showed enhanced global ^{123}I-MIBG uptake compared with those with poorly controlled disease. Such differences were not observed with CART. Similar results have been reported by using carbon-11 hydroxyephedrine (^{11}C-HED) [42, 51]. Recently, it was reported that DM patients with severe systolic HF show lower ^{123}I-MIBG cardiac uptake than matched HF patients without DM and DM patients without HF, and that ^{123}I-MIBG uptake independently correlates with glycemic control (assessed by hemoglobin A1C [HbA_{1c}] levels) over the previous 1 to 2 months, as may be seen here. Multivariate analysis identified HbA_{1c} as the only significant predictor of late H/M ratio (Adapted from Paolillo et al. [52]).

Other Neuropathies

Orthostatic intolerance (OI) may be defined as the development of symptoms (dizziness, presyncope, or syncope) during standing that are relieved by recumbency. It encompasses any condition with inadequate regulation of blood flow, heart rate, and BP and is demonstrated most easily during orthostatic stress, although it may be present in any position. OI has a diverse underlying pathophysiology, with impairment in integrative neurovascular physiology.

"Initial OH" on rapid standing is a normal form of OI. However, in some people, OI seriously interferes with quality of life, either as recurrent acute OI in the form of neurocardiogenic syncope (or postural vasovagal syncope [VVS]) or as chronic OI in the form of postural tachycardia syndrome (POTS). Less common is neurogenic OH, present in PAF. VVS presents as a transient and abrupt loss of consciousness and postural tone followed by rapid recovery. POTS is characterized by an excessive rise in heart rate upon standing and is associated with symptoms of presyncope [53]. The pathophysiologic mechanism of OI usually remains obscure after exhaustive medical evaluation excluding identifiable causes such as blood volume depletion, anemia, arrhythmias, seizures, adrenal insufficiency, and medications that impair autonomic regulation (e.g., vasodilators, diuretics, antidepressants, or anxiolytic agents). Maintenance of arterial pressure under conditions of reduced central blood volume during orthostasis is accomplished in large part through sympathetic efferent nerve traffic to the peripheral vasculature; thus, it seems reasonable to consider the occurrence of sympathetic dysfunction in the pathophysiology of OI.

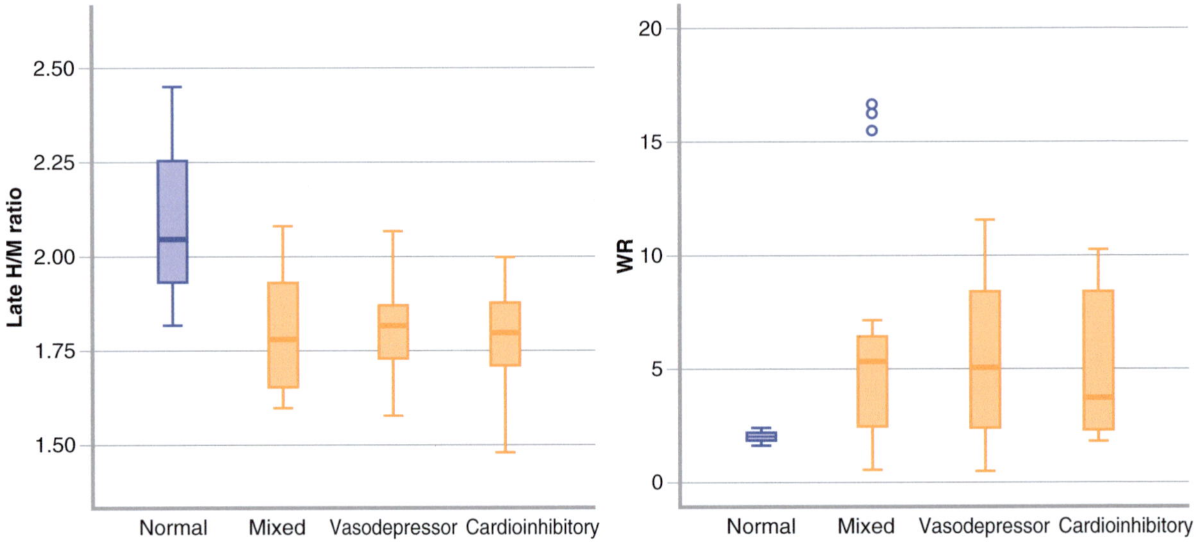

Figure 9-15. Some studies show a significantly lower H/M ratio in patients with VVS who had a positive tilt test compared with healthy control patients. These reports also indicate that most patients with syncope have LV ^{123}I-MIBG defects, suggesting a persistent dysfunction of myocardial adrenergic innervation [54]. However, in pediatric patients, Olguntürk et al. [55] reported higher H/M ratios and plasma norepinephrine (NE) levels in those who had a positive head-up tilt test than in those with a negative test, which may reflect a greater cardiac neuronal capacity of NE storage, playing a potential role in the generation of a paradox reflex in this population (Adapted from Kochiadakis et al. [56]).

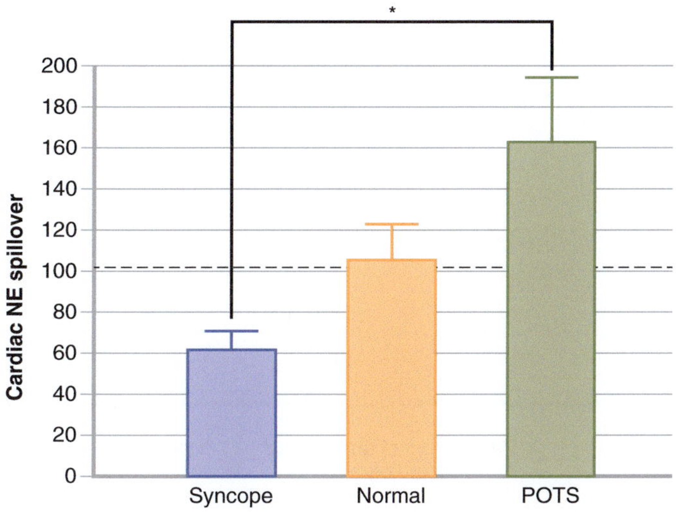

Figure 9-16. Goldstein et al. [57] examined cardiac sympathetic innervation and function in patients with POTS and those with repeated VVS. They measured neurochemical indices of cardiac release, reuptake, and synthesis of NE based on NE entry into the cardiac venous drainage (cardiac NE spillover), cardiac extraction of circulating ^{3}H-NE, and cardiac production of dihydroxyphenylalanine. They also measured LV myocardial innervation density using fluorine-18 (^{18}F)-fluorodopamine PET. Mean cardiac NE spillover was higher in patients with POTS and lower in those with VVS compared with a large group of healthy volunteers, as well as in a subgroup of age-matched healthy women. In both patient groups cardiac extraction of ^{3}H-NE, cardiac production of dihydroxyphenylalanine, and myocardial ^{18}F-fluorodopamine uptake were normal, but the groups differed regarding tonic cardiac sympathetic function, with increased cardiac NE release in POTS and decreased release in VVS, with normal values for indices of function of the cell membrane NE transporter, NE synthesis, and density of myocardial sympathetic innervation in both entities. Tachycardia in the upright position in POTS therefore may partly reflect increased NE delivery to adrenoceptors on myocardial pacemaker cells. Conversely, reduced myocardial ^{123}I-MIBG uptake, indicating reduced cardiac sympathetic neuronal uptake function, has been reported in 20% of patients with POTS, suggesting that cardiac sympathetic denervation may be present in this condition [58]. In a subset of patients with POTS, it also was shown that reduced myocardial ^{123}I-MIBG uptake correlated with the density of sympathetic and somatic C-fiber innervation measured from skin biopsies and suggested that loss of distal sympathetic innervation may produce an exaggerated sympathetic response in innervated tissues such as the heart, resulting in tachycardia [59]. The inconsistency among these studies may reflect the highly recognized heterogeneity of patients with POTS, which is actually a syndrome, likely of various causes, and not a single disease. *$P = 0.001$.

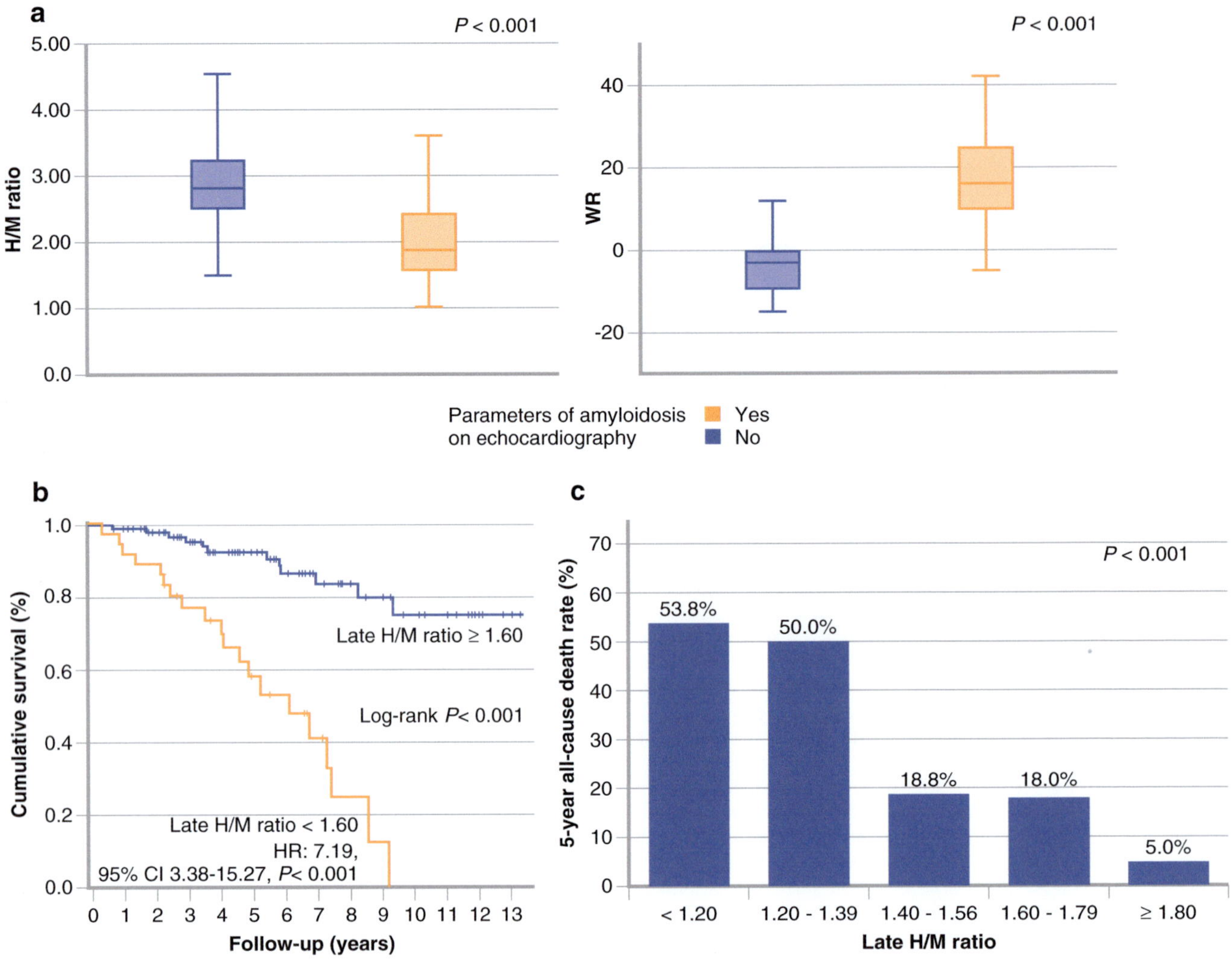

Figure 9-17. Amyloidosis is a disease characterized by deposition in the extracellular space of various insoluble serum protein fibrils (amyloid) that are improperly metabolized. Amyloidoses are defined based on the biochemical nature of the fibril-forming protein, and classified depending on whether deposition is localized (or organ limited) or systemic. Amyloidoses may be hereditary or acquired. Clinical manifestations depend on the anatomic location and extent, as well as the intensity, of amyloid deposition. Transthyretin (TTR) amyloidosis may be hereditary, in the form of familial amyloid polyneuropathy (FAP), with nerve deposits of a genetic TTR variant, or acquired, in the form of senile systemic amyloidosis (SSA), with systemic deposits of wild-type or nonvariant TTR. FAP is characterized by both sensorimotor and autonomic neuropathy. LV dysfunction is rare, but conduction disturbances and SCD may occur, and although not frequent, it is a severe form of amyloidosis. SSA, common after 80 years of age, may produce a clinical syndrome similar to that of FAP. (**a**), Patients with early-stage FAP (before the development of clinical, echocardiographic, and technetium-99 m [^{99m}Tc]-pyrophosphate myocardial scintigraphic changes) have a high incidence of myocardial adrenergic denervation, as shown by reduced myocardial ^{123}I-MIBG uptake [60, 61]. In addition, H/M ratio is lower and WR higher in patients with echocardiographic signs of amyloidosis (Adapted from Noordzij et al. [62]). (**b**, **c**), In addition, ^{123}I-MIBG can detect cardiac denervation in patients with TTR amyloidosis before signs are evident on echocardiography [62]. Furthermore, in a recent study assessing the prognostic value of ^{123}I-MIBG imaging, H/M ratio was an independent predictor of survival in patients with TTR amyloidosis (Adapted from Coutinho et al. [63]).

Conclusions

Cardiac neurotransmission imaging allows in vivo noninvasive assessment of cardiac sympathetic innervation, which has shown utility in evaluating patients with dysautonomia. It has especially added value to the differential diagnosis of diverse parkinsonian syndromes, and in the differential diagnosis between DLB and AD. It also provides a sensitive tool for the early detection of CADN and TTR amyloidosis, even though it may predict an adverse outcome.

References

1. Somsen GA, Verberne HJ, Fleury E, Righetti A. Normal values and within subject variability of cardiac I-123 MIBG scintigraphy in healthy individuals: implications for clinical studies. J Nucl Cardiol. 2004;11:126–33.
2. Wakabayashi K, Takahashi H. Neuropathology of autonomic nervous system in Parkinson's disease. Eur Neurol. 1997;38 suppl 2:2–7.
3. Cersosimo MG, Benarroch EE. Central control of autonomic function and invbolvement in neurodegenerative disorders. Handb Clin Neurol. 2013;117:45–57.
4. Kashihara K, Ohno M, Kawada S, Okumura Y. Reduced cardiac uptake and enhanced washout of 123I-MIBG in pure autonomic failure occurs conjointly with Parkinson's disease and dementia with Lewy bodies. J Nucl Med. 2006;47:1099–101.
5. Nagayama H, Hamamoto M, Ueda M, Nagashima J, Katayama Y. Reliability of mIBG myocardial scintigraphy in the diagnosis of Parkinson's disease. J Neurol Neurosurg Psychiatry. 2005;76:249–51.
6. McKeith I, Mintzer J, Aarsland D, Burn D, Chiu H, Cohen-Mansfield J, et al. Dementia with Lewy bodies. Lancet Neurol. 2004;3:19–28.
7. Ferman TJ, Boeve BF. Dementia with Lewy bodies. Neurol Clin. 2007;25:741–7.
8. Zaccai J, McCracken C, Brayne C. A systematic review of prevalence and incidence studies of dementia with Lewy bodies. Age Ageing. 2005;34:561–6.
9. McKeith IG, Dickson DW, Lowe J, Emre M, O'Brien JT, Feldman H, et al. Diagnosis and management of dementia with Lewy bodies: third report of the DLB Consortium. Neurology. 2005;65:1863–72.
10. Watanabe H, Ieda T, Katayama T, Takeda A, Aiba I, Doyu M, et al. Cardiac 123I-meta-iodobenzylguanidine (mIBG) uptake in dementia with Lewy bodies: comparison with Alzheimer's disease. J Neurol Neurosurg Psychiatry. 2001;70:781–3.
11. Yoshita M, Taki J, Yokoyama K, Noguchi-Shinohara M, Matsumoto Y, Nakajima K, et al. Value of 123I-mIBG radioactivity in the differential diagnosis of DLB from AD. Neurology. 2006;66:1850–4.
12. Camacho V, Marquié M, Lleó A, Alvés L, Artigas C, Flotats A, et al. Cardiac sympathetic impairment parallels nigrostriatal degeneration in Probable Dementia with Lewy Bodies. Q J Nucl Med Mol Imaging. 2011;55:476–83.
13. Kobayashi S, Tateno M, Morii H, Utsumi K, Saito T. Decreased cardiac MIBG uptake, its correlation with clinical symptoms in dementia with Lewy bodies. Psychiatry Res. 2009;174:76–80.
14. Estorch M, Camacho V, Paredes P, Rivera E, Rodríguez-Revuelto A, Flotats A, et al. Cardiac (123) I-metaiodobenzylguanidine imaging allows early identification of dementia with Lewy bodies during life. Eur J Nucl Med Mol Imaging. 2008;35:1636–41.
15. Tateno M, Kobayashi S, Saito T. Imaging improves diagnosis of dementia with Lewy bodies. Psychiatry Invest. 2009;6:233–40.
16. Spallone V, Ziegler D, Freeman R, Bernardi L, Frontoni S, Pop-Busui R, et al; on behalf of the Toronto Consensus Panel on Diabetic Neuropathy. Cardiovascular autonomic neuropathy in diabetes: clinical impact, assessment, diagnosis, and management. Diabetes Metab Res Rev 2011. doi:10.1002/dmrr.1239.
17. Dimitropoulos G, Tahrani AA, Stevens MJ. Cardiac autonomic neuropathy in patients with diabetes mellitus. World J Diabetes. 2014;5:17–39.
18. Maser RE, Mitchell BD, Vinik AI, Freeman R. The association between cardiovascular autonomic neuropathy and mortality in individuals with diabetes: a meta-analysis. Diabetes Care. 2003;26:1895–901.
19. Soedamah-Muthu SS, Chaturvedi N, Witte DR, Stevens LK, Porta M, Fuller JH. Relationship between risk factors and mortality in type 1 diabetic patients in Europe: the EU RODIAB Prospective Complications Study (PCS). Diabetes Care. 2008;31:1360–6.
20. Orchard TJ, Lloyd CE, Maser RE, Kuller LH. Why does diabetic autonomic neuropathy predict IDDM mortality? An analysis from the Pittsburgh Epidemiology of Diabetes Complications Study. Diabetes Res Clin Pract. 1996;34:S165–71.
21. Lee KH, Jang HJ, Kim YH, Lee EJ, Choe YS, Choi Y, et al. Prognostic value of cardiac autonomic neuropathy independent and incremental to perfusion defects in patients with diabetes and suspected coronary artery disease. Am J Cardiol. 2003;92:1458–61.
22. Valensi P, Sachs RN, Harfouche B, Lormeau B, Paries J, Cosson E. Predictive value of cardiac autonomic neuropathy in diabetic patients with or without silent myocardial ischemia. Diabetes Care. 2001;24:339–43.
23. De Lorenzo A, Lima RS, Sequeira-Filho AG, Pantoja MR. Prevalence and prognostic value of perfusion defects detected by stress technetium-99 m sestamibi myocardial perfusion singlephoton emission computed tomography in asymptomatic patients with diabetes mellitus and no known coronary artery disease. Am J Cardiol. 2002;90:827–32.
24. Katz A, Liberty IF, Porath A, Ovsyshcher I, Prystowsky EN. A simple bedside test of 1-minute heart rate variability during deep breathing as a prognostic index after myocardial infarction. Am Heart J. 1999;138:32–8.
25. Carrió I. Cardiac neurotransmission imaging. J Nucl Med. 2001;42:1062–76.
26. Flotats A, Carrió I. Cardiac neurotransmission SPECT imaging. J Nucl Cardiol. 2004;11:587–602.
27. Bengel FM, Schwaiger M. Assessment of cardiac sympathetic neuronal function using PET imaging. J Nucl Cardiol. 2004;11:603–16.
28. Schnell O, Hammer K, Muhr-Becker D, Ziegler A, Weiss M, Tatsch K, et al. Cardiac sympathetic dysinnervation in Type 2 diabetes mellitus with and without ECG-based cardiac autonomic neuropathy. J Diabetes Complications. 2002;16:220–7.
29. Hattori N, Tamaki N, Hayashi T, Masuda I, Kudoh T, Tateno M, et al. Regional abnormality of iodine-123-mIBG in diabetic hearts. J Nucl Med. 1996;37:1985–90.
30. Kim SJ, Lee JD, Ryu YH, Jeon P, Shim YW, Yoo HS, et al. Evaluation of cardiac sympathetic neuronal integrity in diabetic patients using iodine-123 mIBG. Eur J Nucl Med. 1996;23:401–6.

31. Scholte AJ, Schuijf JD, Delgado V, Kok JA, Bus MTJ, Maan AC, et al. Cardiac autonomic neuropathy in patients with diabetes and no symptoms of coronary artery disease: comparison of 123I-metaiodobenzylguanidine myocardial scintigraphy and heart rate variability. Eur J Nucl Med Mol Imaging. 2010;37:1698–705.
32. Yufu K, Takahashi N, Okada N, Shinohara T, Nakagawa M, Hara M, et al. Cardiac iodine-123 metaiodobenzylguanidine (123I-MIBG) scintigraphy parameter predicts cardiac and cerebrovascular events in type 2 diabetic patients without structural heart disease. Circ J. 2012;76:399–404.
33. Murozono Y, Yufu K, Takahashi N, Okada N, Shinohara T, Nakagawa M, et al. Combined assessment of baroreflex sensitivity with iodine 123 metaiodobenzylguanidine scintigraphic findings strengthens the power of predictive value for cerebral and cardiovascular events in type 2 diabetic patients. Circ J. 2013;77:130–6.
34. Nagamachi S, Fujita S, Nishii R, Futami S, Tamura S, Mizuta M, et al. Prognostic value of cardiac I-123 metaiodobenzylguanidine imaging in patients with non-insulin-dependent diabetes mellitus. J Nucl Cardiol. 2006;13:34–42.
35. Takahashi N, Anan F, Nakagawa M, Yufu K, Ooie T, Nawata T, et al. Microalbuminuria, cardiovascular autonomic dysfunction, and insulin resistance in patients with type 2 diabetes mellitus. Metabolism. 2004;53:1359–64.
36. Anan F, Yonemochi H, Masaki T, Takahashi N, Nakagawa M, Eshima N, et al. Homocysteine levels are associated with the results of 123I-metaiodobenzylguanidine myocardial scintigraphy in type 2 diabetic patients. Eur J Nucl Med Mol Imaging. 2007;34:28–35.
37. Anan F, Masaki T, Yonemochi H, Takahashi N, Nakagawa M, Eshima N, et al. Hepatocyte growth factor levels are associated with the results of 123I-metaiodobenzylguanidine myocardial scintigraphy in patients with type 2 diabetes mellitus. Metabolism. 2009;58:167–73.
38. Gustafsson I, Brendorp B, Seibaek M, Burchardt H, Hildebrandt P, Kober L, et al. DIAMOND Study Group. Influence of diabetes and diabetes-gender interaction on the risk of death in patients hospitalized with congestive heart failure. J Am Coll Cardiol. 2004;43:771–7.
39. Gerson MC, Caldwell JH, Ananthasubramaniam K, Clements IP, Henzlova MJ, Amanullah A, et al. Influence of diabetes mellitus on prognostic utility of imaging of myocardial sympathetic innervation in heart failure patients. Circ Cardiovasc Imaging. 2011;4:87–93.
40. Sivieri R, Veglio M, Chinaglia A, Scaglione P, Cavallo-Perin P. Prevalence of QT prolongation in a type 1 diabetic population and its association with autonomic neuropathy. The Neuropathy Study Group of the Italian Society for the Study of Diabetes. Diabet Med. 1993;10:920–4.
41. Veglio M, Borra M, Stevens LK, Fuller JH, Perin PC. The relation between QTc interval prolongation and diabetic complications. The EURODIAB IDDM Complication Study Group. Diabetologia. 1999;42:68–75.
42. Vinik AI, Ziegler D. Diabetic cardiovascular autonomic neuropathy. Circulation. 2007;115:387–97.
43. Bellavere F, Ferri M, Guarini L, Bax G, Piccoli A, Cardone C, et al. Prolonged QT period in diabetic autonomic neuropathy: a possible role in sudden cardiac death? Br Heart J. 1988;59:379–83.
44. Wei K, Dorian P, Newman D, Langer A. Association between QT dispersion and autonomic dysfunction in patients with diabetes mellitus. J Am Coll Cardiol. 1995;26:859–63.
45. Schnell O, Kirsch CM, Stemplinger J, Haslbeck M, Standl E. Scintigraphic evidence for cardiac sympathetic dysinnervation in long-term IDDM patients with and without ECG-based autonomic neuropathy. Diabetologia. 1995;38:1345–52.
46. Langen KJ, Ziegler D, Weise F, Piolot R, Boy C, Hübinger A, et al. Evaluation of QT interval length, QT dispersion and myocardial m-iodobenzylguanidine uptake in insulin-dependent diabetic patients with and without autonomic neuropathy. Clin Sci (Lond). 1997;93:325–33.
47. Claus D, Meudt O, Rozeik C, Engelmann-Kempe K, Huppert PE, Wietholtz H. Prospective investigation of autonomic cardiac neuropathy in diabetes mellitus. Clin Auton Res. 2002;12:373–8.
48. Suarez GA, Clark VM, Norell JE, Kottke TE, Callahan MJ, O'Brien PC, et al. Sudden cardiac death in diabetes mellitus: risk factors in the Rochester diabetic neuropathy study. J Neurol Neurosurg Psychiatry. 2005;76:240–5.
49. Muhr-Becker D, Weiss M, Tatsch K, Wolfram G, Standl E, Schnell O. Scintigraphically assessed cardiac sympathetic dysinnervation in poorly controlled type 1 diabetes mellitus: one-year follow-up with improved metabolic control. Exp Clin Endocrinol Diabetes. 1999;107:306–12.
50. Ziegler D, Weise F, Langen KJ, Piolot R, Boy C, Hubinger A, et al. Effect of glycaemic control on myocardial sympathetic innervation assessed by [123I]metaiodobenzylguanidine scintigraphy: a 4-year prospective study in IDDM patients. Diabetologia. 1998;41:443–51.
51. Stevens M, Raffel D, Allman K, Schwaiger M, Wieland D. Regression and progression of cardiac sympathetic dysinnervation complicating diabetes: an assessment by C-11 hydroxyephedrine and positron emission tomography. Metabolism. 1999;48:92–101.
52. Paolillo S, Rengo G, Pagano G, Pellegrino T, Savarese G, Femminella GD, et al. Impact of diabetes on cardiac sympathetic innervation in patients with heart failure: a 123I metaiodobenzylguanidine (123I MIBG) scintigraphic study. Diabetes Care. 2013;36:2395–401.
53. Raj SR. Postural tachycardia syndrome (POTS). Circulation. 2013;127:2336–42.
54. Lorincz I, Garai I, Varga E, Barta K, Simkó J, Szabó Z, et al. Myocardial adrenergic innervation in patients with vasovagal syncope measured with 123I-MIBG uptake. Nucl Med Commun. 2009;30:134–9.
55. Olguntürk R, Turan L, Tunaoglu FS, Kula S, Gökçora N, Karabacak NI, et al. Abnormality of the left ventricular sympathetic nervous function assessed by I-123 metaiodobenzylguanidine imaging in pediatric patients with neurocardiogenic syncope. Pacing Clin Electrophysiol. 2003;26: 1926–30.
56. Kochiadakis G, Marketou M, Koukouraki S, Parthenakis F, Chlouverakis G, Karkavitsas N, et al. Cardiac autonomic disturbances in patients with vasovagal syndrome: comparison between iodine-123-metaiodobenzylguanidine myocardial scintigraphy and heart rate variability. Europace. 2012;14:1352–8.
57. Goldstein D, Holmes C, Frank SM, Dendi R, Cannon III RO, Sharabi Y. Cardiac sympathetic dysautonomia in chronic orthostatic intolerance syndromes. Circulation. 2002;106:2358–65.
58. Haensch CA, Lerch H, Schlemmer H, Jigalin A. Isenmann S.J Cardiac neurotransmission imaging with 123I-metaiodobenzylguanidine in postural tachycardia syndrome. Neurol Neurosurg Psychiatry. 2010;81:339–43.
59. Haensch CA, Tosch M, Katona I, Weis J, Isenmann S. Small-fiber neuropathy with cardiac denervation in postural tachycardia syndrome. Muscle Nerve. 2014;50:956–61.
60. Tanaka M, Hongo M, Kinoshita O, Takabayashi Y, Fujii T, Yazaki Y, et al. Iodine-123 metaiodobenzylguanidine scintigraphic assessment of myocardial sympathetic innervation in patients with familial amyloid polyneuropathy. J Am Coll Cardiol. 1997;29:168–74.
61. Delahaye N, Dinanian S, Slama MS, Mzabi H, Samuel D, Adams D, et al. Cardiac sympathetic denervation in familial amyloid polyneuropathy assessed by iodine-123 metaiodobenzylguanidine scintigraphy and heart rate variability. Eur J Nucl Med. 1999;26:416–24.

62. Noordzij W, Glaudemans AW, van Rheenen RW, Hazenberg BP, Tio RA, Dierckx RA, et al. (123)I-Labelled metaiodobenzylguanidine for the evaluation of cardiac sympathetic denervation in early stage amyloidosis. Eur J Nucl Med Mol Imaging. 2012;39:1609–17.

63. Coutinho MC, Cortez-Dias N, Cantinho G, Conceição I, Oliveira A, Bordalo e Sá A, et al. Reduced myocardial 123-iodine metaiodobenzylguanidine uptake: a prognostic marker in familial amyloid polyneuropathy. Circ Cardiovasc Imaging. 2013;6:627–36.

10 Cardiac Transplantation: Denervation, Reinnervation, and Myocardial Blood Flow

Avishay Grupper, Henry Gewirtz, and
Sudhir S. Kushwaha

Cardiac Denervation during Heart Transplantation

The intact heart is innervated by the parasympathetic and sympathetic fibers of the autonomic nervous system. Cardiac transplantation results in transection of the postganglionic neural axons innervating the heart. Axonal degeneration develops within days after transplantation and leads to total depletion of cardiac norepinephrine stores and eventual disappearance of nerve terminals in the transplanted tissue, resulting in total cardiac denervation [1].

Loss of afferent innervation alters cardiovascular homeostasis by impairing the normal vasoregulatory response to changing cardiac filling pressures. Efferent denervation results in the loss of sympathetic and parasympathetic regulation, leading to an increase in resting heart rate and blunting the rapid changes in heart rate and contractility during exercise [2–7].

V. Dilsizian, J. Narula (eds.), *Atlas of Cardiac Innervation*, DOI 10.1007/978-3-319-45800-7_10

Table 10-1. Methods to evaluate posttransplant cardiac reinnervation.

Invasive procedures		Noninvasive methods		
Intracoronary injection of tyramine	Invasive evaluation of the response to exercise	Radiolabeled catecholamine analogues		Radiolabeled receptor antagonist
		Guanethidine analogue ^{123}I-MIBG	Catecholamine analogue ^{11}C-HED	β-Adrenergic receptor antagonist ^{11}C-CGP-12177

Invasive procedures to determine catecholamine concentrations involve induction of myocardial sympathetic nerve fiber activation either with intracoronary injection of tyramine (an agent that causes norepinephrine release from intact sympathetic nerve terminals) or with exercise, such as handgrip maneuver, with subsequent evaluation of the response by invasive measurement of cardiac spillover of norepinephrine, left ventricular (LV) pressure, and coronary blood flow velocity [8–11]. Noninvasive methods to delineate sympathetic nerve terminals of the heart have become possible with the introduction of radiolabeled catecholamine analogues. One option is to use the guanethidine analogue iodine-123 metaiodobenzylguanidine (^{123}I-MIBG), which is taken up by presynaptic nerve terminal norepinephrine transporters and retained in norepinephrine storage vesicles [12, 13]. *^{11}C-HED* carbon-11 hydroxyephedrine

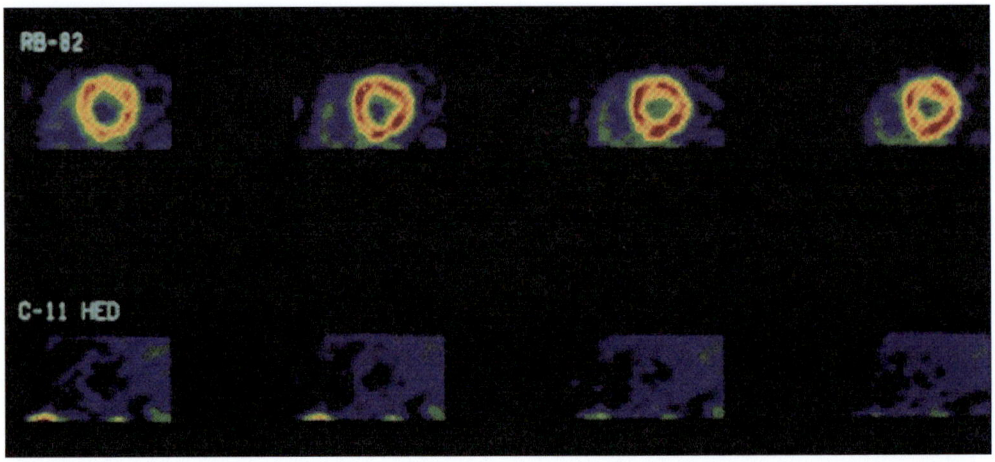

Figure 10-1. Positron emission tomography (PET) imaging with the catecholamine analogue ^{11}C-HED may be used to trace and quantitate norepinephrine uptake and storage in the presynaptic adrenergic nerve terminals [14–18]. Shown here are cross-sectional PET images from a patient with recent cardiac transplantation: rubidium-82 (Rb-82) presents homogeneous blood flow. Myocardial retention of ^{11}C-HED 30 min after tracer injection is markedly reduced compared with that of Rb-82. A PET tracer that can image cardiac β-adrenergic receptor density also is available in the form of ^{11}C-CGP-12177, a β-adrenergic receptor antagonist [19–21]. Similarly, PET imaging of parasympathetic (muscarinic) nerve function also has been used in evaluating the extent and time course of parasympathetic reinnervation of the transplanted heart [22, 23] (From Schwaiger et al. [18]; with permission).

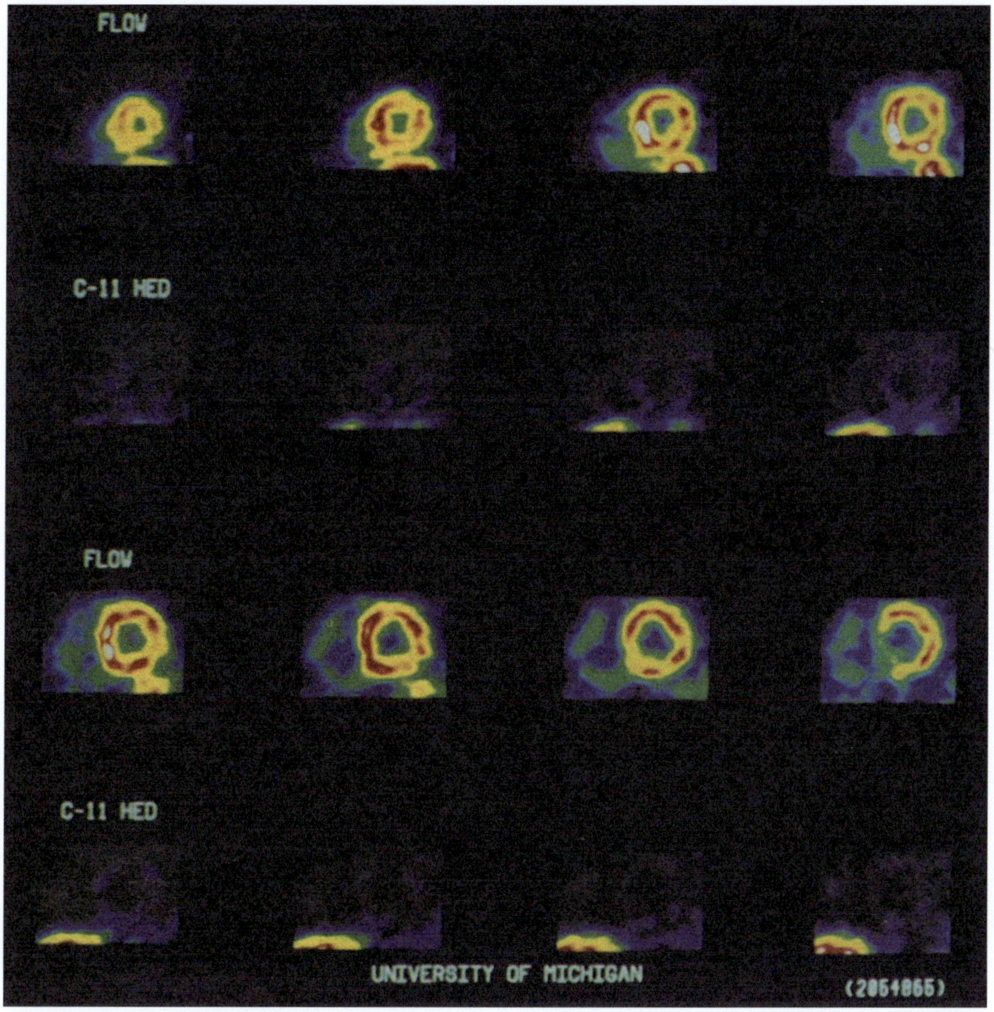

Figure 10-2. Most studies have confirmed complete denervation within the first 6–12 months after transplantation. Show here are ^{11}C-HED and Rb-82 short-axis PET images obtained from a patient with recent cardiac transplant (3 months after cardiac transplantation). The blood flow images show homogeneous blood flow throughout the left ventricle, whereas the ^{11}C-HED images below indicate a marked reduction of tracer retention that is homogeneous throughout the left ventricle (From Schwaiger et al. [14]; with permission).

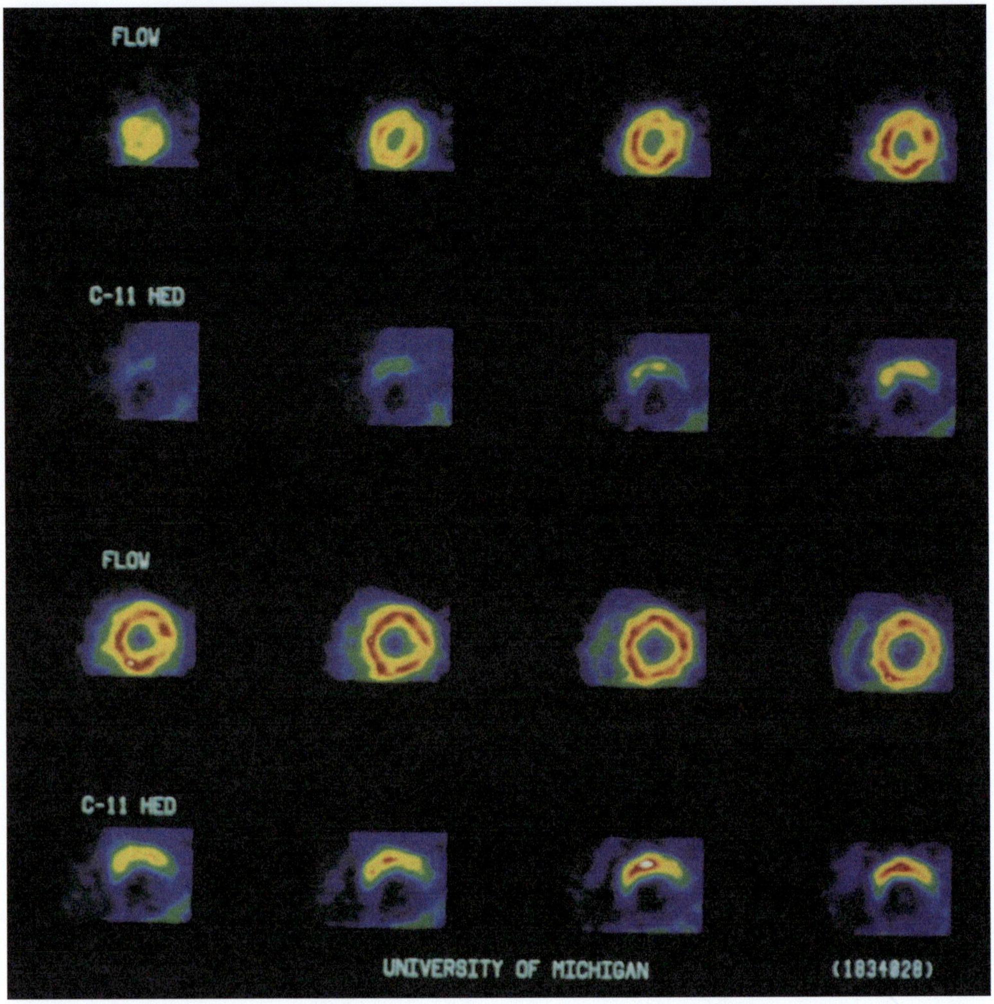

FIGURE 10-3. Myocardial adrenergic reinnervation after heart transplantation is a progressive process with a definitive pattern that usually starts during the second year after transplantation [8–18, 24, 25]. Shown here are short-axis PET images obtained in a patient 55 months after cardiac transplantation. Rb-82 images show homogeneous blood flow throughout the left ventricle. ^{11}C-HED images below indicate tracer retention in the anterior aspects of the left ventricle, increasing from the mid–left ventricle toward the base of the left ventricle (*bottom row*) (From Schwaiger et al. [14]; with permission).

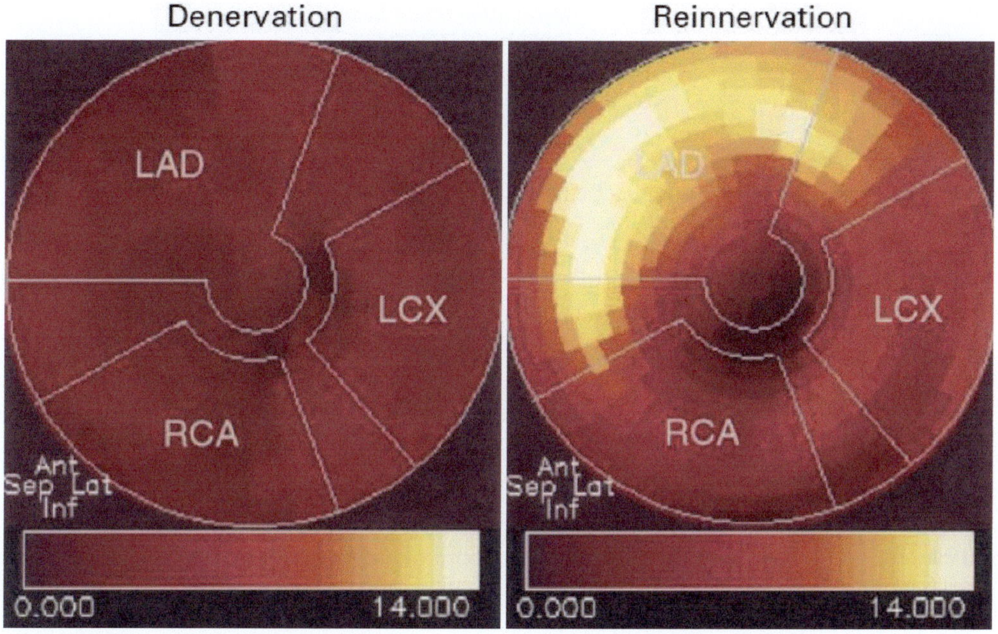

Figure 10-4. The first evidence of myocardial sympathetic reinnervation is found in basal parts of the anterior (*Ant*) wall and subsequently progresses to more distal parts of the myocardium. In addition to the gradient from base to apex, the anterior and septal (*Sep*) walls are reinnervated earlier, whereas the lateral (*Lat*) wall appears to be involved later. The polar maps show the level of ^{11}C-HED retention (percent per minute) in one patient with denervation and one with reinnervation. The apex is in the center, the base in the periphery, the anterior wall on top, the septum on the left, the lateral wall on the right, and the inferior (*Inf*) wall on the bottom. The patient with denervation has low levels of ^{11}C-HED retention in all regions (*dark red*), whereas the patient with reinnervation has a high level of ^{11}C-HED retention (yellow) in the basal anteroseptal wall, indicating partial restoration of catecholamine uptake sites. *LAD* left anterior descending artery, *LCX* left circumflex artery, *RCA* right coronary artery (From Bengel et al. [24]; with permission).

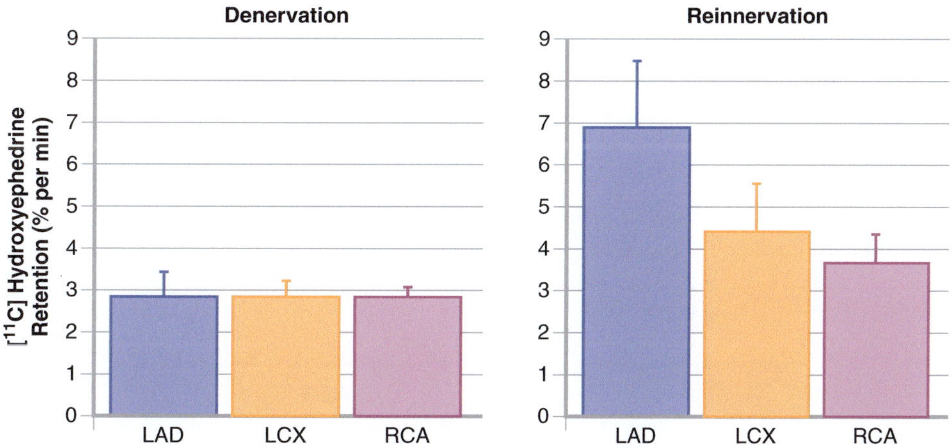

Figure 10-5. The myocardial sympathetic reinnervation process, particularly that involving the anterior and, to a lesser extent, the lateral LV wall, suggests that sympathetic nerves are first restored in the territory of the LAD artery followed later by the LCX territory. In contrast, the territory of the RCA demonstrates little or no reinnervation until late after transplant, when there is only modest, at most, evidence of sympathetic nerve terminals at the apex and inferior wall of the left ventricle [10, 13, 15, 17, 24] (Adapted from Bengal et al. [24]).

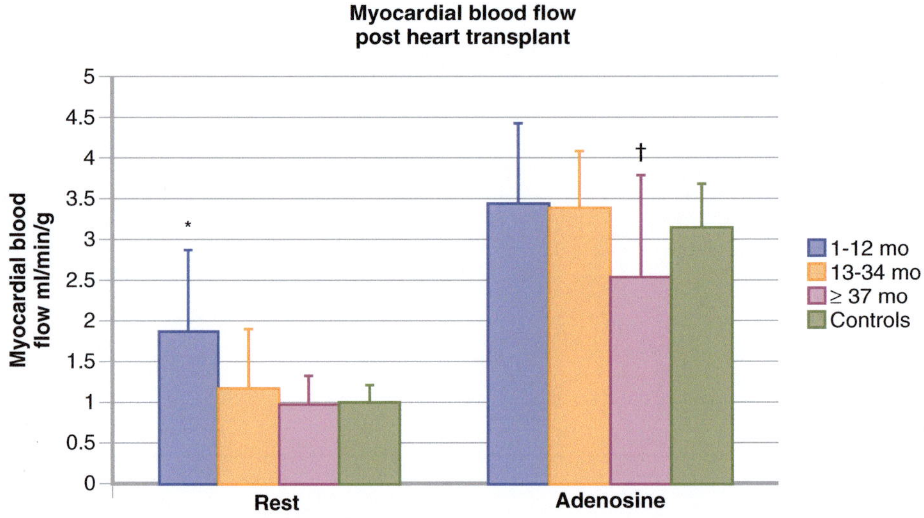

Figure 10-6. Myocardial blood flow after heart transplantation may be quantified by PET imaging with nitrogen-13 (^{13}N)-ammonia or $H_2{}^{15}O$ [21, 26]. Myocardial blood flow at rest and with adenosine is shown for different patient groups according to the interval after heart transplantation, as well as for a healthy control group. Under resting conditions, myocardial blood flow increased in the 1- to 12-month group versus the other groups. Increases in myocardial blood flow in response to adenosine were comparable among transplant recipients 1 and 36 months after transplantation and did not differ significantly from the control group. In contrast, myocardial blood flow with adenosine was reduced in the ≥37-month group versus the other groups. This finding suggests that an immune-mediated mechanism may cause endothelial dysfunction and impairment of microvascular dilator function as posttransplant time increases beyond 3 years. Values are expressed as mean; Error bars represent SD. *$P<0.02$ for the 1- to 12-month group versus all other groups. †$P<0.05$ for the ≥37-month group versus the 1- to 12-month and 13- to 34-month groups, and $P=0.06$ versus controls. (Adapted from Kushwaha et al. [27]).

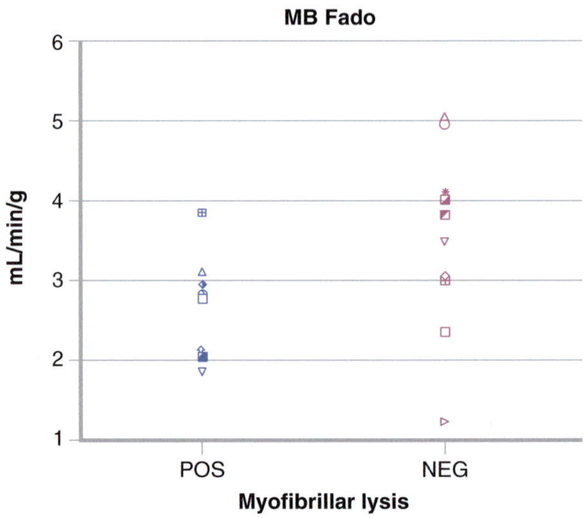

Figure 10-7. Myofibrillar lysis correlated strongly with reduced maximal dilator capacity in response to adenosine (<3 mL/min/g) in all transplant recipients regardless of time interval from transplantation. It appears likely that an immune-mediated mechanism causes both the myofibrillar injury and the impairment of microvascular dilator function [27]. Shown here are individual data values of maximal myocardial blood flow with adenosine (MBFado) for patients after heart transplantation according to the presence (POS) or absence (NEG) of myofibrillar lysis on biopsy. In general, patients with myofibrillar lysis have a maximal myocardial blood flow <3 mL/min/g, whereas those without it have a maximal myocardial blood flow >3 mL/min/g (Adapted from Kushwaha et al. [27]).

Table 10-2. The effect of reinnervation on heart rate response during exercise after cardiac transplantation.

	Normal control	Transplant recipients <6 m	Transplant recipients >1 y		
			Denervated	Mild–moderate reinnervation	Marked reinnervation
Basal HR (bpm)	76±3[a]	88±2	85±3	94±4	87±3
HR at anaerobic threshold (bpm)	151±3[a]	109±4	106±5	121±9[b]	120±3[b]
HR at peak exercise (bmp)	178±4[a]	129±3	126±5	142±7	141±2[b]
Recovery HR (% of peak HR)	64±3[a]	94±1	91±1	87±3[b]	80±2[b]
Change in HR after tyramine injection (bpm)		1.6±0.3	<5	5–14	≥ 15[b]

Transection of the autonomic nerve fibers during heart transplantation results in parasympathetic denervation and loss of the suppression of the sinoatrial (SA) node, leading to a persistent increase in resting heart rate (HR). The sympathetic denervation contributes to a delay in exercise or stress-induced augmentation of SA node automaticity, resulting in diminished maximal heart rate response with exercise, which primarily depends on an increase in plasma catecholamine concentration [2–7, 9, 25]. Heart transplant recipients usually have an elevated resting heart rate and a minimal increase in heart rate during the first few minutes of exercise. The maximal heart rate is reached in the recovery period rather than at peak exercise, returning slowly to the resting values. This may reflect the delayed humoral catecholamine release. In recovery, heart rate falls slowly as plasma catecholamines are metabolized. The major clinical consequence of SA sympathetic reinnervation after cardiac transplantation is partial restoration of a normal heart rate response to exercise, which corresponds to the extent of reinnervation as detected by heart rate response to intracoronary tyramine injection [2, 28] (Adapted from Wilson et al. [2])

[a] $P<0.01$ versus all transplant recipients

[b] $P<0.05$ versus early (<6 months) and late (>1 year) denervated transplant recipients

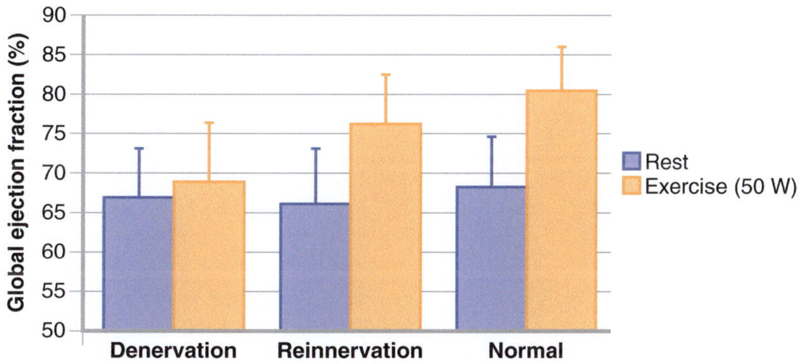

Figure 10-8. Exercise capacity and the maximal heart rate response to exercise are lower in cardiac transplant recipients than in healthy control individuals because of the absence of atrial and SA node innervation. Most of the increase in cardiac output during physical activity in transplant recipients is achieved through an increase in stroke volume (mediated by improvement in the ejection fraction). Typically, the heart rate continues to rise after cessation of exercise as a result of delayed humoral catecholamine release and then returns slowly to resting values [2–7]. Transplant recipients with evidence of restoration of sympathetic innervation performed better on exercise than denervated recipients because of better chronotropic and inotropic response [24, 25] (Adapted from Bengel et al. [24]).

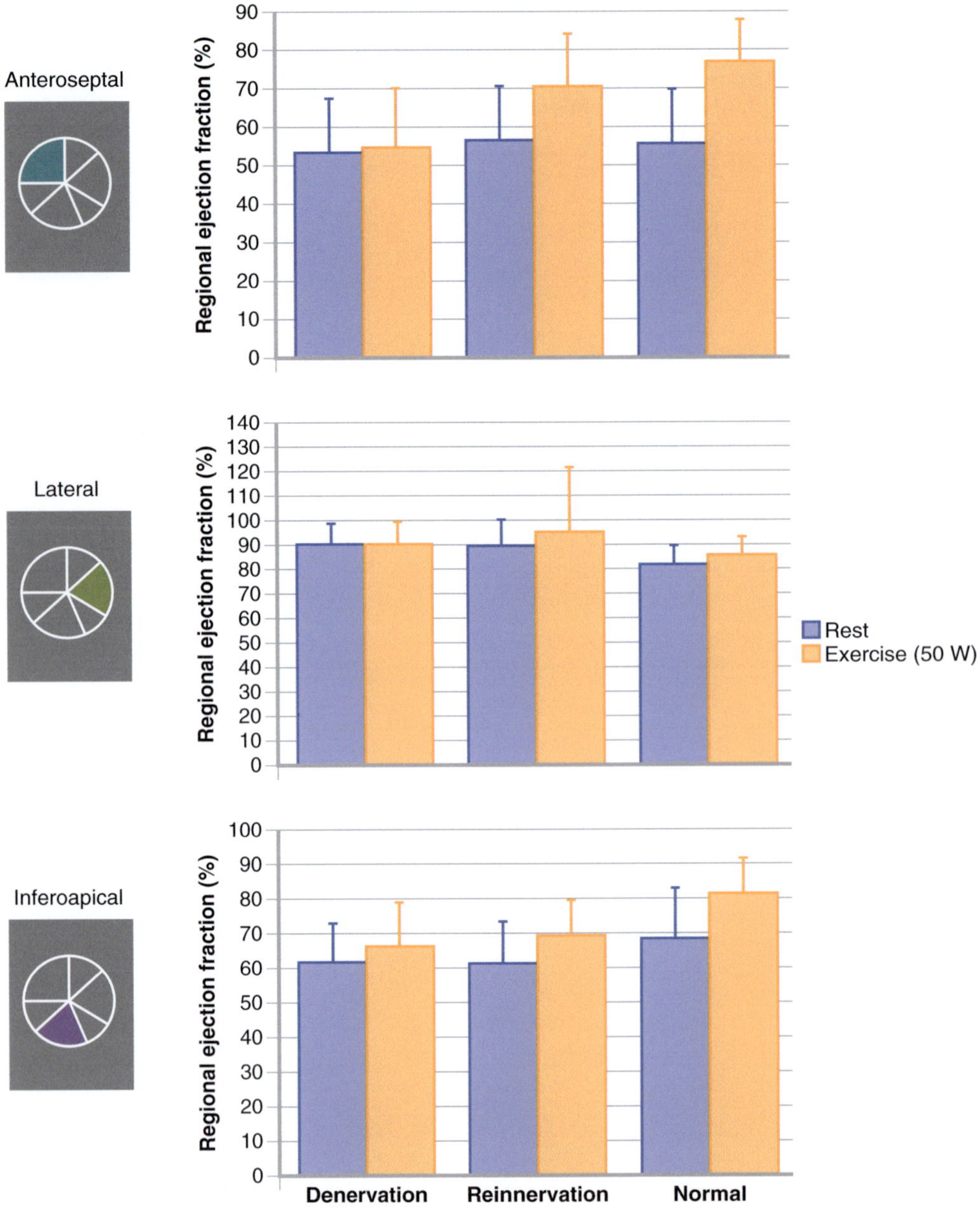

Figure 10-9. There is evidence that the reinnervation process is significantly correlated with an increase in ejection fraction (EF) during exercise [24, 25]. There was no change in EF at rest among transplant patients and the control group; however, during peak exercise, the global EF was significantly lower among denervated than reinnervated recipients, mainly because of improvement in the anteroseptal regional EF in these groups ($P<0.01$). This regional change in EF corresponds to the area of the LAD artery where the reinnervation process begins. The inferoapical region remains denervated in most transplant recipients, and its regional peak EF was lower in all transplant patients compared with the control group ($P<0.03$) [16, 24, 25] (Adapted from Bengel et al. [24]).

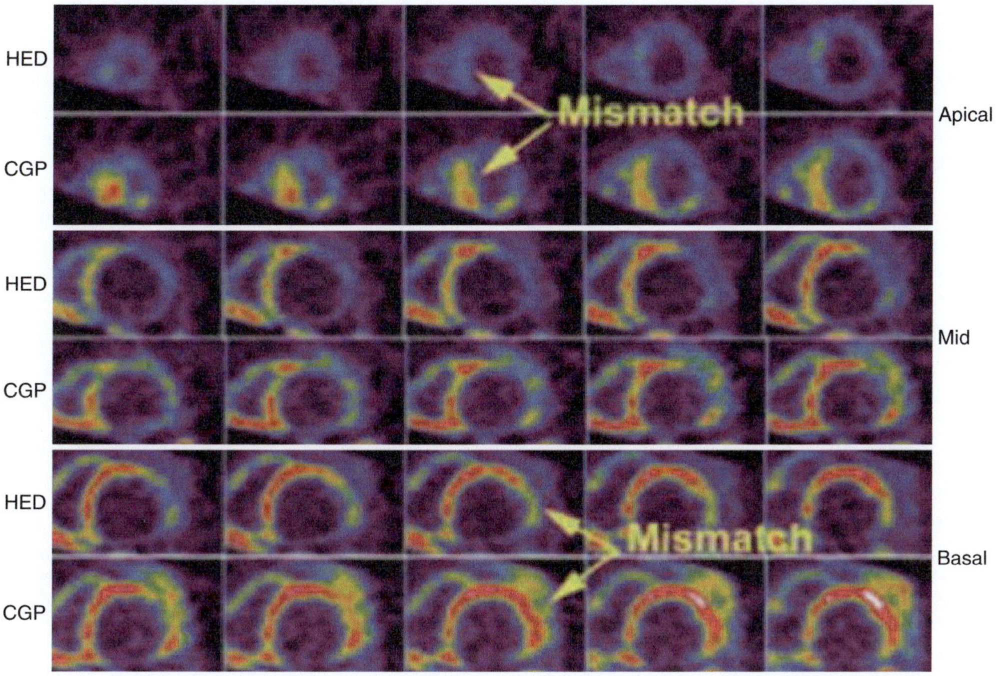

Figure 10-10. β-Blockade has detrimental effects on exercise capacity after heart transplantation as the result of an attenuated increase in heart rate, peak heart rate, and EF during exercise among reinnervated recipients [25, 29]. The fact that the attenuating effects of β-blockade were more pronounced in reinnervated than denervated patients suggests that the beneficial effects of reinnervation and restoration of sympathetic nerve terminals are mediated via β-adrenoceptors [25]. In patients with ischemic cardiomyopathy, preliminary data indicate that "mismatch" between β-receptor density (^{11}C-CGP 12177) and norepinephrine transport function (^{11}C-HED) may portend a worse prognosis because of the propensity for sudden cardiac death (as shown in this image) [30]. The extent to which myocardial β-receptor density and norepinephrine transport function are matched has not been studied in the transplanted human heart (From Fallavollita and Canty [30]; with permission).

Effect of Reinnervation on Outcome

After heart transplantation, cardiac allograft vasculopathy (CAV) is the major limitation to long-term survival of recipients [31, 32]. CAV results from an initial injury to the allograft endothelium causing a chronic inflammatory state, and develops in as many as 50% of heart transplant patients within 5 years after transplantation [33]. Almost no data exist on the relationship between the extent of the reinnervation process and the development of CAV. Estorch et al. [34] evaluated the extent of reinnervation and vasculopathy in 31 heart transplant patients. They reported that patients with established angiographic CAV had less reinnervation than those without CAV, as assessed by ^{123}I-MIBG imaging.

The reinnervation process improves exercise capacity in cardiac transplant recipients and provides them with a better quality of life. Nevertheless, a survival analysis did not reveal a significant association between reinnervation and the occurrence of allograft-related events or survival [35].

References

1. Norvell JE, Lower RR. Degeneration and reinnervation of the nerves of the heart after transplantation. Transplantation. 1973;15:337–44.
2. Wilson RF, Johnson TH, Haidet GC, Kubo SH, Mianuelli M. Sympathetic reinnervation of the sinus node and exercise hemodynamics after cardiac transplantation. Circulation. 2000; 101:2727–33.
3. Kavanagh T, Yacoub M, Mertens D, Kennedy J, Campbell R, Sawyer P. Cardiorespiratory responses to exercise training after orthotopic cardiac transplantation. Circulation. 1988;77:162–71.
4. Banner N, Patel N, Cox A, Patton H, Lachno D, Yacoub M. Altered sympathoadrenal response to dynamic exercise in cardiac transplant recipients. Cardiovasc Res. 1989;23:965–72.
5. Kao AC, Van Trigt 3rd P, Shaeffer-McCall GS, Shaw JP, Kuzil BB, Page RD, Higginbotham MB. Central and peripheral limitations to upright exercise in untrained cardiac transplant receipts. Circulation. 1994;89:2605–15.
6. Quigg RJ, Rocco MB, Gauthier DF, Creager MA, Hartley LH, Colucci WS. Mechanism of the attenuated peak heart rate response to exercise after orthotopic cardiac transplantation. J Am Coll Cardiol. 1989;14:338–44.
7. Paulus WJ, Bronzwaer JG, Felice H, Kishan N, Wellens F. Deficient acceleration of left ventricular relaxation during exercise after heart transplantation. Circulation. 1992;86:1175–85.
8. Wilson RF, Christensen BV, Olivari MT, Simon A, White CW, Laxson DD. Evidence for structural sympathetic reinnervation after orthotopic cardiac transplantation in humans. Circulation. 1991;83:1210–20.
9. Kaye DM, Esler M, Kingwell B, McPherson G, Esmore D, Jennings G. Functional and neurochemical evidence for partial cardiac sympathetic reinnervation after cardiac transplantation in humans. Circulation. 1993;88:1110–8.
10. Wilson RF, Laxson DD, Christensen BV, McGinn AL, Kubo SH. Regional differences in sympathetic reinnervation after human orthotopic cardiac transplantation. Circulation. 1993;88: 165–71.
11. Burke MN, McGinn AL, Homans DC, Christensen BV, Kubo SH, Wilson RF. Evidence for functional sympathetic reinnervation of left ventricle and coronary arteries after orthotopic cardiac transplantation in humans. Circulation. 1995;91:72–8.
12. DeMarco T, Dae M, Yuen GM, Kumar S, Sudhir K, Keith F, Amidon TM, Rifkin C, Klinski C, Lau D. Iodine-123 metaiodobenzylguanidine scintigraphic assessment of the transplanted human heart: evidence for late reinnervation. J Am Coll Cardiol. 1995;25:927–31.
13. Lovrica SS, Avbeljc V, Trobecc R, Zormana D, Rakoveca P, Hojkerb S, Gersakd B, Milcinski M. Sympathetic reinnervation after heart transplantation, assessed by iodine-123 metaiodobenzylguanidine imaging, and heart rate variability. Eur J Cardiothorac Surg. 2004;26:736–41.
14. Schwaiger M, Hutchins GD, Kalff V, Rosenspire K, Haka MS, Mallette S, Deeb GM, Abrams GD, Wieland D. Evidence for regional catecholamine uptake and storage sites in the transplanted human heart by positron emission tomography. J Clin Invest. 1991;87:1681–90.
15. Bengel FM, Ueberfuhr P, Ziegler SI, Nekolla S, Reichart B, Schwaiger M. Serial assessment of sympathetic reinnervation after orthotopic heart transplantation: a longitudinal study using PET and C-11 Hydroxyephedrine. Circulation. 1999;99:1866–71.
16. Di Carli MF, Tobes MC, Mangner T, Levine AB, Muzik O, Chakroborty P, Levine TB. Effects of cardiac sympathetic innervation on coronary blood flow. N Engl J Med. 1997;336:1208–15.
17. Uberfuhr P, Frey AW, Ziegler S, Reichart B, Schwaiger M. Sympathetic reinnervation of sinus node and left ventricle after heart transplantation in humans: regional differences assessed by heart rate variability and positron emission tomography. J Heart Lung Transplant. 2000;19:317–23.
18. Schwaiger M, Kalff V, Rosenspire K, Haka MS, Molina E, Hutchins GD, Deeb M, Wolfe Jr E, Wieland MD. Noninvasive evaluation of the sympathetic nervous system in the human heart by PET. Circulation. 1990;82:457–64.
19. John AS, Mongillo M, Depre C, Khan MT, Rimoldi OE, Pepper JR, Dreyfus GD, Pennell DJ, Camici PG. Pre- and post-synaptic sympathetic function in human hibernating myocardium. Euro J Nucl Med Mol Imaging. 2007;34:1973–80.
20. Caldwell JH, Link JM, Levy WC, Poole JE, Stratton JR. Evidence for pre- to postsynaptic mismatch of the cardiac sympathetic nervous system in ischemic congestive heart failure. J Nucl Med. 2008;49:234–41.
21. Link JM, Stratton JR, Levy W, Poole JE, Shoner SC, Stuetzle W, Caldwell JH. PET measures of pre- and post-synaptic cardiac beta adrenergic function. Nuc Med Biol. 2003;30:795–803.
22. Bucerius J, Joe AY, Schmaljohann J, Gündisch D, Minnerop M, Biersack HJ, Wüllner U, Reinhardt MJ. Feasibility of 2-deoxy-2-[18F] fluoro-D-glucose- A85380-PET for imaging of human cardiac nicotinic acetylcholine receptors in vivo. Clin Res Cardiol. 2006;95:105–9.
23. Mazzadi AN, Pineau J, Costes N, Le Bars D, Bonnefoi F, Croisille P, Porcher R, Chevalier P. Muscarinic receptor upregulation in patients with myocardial infarction: a new paradigm. Circ Cardiovasc Imaging. 2009;2:365–72.
24. Bengel FM, Ueberfuhr P, Schiepel N, Nekolla SG, Reichart B, Schwaiger M. Effect of sympathetic reinnervation on cardiac performance after heart transplantation. N Engl J Med. 2001;345:731–8.
25. Bengel FM, Ueberfuhr P, Karja J, Schreiber K, Nekolla SG, Reichart B, Schwaiger M. Sympathetic reinnervation, exercise

performance and effects of beta-adrenergic blockade in cardiac transplant recipients. Eur Heart J. 2004;25:1726–33.

26. Muzik O, Beanlands RS, Hutchins GD, Mangner TJ, Nguyen N, Schwaiger M. Validation of nitrogen-13-ammonia tracer kinetic model for quantification of myocardial blood flow using PET. J Nucl Med. 1993;34:83–91.
27. Kushwaha SS, Narula J, Narula N, Zervos G, Semigran MJ, Fischman AJ, Alpert NA, Dec GW, Gewirtz H. Pattern of changes over time in myocardial blood flow and microvascular dilator capacity in patients with normally functioning cardiac allografts. Am J Cardiol. 1998;82:1377–81.
28. Uberfuhr P, Frey AW, Fuchs A, Paniara C, Roskamm H, Schwaiger M, Reichart B. Signs of vagal reinnervation 4 years after heart transplantation in spectra of heart tare variability. Eur J Cardiothorac Surg. 1997;12:907–12.
29. Kushwaha SS, Banner NR, Patel N, Cox A, Patton H, Yacoub MH. Effect of beta-blockade on the neurohumoral and cardiopulmonary response to dynamic exercise in cardiac transplant recipients. Br Heart J. 1994;71:431–6.
30. Fallavollita JA, Canty Jr JM. Dysinnervated but viable myocardium in ischemic heart disease. J Nucl Cardiol. 2010;17:1107–15.
31. Weis M, von Scheidt W. Cardiac allograft vasculopathy: a review. Circulation. 1997;96:2069–77.
32. Fang JC, Rocco T, Jarcho J, Ganz P, Mudge GH. Noninvasive assessment of transplant-associated arteriosclerosis. Am Heart J. 1998;135:980–7.
33. O'Neill BJ, Pflugfelder PW, Singh NR, Menkis AH, McKenzie FN, Kostuk WJ. Frequency of angiographic detection and quantitative assessment of coronary arterial disease one and three years after cardiac transplantation. Am J Cardiol. 1989;63:1221–6.
34. Estorch M, Campreciós M, Flotats A, Marí C, Bernà L, Catafau AM, Ballester M, Narula J, Carrió I. Sympathetic reinnervation of cardiac allografts evaluated by 123I-MIBG imaging. J Nucl Med. 1999;40:911–6.
35. Bengel FM, Ueberfuhr P, Hesse T, Schiepel N, Ziegler SI, Scholz S, Nekolla SG, Reichart B, Schwaiger M. Clinical determinants of ventricular sympathetic reinnervation after orthotopic heart transplantation. Circulation. 2002;106:831–5.

Index

V. Dilsizian, J. Narula (eds.), *Atlas of Cardiac Innervation*, DOI 10.1007/978-3-319-45800-7

MIX
Papier aus verantwortungsvollen Quellen
Paper from responsible sources
FSC® C105338

If you have any concerns about our products,
you can contact us on
ProductSafety@springernature.com

In case Publisher is established outside the EU,
the EU authorized representative is:
Springer Nature Customer Service Center GmbH
Europaplatz 3, 69115 Heidelberg, Germany

Printed by Libri Plureos GmbH
in Hamburg, Germany